THE BODY UNDER STRESS
Developing Skills for Keeping Healthy

THE BODY UNDER STRESS

Developing Skills for Keeping Healthy

Ed Conduit

LEA **LAWRENCE ERLBAUM ASSOCIATES, PUBLISHERS** LEA
Hove (UK)   Hillsdale (USA)

Lawrence Erlbaum Associates Ltd., Publishers
27 Palmeira Mansions
Church Road
Hove
East Sussex, BN3 2FA
UK

British Library Cataloguing in Publication Data

A catalogue record for this book is available from the British Library.

   ISBN: 0-86377-360-5 (Hbk)
   ISBN: 0-86377-361-3 (Pbk)

Printed in Great Britain by BPC Wheatons Ltd, Exeter

Contents

II
BODY SYSTEMS

Preface

Prevention rather than cure has long been recognised as the most effective approach to maintaining health. The World Health Organisation adopted a philosophy of positive health at its inception, and public health services give appropriate importance to clean water, immunisation, and other proactive measures. The identification of AIDS in the 1980s gave an impetus to preventive health concerns in the realm of individual behaviour. Yet great problems are posed when the behaviour of large numbers of individuals needs to conform to health ideals. Work, recreation, food and drink, and sex each have major implications for health but are not intrinsically closely related to provision of health care. Behaviour that is not currently usual would need to become the consensus for most people, and such behaviour change would have costs—for example, safer sexual behaviour creates requirements to communicate well and delay desire, and abstinence from smoking means that other methods of achieving a sense of well-being have to be developed.

Most people have some kind of belief in positive health in addition to the absence of illness. The most commonly held conceptions concern some idea of fitness and psychosocial well-being. Strictly speaking, the term "fitness" refers to stamina, but it can be used more generally to refer to skills and knowledge that enable each individual to manage demands. The ability to manage time and to plan ahead can prevent later agitation, and good eating habits can prevent later problems of excess. In chapter 1, a number of such habits are suggested as the "skills of a fit person". Just over two dozen such skills are postulated. These focus discussion and provide a framework for evaluation. If adopted elsewhere, the list would undoubtedly need revision over years of use and evaluation.

The first part of the book examines those aspects of lifestyle that the individual can modify to achieve better control of health. Behaviour that enables us to deal with demands is discussed in chapters 2, 3, and 4. Environmental demands that can be altered by behaviours such as assertion and time management are described in chapter 2. For other demands, constructive withdrawal, and seeking comfort and support are more useful. Such issues are described in chapter 3—"Coping with Life Events". These two approaches subsume much of what has been known historically as "psychosomatic illness". Some other mind–body issues remain, and these are discussed in chapter 4. Food has been implicated as a contributor to many physical illnesses, and the possibilities for improving health through better use of food and self-administered drugs are reviewed in chapter 5. Other aspects of lifestyle that maintain health include exercise, sex, and some aspects of work behaviour, and these are reviewed briefly in chapter 6. Being able to use medical services for health advice and prescriptions is also a skilled behaviour, and some of the skills are described in chapter 7.

The structure of the second part of the book is based on maintaining organ systems—circulation, digestion, breathing, movement, and immunity. The circulatory system is particularly prone to psychological influences, operating through the autonomic nervous system and stress hormones. Stress-coping skills and other lifestyle issues in the primary and secondary prevention of heart disease warrant two chapters, 8 and 9. Breathing and digestion have attracted less research and preventive health attention, but fit behaviours can substantially reduce illnesses of the lungs and digestive tract. Back care and suppleness of the body are described in chapter 12, and the related issue of activity alternative to the emotion of pain is described in 13. Immunity is a further system that is now seen to be influenced by psychophysiology, though whether fit behaviours can be prescribed to confer resistance to disease remains to be established. Other organ systems such as the skin are mentioned only briefly, as the research on this is relatively limited at present. The reproductive system is also susceptible to psychophysiological influences, but these problems are sufficiently complex to warrant a book of their own.

An attempt has been made to organise material in part II with a positive, preventive focus. Breathing is an example of a habitual activity that can have significant adverse effects on health if performed inappropriately, and prevention of panic and wheezing can be achieved by good use of respiration. There are systems of thought and behaviour, such as the Alexander technique or yoga, which maintain a consistent focus on positive health, but claims for their efficacy are not well researched as yet. It is hard to escape an illness focus at times, as nearly all our knowledge about circulatory health is actually about the risk of specific illnesses. Consequently the illness-focused research is presented in order to infer a health focus. For example, the evidence on the harmful effects of smoking seems to imply the need to achieve emotional intimacy and well-paced daily activity.

Research on preventive health behaviours is sometimes called "health psychology", and most of the material in this book falls under that umbrella. The task of disseminating health behaviour falls to a variety of healthcare providers, including nurses, doctors, remedial therapists of several disciplines, and health promotion workers. Clinical psychologists working in the prevention of recurrence of physical illness in the United Kingdom make up a small number of skill disseminators but bring a "scientist–practitioner" approach to the task. Skilled behaviour has to be acquired through knowledge, paced practice, and feedback, and learning curves occupy months or years. Although crash diets and quick relaxation courses may have some benefit, the achievement of good eating habits or of good management of time are skills developed over several years. The extent to which any professional intervention leads to long-term practice of health behaviours in its clients is an essential part of such professional activity. For example, chapter 9 describes a national blood pressure education project in the United States. The extent of knowledge about hypertension and the adherence to effective remedies were monitored over several years, and this provides a useful model for assessing other health behaviour services.

The present book was developed from a lecture course in health psychology to final-year undergraduates at Aston University in Birmingham. The contributions of students to debugging and challenging various embedded assumptions has been invaluable. The material in this book will be most accessible to readers with some background in higher education in both psychology and physiology. The research concepts are derived from those practised by psychologists, and to a lesser extent by epidemiologists. Normal physiology of each organ system in part II is summarised in the text and should be moderately accessible to most readers. Readers without a background in physiology may find occasional use of the glossary helpful, supplemented by recourse to a medical dictionary or textbook of physiology.

The second factor influencing this book is the author's professional practice as a clinical psychologist with patients who have had a major physical illness. The author has nearly two decades of experience in practice, the last seven of which have involved treating patients with cardiovascular, respiratory, pain, and other problems. The present book indicates the most important health behaviours for primary or secondary prevention of particular illnesses. However, it cannot by itself be sufficient for the achievement of such skills. Several healthcare professions and paraprofessions use educational approaches to health maintenance. Each discipline has its own basis of skills, which take at least three, and sometimes as many as ten, years of higher education to acquire. In principle it is possible for the lay person to acquire health maintenance skills, but the learning process involved should not be underestimated. The process of acquiring expertise in the dissemination of healthcare skills also has requirements for acquiring a large body of knowledge and supervised practice in the relevant interpersonal skills. Readers are encouraged to pursue the comprehensive references, and to find skill development opportunities for themselves.

This book presents a model of fitness as a repertoire of personal health behaviours. This novel approach may, in the future, be a measure of the success of healthcare systems and the health of populations.

Acknowledgements

This book could not have been written without the information and suggestions of many experienced professionals, but any excesses or misunderstandings are mine rather than theirs. I would like particularly to thank:

Jacky Conduit and Moya Horton at Wolverhampton School of Physiotherapy; Norman Stentiford, Marion Joshi, and Ev Fogarty at Russells Hall Coronary Care Unit; exercise physiologists Russell Tipson, Anne Welsh, and Jenny Bell; A.K. Biswas and Marie Jones, GUM specialists; Gina Cuthbertson, clinical psychologist; Ingrid Turner, assistant psychologist; Madeline Atherden, speech therapist; Barbara Bolton, librarian; Sallyanne Hathaway, my secretary; Rob Stammers and Lorna Debney, psychology lecturers; Trisha Steele, Andy Pritchard, and other students of Aston University.

LIMITATION OF LIABILITY

This book has been compiled with every care to reflect current medical and healthcare research on preventive health. Individuals who are interested in preventing a recurrence of their own illness may read advice that is valid for most people, but may be wrong in particular cases. No book can substitute for detailed assessment by medical and other practitioners. Healthcare professionals who wish to use particular methods described within are urged to seek face-to-face training in the methods described and to read the original references. The author and publishers cannot be held liable for adverse health effects of using the present book.

I

LIFESTYLE

1

Health and Illness

PREVENTIVE HEALTH: PUBLIC AND PRIVATE

In the twentieth century, scientific medicine has made enormous progress in treating illnesses: Most bacterial illnesses can be cured by antibiotics, many more can be prevented by immunisation, and feared diseases such as cancer are relentlessly being pushed back. The models of the human being used in medicine have produced results. The body has been seen as a set of subsystems, obeying precise laws; identification of disease categories is followed by the search for discrete causes; once the deviation from ideal function has been identified, the doctor can intervene with some agent to restore the balance. Health systems tend in practice to be illness systems, to which people come when they have an overt problem. It has often been remarked that the National Health Service in Britain might better be called a "National Illness Service".

Yet most of the huge gains in health in Britain and other industrialised countries have come not from medical treatments but, rather, from improvements in the environment. The great achievement of the nineteenth century was clean drinking water. Piped water, town sewers, and the water closet in late Victorian England led to a huge cut in infant mortality and in epidemics of infectious disease. Many of the health gains of the early twentieth century are attributable to improved nutrition—for example, tuberculosis was already declining rapidly before effective drugs for its treatment were found around 1940. Reduction of exposure to coal dust and asbestos at work and control of smoke emissions in towns made dramatic reductions in the level of lung disease. Control of our exposure to hazardous chemicals, noise, sunlight, tobacco smoke, and alcohol all make substantial contributions. Public health and occupational health services have thus made huge contributions to the maintenance of health. The pattern of illness in industrialised countries in the 1990s is now much less modifiable by such public health policy, and individual behaviour plays a correspondingly increased role. Personal behaviour to maintain health includes nutrition, stress management, and exercise.

Probably the most comprehensive statement of a preventive health strategy for health behaviours is *Healthy people 2000*, the disease-prevention objectives of the US Department of Health and Human Services Public Health Service (1992). A similar report in the United Kingdom may be found in the document *The nation's health* (Jacobson, Smith, & Whitehead, 1992). The US report uses comprehensive epidemiological data but goes on to specify "targets" for reducing diseases, and the precision of this approach is worth further elaboration. The example of high blood pressure will be chosen, and we shall return to this problem at several points in the book.

Cerebro-vascular accidents are a major source of disability, and the following examples from *Healthy people 2000* illustrate the way a large-scale preventive strategy devolves into many small-scale healthcare activities:

> 15.2   Reduce stroke deaths to no more than 20 per 100,000 people. (Age-adjusted baseline: 30.3 per 100,000 in 1987.)

The goal of reducing a particular disease then reduces to reduction of risk factors. In this case, the goals are control of blood pressure and reduction of smoking. Certain sub-groups may be special targets for risk reduction; for example, black Americans have a higher risk of stroke than do white Americans:

> 15.4   Increase to at least 50% the proportion of people with high blood pressure whose blood pressure is under control. (Baseline: 11% controlled among people aged 18 through 74 in 1976–80: an estimated 24% for people aged 18 and older in 1982–84.)

Most people with blood pressure above the hypertensive threshold (140 mm of mercury systolic, and 90 mm Hg diastolic) are not aware that this is a problem. As many as 50% of those with high blood pressure drop out of treatment in the first year, and only two-thirds who continue in care take enough medication to achieve adequate blood pressure reduction. Effective long-term prevention of stroke therefore requires that most of the population know their blood pressure, can eat and drink appropriately, and can adhere to drugs if prescribed. The strategy thus devolves into an adherence target:

15.5 Increase to at least 90% the proportion of people with high blood pressure who are taking action to help control their blood pressure. (Baseline: 79% of aware hypertensives aged 18 or over were taking action to control their blood pressure in 1985.)

There is usually a large gap between political intention to improve health and effective strategies for increasing health behaviours. Many health promotion campaigns that simply give information have little or no effect on health behaviour. This will be seen most clearly in the discussion of HIV prevention in the chapter on "Work and Play". In some cases public policy initiatives even have a negative effect—for example, in Edinburgh a police strategy for controlling drug trafficking by searching users for syringes may have led to an increase in needle sharing. The most general reason for people not heeding health promotion messages is competing beliefs; they have good reasons for continuing to smoke, to eat high-fat foods, or to contain anger. Most smokers know of the association between cigarettes and cancer or heart disease, but they continue to smoke. For teenagers the prospect of death in mid-life may be less of a threat than being seen as immature by their peers, and the older adult may see increased irritability and gain in weight in the short term as greater hazards than a hypothetical disease in the long term. Only by engaging with people's health beliefs can new healthy habits be established. Effective strategies for achieving such "health behaviours" are the subject of this book.

POSITIVE HEALTH

Attempts to define health usually start with absence of illness. Definitions of health as a positive state rapidly become controversial, as they invoke various abstract principles derived from philosophy and even from economics. Four conceptions may be contrasted in order to develop a working definition of positive health:

- *An ideal state:* Plato used health in this sense, to mean perfection. The World Health Organisation offered a famous definition of health in its 1946 constitution: "Health is a state of complete physical, mental and social well-being, and not merely the absence of disease or infirmity." The WHO's *Health for all by the year 2000* envisages, among other things, the complete cessation of war. This is unlikely to be achieved, and definitions of health as ideal states tend to suffer from a lack of pragmatic strategy to accompany them.

- *A commodity* that may be bought, given, gained, or lost. This has the implication that the commodity exists apart from the individual but can be supplied—for example, via drugs. At other times, the commodity approach regards health as an ideal state, which needs to be maintained by input of medical services. Seedhouse (1986) distinguishes this as one of four theories of positive health. This view of health as a commodity has become increasingly influential as costs of providing health care have increased at the same time as budgets for public expenditure have fallen.

- *A level of fitness* necessary to perform the tasks of a normal person in society. The American sociologist Talcott Parsons advocates this approach and defines health as ". . . the state of optimum capacity of an individual for the effective role and tasks for which he has been socialized". Parsons contrasts this with the "sick role", which allows the person to be excused from duties and to seek professional care. Health and sickness tend to be polar opposites in this theory. Other aspects of fitness include athleticism and physiological measures.

- *A personal strength or ability*: One of the best-known views of this type comes from the neurologist Oliver Sacks, who regards health as a metaphysical strength. This view was influenced by Sacks's work with patients suffering from the long-term effects of encephalitis lethargica, some of whom fought back from inside huge handicaps. In some cases the sufferer had remained in an indifferent lethargic state for nearly 50 years, but a person somehow managed to emerge during treatment by L-DOPA. Lay theories of health often contain a similar view of health as a reserve of physical and mental strength.

Seedhouse's definition of positive health tends to be weighted towards the environment:

A person's health is equivalent to the state of the set of conditions which fulfil or enable a person to work to fulfil his or her realistic chosen and biological potentials.

Horton (1993), in a critique of Seedhouse's view, emphasises the role of homeostatic processes within the individual, which can allow an optimum state to be maintained even under adverse conditions. Writing from her perspective as a physiotherapy tutor, she suggests the following alternative definition:

Health is that property which enables the individual to make continuously appropriate responses to changes occurring in both his internal and his external environment so that optimum function is preserved.

This inclusion of internal regulatory processes takes us one step further towards the definition of health as a state of fitness, which will be needed for effective programmes of prevention.

Lay concepts of health and lifestyles include notions of fitness and psychosocial well-being. A comprehensive survey was undertaken by Professor Cox and colleagues at Cambridge and reported by Blaxter (1990). The first interview produced a sample of 9,003 people in three age ranges; the subsequent visit by a nurse produced physiological data for 7,414 people, and a psychological schedule was returned for 6,572. The authors analysed lay conceptions of health according to four dimensions, whose poles included two positive states and two absence-of-illness states:

- *Fitness:* Among younger respondents this tended to mean being athletic, and in older respondents to mean having energy. This concept was more frequently applied to males, because of the link with athleticism. In the survey it was mainly equated with physiological measurements of blood pressure, body mass, etc.

- *Psychosocial well-being:* Freedom from mainly psychological problems, such as sleep disturbance, worry, etc. was measured with the "General Health Questionnaire". This concept was rarely used by men, in contrast to the fitness concept.

- *Absence of disease and impairment:* This concept entailed the respondent declaring a medically defined condition, which might not be currently troublesome. It also included the notion of a personal threat.

- *Freedom from symptoms:* Absence of 16 common symptoms, such as "trouble with eyes", "bad back", "trouble with feet", headache, etc., during the past month.

The main aim of this book is the prevention of disability from conditions such as myocardial infarction, gastric ulcer, lower-back injury, or bronchial asthma. In most such cases there will be an ongoing physical weakness corresponding to the "disease and impairment" concept used by Blaxter. A history of such an episode is still compatible with fitness, freedom from symptoms, and psychosocial well-being. Indeed, motivation to maintain health increases significantly after such an event, and much of the material in this book is based on recurrence prevention. Fitness will be used as the most general synonym for positive health. In chapter 2, on "Optimum Arousal", we will see that skills such as assertion and relaxation ability are states of fitness that reduce psychological problems. Similarly, in chapters 12 and 13, on "Movement" and "Alternatives to Pain", evidence will be presented that skilful use of the body reduces the level of physical symptoms. We will also see that psychological states such as good self-esteem and assertiveness are linked with physical states such as lower blood pressure and better weight control. No sharp distinction can be drawn between physiological and psychological well-being.

With this in mind, it is now possible to specify more precisely some components of fitness as discrete health behaviours. As these components depend partly on the current research consensus, they might best be thought of as "hypotheses" (at the present time, alcohol is thought to make some positive contribution to fitness, whereas tobacco smoking is thought to be totally incompatible with fitness, though this consensus might change with further research). The first digit before each of the fitness statements listed below indicates the chapter in which more evidence can be found.

Skills of the fit person

2.1 can readily achieve low arousal by using a relaxation skill

2.2 can be appropriately assertive and thus achieve optimum level of arousal

2.3 manages time and uses problem-solving approaches for moderate arousal

2.4 maintains autonomy (internal control) for most adult tasks, but can yield to external control when appropriate

3.1 expresses necessary distress, anger, and other feelings in constructive ways

3.2 maintains self-esteem to prevent anger

3.3 achieves social support during bereavement and other traumas

3.4 achieves respite from sustained stress by distraction and perspective-taking

3.5 makes life transitions with appropriate awareness, and adjusts goals and relationships appropriately

5.1 eats food with about the right calorific content, low in total fats, high in fibre, and with adequate vitamins, oils, etc.

5.2 eats in social contexts with pleasure, relaxation, and social exchange

5.3 abstains from tobacco smoking

5.4 drinks alcohol in moderation, or abstains, and enjoys social contexts

5.5 uses recreational drugs, if at all, in moderation and with knowledge of their effects

6.1 maintains a high exercise tolerance by regular aerobic exercise

6.2 maintains good range of joint movement and tone in voluntary muscles

6.3 maximises opportunities for self-actualisation and self-esteem in the work context

6.4 practises safer sex, or abstains from penetrative sex

7.1 has sufficient awareness of human biology to maintain personal health

7.2 consults medical and other practitioners for expert advice if this is suggested, or if personal health behaviours appear ineffective

7.3 uses prescribed drugs with knowledge of their actions

7.4 complies with surgical procedures entailing discomfort or embarrassment

10.1 breathes in a relaxed way with good flow under demand conditions such as public performance, or partial airway obstruction

12.1 uses good postural support, especially of the lower back

12.2 uses ergonomically optimum workspaces most of the time

13.1 has effective strategies to reduce pain and maintain social commitments

14.1 uses palliative and some other strategies when immunity is compromised

These definitions of health enable us to define illness as the absence of fitness factors. The strongest example is that of myocardial infarction: Its statistical probability decreases in proportion to several of the fitness factors above—smoking abstinence, food low in fat, good exercise tolerance, assertiveness, anger expression, relaxation. The cardiovascular system is particularly prone to lifestyle influences, and this will warrant two chapters in part II.

SKILL ACQUISITION

Educationalists traditionally distinguish between knowledge, attitude and skill. A few of the statements above, such as 7.1 and 7.2, refer mainly to knowledge, but the majority are appropriately described as "skills". Some consideration of how skills are learned is needed at this point.

Learning curves. The acquisition of a new skill tends to start with a high proportion of errors, followed by a phase of useful but slow competence, and eventually the achievement of a flat phase on the learning curve, when small increases in speed alone are achieved. Many of the programmes led by clinical psychologists, speech therapists, or physiotherapists involve skills of this kind. Such therapies typically occupy 5, 10, or 15 sessions, spaced at weekly intervals. However, this distribution of time is largely a matter of tradition and convenience, and patterns of greater or lesser intensity may be more effective for particular skills.

Feedback. It is possible to some extent to learn from books or role-models, but some element of dilution or distortion often creeps in. For example, "relaxation" tends to come to mean leisure activities that may involve quite high arousal, and "assertiveness" tends to be thought of as being loud and aggressive. The adoption of a comfortable posture to relieve back pain is often the opposite of one that a physiotherapist would recommend. The development of good posture, vocal hygiene, or assertiveness usually requires detailed individual feedback by a competent practitioner, and the availability of such trained practitioners forms one limit on the process of skill generalisation. To some extent the use of modelling, perhaps including video material and manuals, can reduce the need for feedback.

Generalisation. The achievement of skill in a clinical situation needs to be followed by generalisation in the use of that skill elsewhere. Cues are needed for the new habit, which may be inside the body or in the environment. Old cues in the home or work environment may mean that the old unhealthy habit continues. For example, the person who has had bronchial asthma for many years may achieve diaphragmatic breathing in front of the therapist but return to the use of upper-thorax breathing in difficult situations elsewhere. New cues need to be explicitly sensitised to help generalisation. Kinaesthetic cues such as shoulder tension or pulse in the ears can be used as reminders; thoughts linked with cravings for drugs can be made explicit by keeping diaries during therapy; and environmental cues, such as availability of ashtrays, may have to be replaced.

EVALUATION

A great variety of mainstream and complementary approaches to the maintenance of health is on offer. Eating garlic pearls to prevent heart attacks, acupuncture of the ear as a cure for the urge to smoke, or taking large doses of vitamin C to prevent colds, each have their adherents. There is little evidence either for or against such beliefs. Many mainstream medical practices, such as the use of cholesterol-reducing drugs to prevent heart attacks or the prescription of antibiotics during a viral chest infection, are equally poorly supported by scientific evidence. Some may eventually be found to be beneficial, though most will probably have little effect, either positive or negative. Some may turn out to be positively harmful, particularly those involving severe dietary restrictions or those that focus on "natural" herbal remedies, which may contain powerful toxins. Scientific study of the long-term effects of each practice is necessary. A short summary of some principles of behavioural science is needed here.

Disproof. Scientific method requires us to try to disprove what we believe to be true. Karl Popper advocated "falsifiability" as the criterion of a proper scientific statement. If repeated dispassionate attempts to disprove the theory fail to do so, the belief becomes more probable, though still not certain. Some health theories that are implausible to scientific thinking continue to show above-chance levels of effect and have to be considered seriously. For example, homeopathic theory proposes that diluting an active ingredient by millions of times increases the potency of the remedy. This is directly at odds with chemical principles, but nonetheless some remedies are associated with higher levels of recovery in those taking the remedy than in control patients. Chinese astrology predicts some particularly unhealthy combinations, and these predictions failed to be disproved in research by Phillips to be described in chapter 4.

Control. In order to study the effect of a treatment on future health, scientists require to know as far as practically possible that no other variable could have brought about any effect that has been observed. The usual way to do this is to arrange that one group of people receive the treatment, while a second group people who are similar in every other possible way do not receive it. In the case of preventive health strategies, attendance at a course of training or adherence to a particular diet or pattern of drug use are likely treatment variables. Ideally, people are "randomly assigned" to treatment or control, but this is often impractical or unethical, so comparisons between two series present the next-best alternative. The exact comparability of such series was particularly important in the case of people attending the Bristol Cancer Help Centre, which is described in chapter 14. Audit is becoming an increasingly important concept and usually means establishing the extent to which an intended service has actually been delivered. Audit does not require control groups and is appropriate where cost and benefit rather than true cause–effect relationships are to be studied.

Adherence. Most of the strategies described in this book feature skill acquisition. Research that follows the drug trial model tends to regard attendance at a course as equivalent to the administration of a drug. In practice, some people acquire skills very rapidly and some not at all. The Lifestyle Heart Trial, described in chapter 9, included a measure of the extent to which participants achieved the recommended targets. Such adherence measures are probably a better measure of skill, though more subject to therapist bias, than measures of therapist input.

Blindness. We tend to seek confirmation of our beliefs, in the form of testimonials or positive cases of recovery. There have been many scientific claims, including Martian canals and Z-rays, which turned out to be linked to the enthusiasm of the scientists for their beliefs. To counteract the effect of biasing beliefs, drug trials require that the person who gives the medicine and the person who assesses the patient should both be "blind"—that is, ignorant of what drug each patient has taken. Such blindness to the treatment conditions cannot in principle be achieved in behavioural research, but the inclusion of an assessor who does not know the subject's history reduces one source of bias.

CONCLUSION

Health improvements over the last century owe more to public health programmes than treatment of established disease. Personal behaviour can now make a substantial contribution to illness prevention. Governments are giving attention to prevention, but strategies are often poorly elaborated. Concepts of positive health include various notions of fitness, energy reserve, and psychosocial well-being. A set of behaviours for the maintenance of positive health are presented, using "fitness" as the most general framework. Many physical illnesses may be directly influenced by emotions and other brain states; others may be indirectly influenced by behaviours such as eating, drinking, or knowledge and attitudes towards medicine. Principles of skill acquisition and research evaluation are summarised.

REFERENCES

Blaxter, M. (1990). *Health and lifestyles.* London: Routledge, Chapman & Hall.

Horton, M. (1993). *What is health?* Unpublished M.Sc. Thesis, Dept. of General Practice, Liverpool University.

Jacobson, B., Smith, A., & Whitehead, M. (1992). *The nation's health: A strategy for the 1990s.* London: King's Fund Centre.

Seedhouse, D. (1986). *Health: The foundation for achievement.* London: John Wiley.

US Department of Health and Human Services Public Health Service (1992). *Healthy people 2000: National health promotion and disease prevention objectives.* Boston: Jones & Bartlett.

2

Optimum Arousal

Stress may be thought of as unpleasant mental and physical states, associated with environmental demands with which the individual cannot cope adequately. High-demand situations such as an examination or a new job last hours or days and involve heightened arousal. The effects of mental arousal on the body are mediated by the Sympathetic Adrenal–Medullary (SAM) system. Human beings need to adapt to demands that vary from sleep to life-threatening emergency. There is an optimum level of physiological arousal for each demand situation and coping skills appropriate to the level of demand. Arousal has direct effects on the body through the autonomic nervous system. Instrumental coping skills such as assertion and time management can affect the demands and hence reduce arousal. Methods of achieving optimum arousal in relation to demand are discussed in this chapter. The main determinants of physiological arousal may be summarised in the following behavioural skills:

2.1 can readily achieve low arousal by using a relaxation skill

2.2 can be appropriately assertive and thus achieve optimum level of arousal

2.3 manages time and uses problem-solving approaches for moderate arousal

2.4 maintains autonomy (internal control) for most adult tasks, but can yield to external control when appropriate

Some challenging events—for example, bereavement—are longer-term and not easily alterable: The person suffering from grief can produce no useful change in the external world to reduce stress. In such situations, withdrawal and sadness are appropriate, and a second system of stress hormones comes into play. This system is the Hypothalamic–Pituitary–Adrenocortical (HPAC) system, which is described in greater detail in chapter 3. These two main physiological systems and the two classes of coping skills are shown in Figure 2.1. A broad parallel between coping and hormone systems is as follows: Palliative coping skills tend to evoke HPAC activity, whereas instrumental coping skills achieve a level of SAM activity appropriate to demand.

STRESS AND COPING

The word "stress" is very widely used, but to refer sometimes to factors in the environment and at other times to factors in the individual. Any model of stress that purports to explain how it causes physical illness must include at

Stress hormone systems

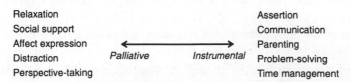

HPAC
system

Corticotrophin-releasing
hormone

↓

ACTH
↓
Glucocortoids

→ Heart & arteries ←
→ Gut ←
→ Lungs ←
→ Immune system ←

SAM
system

Sympathetic adrenal medullary system
Locus ceruleus

↓

Adrenalin
Noradrenalin

Cognitive-behavioural processes

Relaxation
Social support
Affect expression
Distraction
Perspective-taking

Palliative ←——————→ *Instrumental*

Assertion
Communication
Parenting
Problem-solving
Time management

Figure 2.1. Stress hormone systems and cognitive-behavioural processes

least three elements. At present, definitions of stress may include any or all of these in their definition, so it will not be possible to give a "lowest common denominator" in the following models. Three components of stress, and well-known theorists who focus on that aspect, are:

1. *Demand factors* in the environment or self: *stimuli* (e.g. Holmes & Rahe, 1967; Eysenk, 1990)

2. *Perceptual processes* in the individual: *appraisal* (e.g. Lazarus, 1966)

3. *Undesirable moods* or lesions in the individual: *responses* (e.g. Selye, 1956; Chrousos & Gold, 1992)

Eysenck (1990) equates stress with demands, using the etymology of the words "stress" and "strain" in physics: "Stress" refers to the applied force, "strain" to the consequent movement. He therefore defines the three aspects of stress as follows: "Stress" equates with demands, "strain" with undesirable states, "appraisal" with personality. Selye also borrowed the word "stress" from physics, but he used it to refer to the internal state; he coined the term "General Adaptational Syndrome" for the internal homeostatic mechanisms. Writers with a predominantly medical background, such as Chrousos and Gold (1992), define stress as a "threatened homeostasis" or disequilibrium of the internal physiological state of the organism. Lazarus (1966) gives one of the best-known statements of the appraisal approach and defines stress in terms of processes inside the individual; "Stress occurs when there are demands on the person which tax or exceed his adjustive coping resources". In this book external factors will generally be referred to as "demands" or "life events", and undesirable internal physiological states as "overarousal".

THE AUTONOMIC NERVOUS SYSTEM (ANS)

Arousal in all animals including humans is mainly mediated by a control system that shifts priorities between activities: Acquiring food is the usual priority, but self-preservation needs to override this; courtship is another crucial behaviour that uses the same system.

The ANS consists of efferent neurons that extend from the central nervous system to effector structures other than skeletal muscle—which, therefore, means smooth and cardiac muscle. The sympathetic division is involved most heavily in preparation for emergencies, and the parasympathetic division is active during digestion and repair (see Table 2.1). The locus ceruleus in the brain stem initiates activation of the sympathetic division. Fibres leave the spinal cord in the central region of the spine and synapse with postganglionic fibres which reach the effector. Whereas sympathetic postganglionic fibres

Table 2.1 The SAM system

	Division of ANS	
	Sympathetic	Parasympathetic
adaptive function	fight or flight	digestion and repair
	all functions in sympathy	elimination, sexual arousal, etc. are independent of digestion
cardiovascular subsystem	increase in heart rate and dilation of coronary arteries; constriction in skin and viscera	decrease in HR, BP; dilation in external genitalia and salivary glands
respiratory subsystem	dilation of bronchioles	contraction of bronchioles
sense organs	pupil dilation, close focus; lacrimation	pupil constriction, distant focus
digestive subsystem	stimulation of glycogen breakdown; inhibition of stomach and bile; secretion of salivary mucus	stimulation of gastric motility; increased bile secretion; secretion of watery saliva
elimination	urination inhibited; sweat increased	stimulation of urination
immunity	redistribution of lymphocytes	
anatomy	efferent fibres leave cord in thoracic and lumbar regions; adrenal medulla produces adrenalin and noradrenalin	vagus nerve and fibres emerging in sacral region

secrete noradrenalin as a transmitter, preganglionic fibres release acetylcholine at their synapses. The parasympathetic division has preganglionic fibres emerging in the sacral region at the bottom of the spine, and via the vagus nerve from the brain stem. The ganglia are very near the effectors, and postganglionic fibres are very short. Acetylcholine is the transmitter at all parasympathetic synapses.

The end-effects of sympathetic nervous activity are through noradrenalin, but the same results in the effector are achieved by the hormones adrenalin and noradrenalin, which come from a quite different structure, the adrenal gland. The word "adrenalin" means "near kidney"; in the United States the word "epinephrine" is used, which means the same thing in Greek instead of Latin. These two catecholamines have very similar effects in stimulating circulation and respiration, except that noradrenalin does not cause blood to flow to skeletal muscle and causes heart-rate slowing. For further details see Raynor (1977) or another general textbook of physiology. The sympathetic system usually acts in a mass way with all effectors in sympathy, but parasympathetic activity can create specific effects such as tear production or urination.

The adrenal gland

Hormones are chemicals secreted into the bloodstream from ductless glands. The most important are adrenalin and noradrenalin, but the sex hormones testosterone and oestrogen are also influential. Hormonal control of behaviour by catecholamines functions in parallel to that of the sympathetic system, but at a slower rate. The human adrenal comprises an inner medulla, which synthesises, stores, and secretes catecholamines, and an outer cortex producing steroids. Adrenal steroids tend to be chemically very similar and include androgens, which have relatively weak effects in producing male characteristics, and aldosterone and other mineralocorticoids, which affect the sodium/potassium balance in the kidney. The most interesting psychological effects are mediated by a third group of steroids, the glucocorticoids, including cortisol. These produce many effects, including changes in fat and glucose availability and reduced immunity. Glucocorticoid production by the adrenal is under hypothalamic/pituitary control. Corticotrophin-releasing factor (CRF) is produced by the hypothalamus in response to circadian rhythm and stress, and this, in turn, stimulates the pituitary to produce adrenocorticotrophic hormone (ACTH). CRF/ACTH release causes cortisol secretion, but a negative feedback loop promptly inhibits further secretion of ACTH.

The term "autonomic" reflects an older view that this branch of the nervous system functions independently of voluntary control. However, it has been repeatedly shown since the 1960s that functions such as heart rate, peripheral blood flow, or gastric motility can be conditioned by operant means. Moreover, biofeedback enables humans to alter these functions by voluntary means. Although the sympathetic system tends to engage in mass action, some very specific effects have been shown—for example, blood flow in one ear of a cat could be conditioned; another was constriction of blood vessels in one arm to a tone, which had followed the application of iced water to the other arm. The extent and specificity of central nervous control through the ANS is, in principle, considerable, but it remains to be seen how powerful these mechanisms are in each specific disorder.

Noradrenalin and birth stress

Some fascinating research into the development of the adrenal gland has been provided by Lagercrantz and Slotkin (1986) on what they call the "stress" of being born. They started from the observation that infants of various species produce unusually large amounts of adrenalin and noradrenalin during the hypoxia associated with birth. The level of these catecholamines in the foetal umbilical cord was 20 times higher on the average than that in the venous blood of adults. In infants who were asphyxiated, the catecholamine levels soared to levels that would cause a stroke in an adult. This huge level of stress hormones seems to enable the infant to survive asphyxiation, by shunting oxygenated blood to the brain, heart, adrenals, and placenta. This effect mimics the diving reflex found in sea-living mammals, in which cold water on the face reflexively causes shunting of the blood. This reflex persists in humans and is thought to account for the apparently miraculous survival of children who have fallen through ice on frozen ponds; cases are on record where children have recovered after nearly 45 minutes of being submerged in freezing water.

In the foetus, the adrenal glands are not yet innervated by the ANS but respond directly to circulating hormones. At this stage, the adrenals produce mainly noradrenalin, and the level of this hormone is supplemented by secretions from paraganglia, which later disappear. A surge of noradrenalin during labour serves to protect the vital organs from hypoxia. After birth, the proportion of adrenalin from the adrenals rises rapidly. Lagercrantz also notes the wide eyes and alertness in the neonate caused by stress hormones and speculates that this promotes bonding to the parents.

The SAM and HPAC systems

The ANS and adrenal glands work in parallel, but their numerous effects in response to stress seem to fall into two functions: the sympathetic adrenal-medullary (SAM) system, and the hypothalamic–pituitary–adrenocortical (HPAC) system. The argument for two such systems is well presented by O'Leary (1990). In psychological terms, SAM and HPAC have been described as the "effort" and "distress" systems, respectively, or as the fight-or-flight and conservation–withdrawal systems. The sympathetic nervous system is engaged most strongly in connection with fear and anger, as well as with other acute emotional states, such as excitement. Activation of the pituitary-adrenocortical system is thought to occur during threats appraised as more overwhelming and less readily coped with, and often accompanies chronic stress, as well as clinical depression. SAM activation is accompanied by the release of adrenalin, noradrenalin, and other catecholamines into the bloodstream, whereas HPAC activation results in the release of adrenocorticotrophic hormone (ACTH) and corticosteroids (cortisol in humans and other primates). This two-system approach may be overly simplistic, however, because both stress systems are often engaged during stressful encounters.

Freeze rather than flight occurs in animals that depend on camouflage, such as partridge or deer.

AROUSAL AND PERFORMANCE

The U-curve relating arousal and performance is one of the best-known principles in psychology and was popularised by Donald Hebb (1955). It is intended to show that humans work most effectively when moderately aroused. Performance deteriorates if we are too casual—but also if we are too anxious. This rule is somewhat idealised, and the empirical evidence for it is actually quite limited. Experiments on avoidance of electric shock by mice, conducted by Yerkes and Dodson at the turn of the century, gave the first experimental results.

The U-curve model shown in generalised form in Figure 2.2 views arousal as a normal adaptation to demand. Consequently, excessive anxiety may be seen as arousal that is out of proportion to the demands being faced. The biological system has adapted to prepare the body for fight or flight in the face of life-threatening demands such as predation, but in industrialised societies threats are more likely to be symbolic than physical. Flight is only rarely appropriate—perhaps for the walker who must avoid oncoming traffic

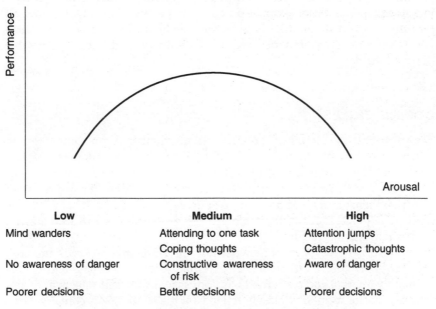

Low	Medium	High
Mind wanders	Attending to one task	Attention jumps
	Coping thoughts	Catastrophic thoughts
No awareness of danger	Constructive awareness of risk	Aware of danger
Poorer decisions	Better decisions	Poorer decisions

Figure 2.2 The U-curve of arousal and performance

Table 2.2 A strategy for achieving optimum arousal for a physical threat

	Excessive arousal	*Optimum arousal*
breathing	rapid (2–3 sec per breath); shallow , stomach not moving	breathe in . . . 2 . . . 3, sigh out 1 . . . 2 . . . 3 (. . . 4)
voluntary muscles	clenching hands; moving continuously	moderate grip: pause to take stock
vision, hearing	attend to any new stimulus	attend to feet and hands only; make safe and close eyes if panicky
self-talk	catastrophic, e.g. "I'll be killed if I slip!"	task-oriented; "left hand, right hand, left foot . . ."
time pressure	"I must get out of here!"	"there's lots of time"

the speed of which has been underestimated. The urge to run is, nonetheless, very strong and is the main behavioural consequence of excessive arousal.

The scheme shown in Table 2.2 was used by the author as part of a mountain leadership training course. Several physical threats are encountered by mountain walkers, including becoming too cold, being at risk of falling, becoming lost or overtaken by darkness, and sustaining injuries. In nearly all of these situations there is plenty of time to consider the best course of action, but the urge to act quickly becomes strong. The cognitive-behavioural sequence in the table can be practised as a way of "inoculating" oneself for future hazard situations. The situation can be imagined as one in which you have sprained your wrist, are feeling shivery, and need to scramble down a hillside.

COPING SKILLS

The psychological literature contains a large number of presumed coping skills; the review of Matheny et al. (1986) is one way of summarising this literature. They undertook a literature search of psychological abstracts, which retrieved a large number of studies on coping skills. The taxonomy of 17 coping behaviours and 5 coping resources presented in Table 2.3 is the result. The percentages in the table are the proportion of the 35 reviewed studies that cite this factor.

The taxonomy becomes somewhat less discriminative towards the end: Social support appears to be mainly external, whereas wellness and beliefs are mainly internal and concerned with physical health; self-esteem and confidence/control seem to be closely related. Of the studies, 74% contained one or more "others" that could not be subsumed into the above 17 categories.

Table 2.3 Coping behaviour and resources

Coping behaviours	Studies mentioning	Definition
cognitive restructuring	71%	includes reframing of demand and of one's own coping resources
problem-solving	80%	action directed at the stressor which reduces its stressfulness, e.g. divorce, changing jobs
tension reduction	51%	lowers hurtful physiological arousal; most importantly relaxation, but also hobbies and exercise
use of social skills	20%	use of negotiation, communication, or humour, but not assertion, which is a separate category
self disclosure/catharsis	31%	the sharing of positive and negative feeling states, either to friends or professionals
structuring	23%	includes (1) assembling and organising coping resources and (2) planning their use
seeking information	23%	gaining additional information about stressors to reduce their threat or increase response
stress monitoring	17%	includes awareness of (1) tension, (2) events or thoughts, (3) one's optimal stimulation range
assertive responses	17%	straightforward expression of what one believes, feels, and wants; this may involve conflict
avoidance/withdrawal	34%	escape by physically removing oneself from the situation
suppression/denial	31%	another escape response, in which the person explains away or ignores the stressor
self-medication	14%	use of tranquillisers, alcohol, or other drugs to reduce arousal

Coping resources		
social support	54%	a network of friends and relatives across whom one can spread the shock of stressful events
beliefs/values	43%	functional beliefs and bio-positive values
confidence/control	34%	faith in one's ability
wellness	37%	overall health, including physical fitness, weight control, absence of smoking and drinking
self-esteem	17%	the feeling that one is a competent and well-intentioned person

From Matheny et al. (1986). Reproduced by permission.

The presumption is that low levels of coping skills entail vulnerability to illness, and that prevention of illness involves teaching such skills. There are considerable methodological difficulties in comparing levels of coping skills with measures of cardiovascular and digestive health, so evidence about presumed mediators such as moods is often the only evidence available. Endogenous opioids may reduce the rise in blood pressure and heart rate which occurs during stress. Bruehl et al. (1994) used a drug that blocks these natural pain-killers and found poorer cardiovascular recovery in subjects at both extremes of behavioural coping—monitoring and blunting. Matheny also undertook a meta-analysis of stress management studies. As we are concerned at the moment mainly with causation rather than with treatment, the question of whether each coping skill was accompanied by freedom from anxiety, pain, and so on is of interest. Such mood states showed an effect size of 0.62 for both relaxation and cognitive restructuring, but stress monitoring alone and wellness alone had negative correlations with effect size.

Extending control

The trait descriptor that probably appears more frequently than any other in health psychology research is locus of control. Rotter (1966) gave one of the best-known accounts of locus of control as a personality trait, viewed as an opposition between internality and externality. Internally oriented individuals were seen as taking responsibility for their own actions, while highly external individuals saw control in the hands of fate or powerful others. The 29-item I-E questionnaire includes items that give the respondent a forced choice between personal responsibility and external influence; for example,

- For a well-prepared student there is never such a thing as an unfair test.
- Exam questions are often so unrelated to course work that studying is really useless.

External control is further divided into "chance" and "powerful others" by writers such as Wallston and Wallston (1982). Their studies on rheumatoid arthritis showed that a mixed locus of control was the most adaptive. This disease involves chronic discomfort at a moderate level, with which the sufferer can cope alone, and exacerbations, when medical help will be needed. Recognising the threshold at which to give up internal coping and consult the "powerful others" is a key skill.

Models of stress and illness in the 1960s favoured the view that too much control led to illness, and this resulted in the popular notion of "executive stress". This notion came directly from the "executive monkey" study of

Brady, Porter, Conrad, and Mason (1958). In this study, pairs of monkeys were placed in an environment where one (the "executive") had to press a lever in response to the onset of a light in order for both monkeys to avoid an electric shock. Only the executive monkeys developed ulcers. However, this finding could not be replicated, and the result might have been an artefact of subject selection: Executives were chosen from those subjects that began to bar-press first, and these may have been more emotional monkeys. A similar study by Weiss (1972) on shock-avoidance using rats produced almost opposite results. One rat could avoid shock by touching its nose to a panel; a second was given exactly the same shock but could do nothing to avoid it. Rats with and without control received the same number of shocks, but those without control developed far more ulcers. The stereotypes of executive illness have been reversed by findings on socio-economic factors, and this may reflect a more egalitarian awareness accompanying the extension of psychological services beyond a rather limited client group.

Steptoe and Appels (1989) have proposed control as a central factor in many physical illnesses. Control may refer to a *situation* that can be perceived as more or less controllable or to a *trait*. Researchers at UCLA Berkeley have undertaken a number of studies examining control and status. Bus drivers seem to be particularly prone to hypertension and gut disorders (see chapters 6, 9, and 11), especially if they are highly governed by timetables. Marmot (1989) suggests that control over the work environment is proportional to socio-economic status and postulates low control and high reactivity as partial explanations for the higher rates of heart disease in lower social classes. Whereas controllability of a situation emerges as a major aspect of health vulnerability, the evidence for a locus of control factor is more equivocal in many areas. Smoking cessation, self-administration of insulin, and uptake of inoculation seem to be easier for highly internal people.

Stress inoculation training

Meichenbaum's (1985) approach is one of the most widely used for stress management and provides a particularly well-defined model. A fundamental distinction is made between palliative and instrumental skills. The former affect the subject's response only, wheras instrumental skills such as assertion may modify the stimulus. The terms emotion-focused and problem-focused are used by other authors to convey the same distinction. Meichenbaum's dichotomy and list of skills is used in this chapter and in chapter 3 to structure the discussion of coping skills that affect arousal. In general, instrumental skills are the ones appropriate to work and social exchange associated with moderate arousal. Relaxation is appropriate for soli-

Table 2.4 Stress-coping profile: Instrumental skills

communication skills	95 %
your ability to assert yourself appropriately	85 %
your ability to manage time	40 %
skills in managing children's behaviour	75 %
problem-solving ability	85 %

tary activities, low demand, and low arousal. The other palliative skills are most applicable to long-term stressors and are discussed further in chapter 3.

Stress inoculation involves an assessment phase, a skill-training phase, and a generalisation phase. Assessment may involve observation by the therapist, image-based reconstruction, or questionnaire. The report in Table 2.4 is generated from a computer-based interview on coping skills that is used by the author as part of a stress-management course for patients after a heart attack. The use of percentages is, of course, arbitrary but rapidly identifies the deficient skills in many cases. The second part, involving palliative skills, appears in chapter 3.

This client was fairly effective at dealing with external demands at work apart from a constant sense of time pressure, but not so good at the palliative skill of leaving these challenges behind. During the skill-training phase, he was taught a system of time management involving setting goals and priorities, as well as a relaxation method. He was able to generalise the relaxation method to high-demand times at work; he also become somewhat better at obtaining constructive support when sharing distress, as practised during the group. Stress inoculation is a relatively efficient form of psychological therapy, but still requires contact with a skilled practitioner over several months for skills such as assertion or anger expression to be achieved.

Time management

Effective allocation of time according to one's priorities is an important skill, which can prevent agitated overarousal and make space for low-arousal activities. Fontana (1993) gives a prescriptive account of techniques for managers to improve organisational efficiency. The present discussion will focus on those techniques that allow the individual to achieve optimum arousal, rather than on improving organisational factors.

- *Objectives.* Specifying the expected outcome is an important part of behavioural psychology. While this may constrain creativity in some contexts, management by objectives (Drucker, 1982) encourages focus on output rather than inputs. Time-on-task can be evaluated where objectives have been specified.

- *Assigning priorities.* Priorities may either be those of time or those of importance. Incoming telephone calls or the visible accumulation of stock tend to have higher demand than tasks with long-term implications, such as training new staff or scheduling planned maintenance. Lakein (1974) advocates giving tasks a priority letter (A, B, or C) in order that importance should not be overwhelmed by urgency.

- *Procrastination.* The tendency to put off decisions is accompanied by a sense that events are outside the individual's control, so Fontana advocates internal locus of control statements. For example, "Where has the day gone?" is replaced by "What have I done with the day?"

- *Delegation.* The purpose of delegation is to free oneself for tasks that others cannot be asked to do. There are several emotional blocks to delegation, including a need to conceal weakness, the sense of being indispensable, or the undervaluation of others' abilities. Fontana concentrates on work delegation issues, but the reluctance to let go of domestic repairs, vehicle maintenance, or child care may arise through the same kind of covert self-esteem factors.

Assertion

Assertiveness allows each individual to put forward personal needs in a way that is likely to lead to these needs being met. It may be contrasted with *aggression* on one side, and *passivity* on the other. The aggressive and passive stances are not stable, as a predominantly passive person is likely eventually to become aggressive. Such aggression is often followed by guilt and a return to passivity. To maintain assertiveness, both assertive cognitions and communicative behaviour must be used. Assertiveness is generally agreed to be both highly desirable and difficult to achieve—substantial practice and feedback are necessary (Dickson, Hargie, & Morrow, 1991). Gilbert and Allan (1994) suggest that assessing one's social rank as inferior is a major reason for submissiveness. Dominance is a crucial aspect of social behaviour in many animals. These authors found that lack of assertiveness was related to unfavourable comparisons of one's rank, and submissiveness was strongly associated with introversion and neuroticism.

- *Cognitions* (thoughts). Assertion aims to achieve one's rights:

    assertion involves the thought "I understand you have needs, but mine are more important";

aggression involves thoughts such as "my needs are the only important issue";

passivity involves saying to oneself, "your needs are more important than mine";

- *Gaze.* Turn-taking in conversation is mainly signalled by eye-contact. The person listening focuses on the speaker most of the time, while the speaker looks at the listener, but also at the imaginary mental focus. To be assertive, a speaker must be able to gain eye-contact from the other person but not yield the floor prematurely.

- *Height.* The physical relationship of the communication situation contributes significantly to assertiveness. A slightly higher position may increase influence; standing over a sitting person may be received as aggression.

- *Distance.* An assertive speaker needs to be able to engage sustained attention from the listeners. In European cultures, face-to-face speech is most engaging between 1 and 2 metres, although in some Arabic-speaking communities closer approach is expected. Moving into the body space of another person is likely to be seen as aggressive, whereas standing further away may not engage the listener sufficiently.

- *Posture.* Sitting facing across a desk or standing face to face are likely to be seen as more formal, and hence more appropriate to communications about rights and power. Sitting or standing at about 45 degrees allows much closer proximity, and hence intimacy.

- *Speech.* Assertive statements should start with "I" and express a need. "You" statements (e.g. "you're trying to . . ."), and complaints are likely to be seen as aggressive.

There are marked gender differences in speech patterns: Women on average use more "relationship-sustaining" utterances, while men use more information-exchanging statements; self-deprecations and rise–fall patterns of voice pitch are used more commonly by women, while factual statements and pitch variation only at the end of an utterance are more common in male speech (Eakins & Eakins, 1978). Communications issued assertively with little preamble and flat pitch by men may be received as aggression by women. Utterances by women that include "you" statements and pitch variation may be received as moving from passive to aggressive by male listeners.

Communication skills are usually regarded as the appropriate expression of emotions that have a positive effect on the other person. This can include positive expressions that one values or loves the other person, but it can also include expression of sadness or disappointment, which evoke a positive response in the listener. The popularity of assertiveness in the United States led to an expansion of the original concept of rights-assertion to include positive affect disclosure. However, the thoughts and non-verbal skills are quite different, so it is probably safer to distinguish between communication and assertion as separate skills (Jacobson, 1982).

RELAXATION

Low arousal, as described on the U-curve above, may be equated with the skill of relaxation. The simplest way of achieving a state of low physical arousal is to move those voluntary muscles associated with defensive posture to their opposite. Laura Mitchell, a physiotherapist, proposes that anatomical systems tend to work in antagonistic pairs—for example, the biceps and triceps muscles of the upper arm. The tense state is predominantly identified anatomically with flexion of the muscles appropriate to a defensive stance. The relaxed state can then be simply defined as its opposite, i.e. an undefended posture and extension of the voluntary muscles.

The Mitchell Method uses self-talk statements that guide the main muscle groups towards the relaxed end-state. This can become very rapid once the pattern of instructions to the self and kinaesthetic cues are learned. Statements include:

"Pull shoulders down towards the feet. Stop."

"Fingers and thumbs stretched out and long. Stop."

"Turns the hips slightly outwards. Stop."

"Breathe in through the nose. Hold it. Sigh out through the mouth."

Jacobsen's (1938) progressive contrast method is more widely used and is probably the most popular and useful coping skill that can be taught. Voluntary muscle groups are first tensed in order to heighten the subsequent relaxation. This has advantages for initial learning but makes it more difficult to generalise to high-demand situations. The focus on breathing is the most important element of relaxation, and Yoga and transcendental meditation concentrate heavily on breathing. Biofeedback is yet another approach, and all involve simple relaxation as their main therapeutic mechanism.

BIOFEEDBACK

Relaxation and low arousal of particular functions may be modified by supplying external feedback in addition to kinaesthetic awareness of that function. The traditional view of the autonomic nervous system is that physiological effects are "autonomous", by contrast with the voluntary nerv-

Table 2.5

Health problem	Cue fed back to subject	Practitioners
migraine (arterial) headache	forehead temperature above frontalis muscle	Tarler-Benlolo, 1978; Blanchard & Andrasik, 1985
tension headache	EMG output of electrical activity of frontalis muscle	Blanchard & Andrasik, 1985
hypertension	audible feedback from blood pressure monitoring cuff	Shapiro, 1977; Blanchard, Martin, & Dubbert, 1988
faecal incontinence	pressure in anal canal	Whitehead, 1992

ous system. However, psychologists such as Miller et al. (1974) showed that some of these functions could be brought under voluntary control with the help of some external feedback. Biofeedback is often described in terms of learning theory, by contrast with the psychoanalytic theory used to describe psychosomatic illnesses. Classical conditioning was defined by the association of an autonomically mediated response, such as salivation, to an external cue. Operant conditioning was thought to involve increasing the probability of responses mediated by the voluntary nervous system by association with external reinforcement. Biofeedback involves the association of a physiological function, an external cue, and a voluntary response. The physiological function may be mediated by the voluntary nervous system—for example, muscle tone in cases of partial paralysis. More usually, functions mediated by the ANS are involved. As the subject becomes able to control the physiological parameter, awareness of one or other kinaesthetic cue allows control to be generalised without the feedback device.

Cardiovascular responses have proved of most interest, though early claims by Shapiro and colleagues for efficacy of biofeedback in reducing hypertension were not replicated (Shapiro, 1977). Some examples are presented in Table 2.5.

SEX HORMONES

Before leaving the topic of arousal and health, some mention must be made of the mediation of a further group of hormones. There are links between eating disorders and female hormones and between smoking and testosterone, as well as some other endocrine links. Heart disease appears to linked to biological masculinity, for reasons that are not well described. Heart attacks in women before the menopause are rare, but their probability rises to male levels as the protective effect of oestrogen diminishes. After the menopause, male secondary sexual characteristics such as facial hair start to emerge in women, and it is likely that cardiovascular changes of a masculine kind also occur (see chapter 8). Hypertrophy of glands adapted for reproductive activity, notably the breasts or prostate, occur with increased frequency when child-bearing and intercourse decline (see chapter 14).

Testosterone is produced by the testes and is usually thought of in terms of male sexual response, but more generally it subserves active, combative behaviour in both sexes. Testosterone also mediates sexual arousal and assertion in females, although serum levels are much higher in the male than in the female. A complex sequence of female hormones includes gonadotrophin-releasing hormone (GnRH), luteinising hormone (LH), follicle-stimulating hormone (FSH), and negative feedback by inhibin. FSH initiates the conversion of androgens into oestrogens, as well as stimulating the follicle. Oestrogens cause follicle ripening, but also feedback on GnRH. The mid-cycle LH surge induces ovulation, and the follicle produces progesterone, which promotes womb growth, and oestradiol (Kumar & Clark, 1990, p. 780).

The relationship between biological sexuality and gender role in industrialised societies is, of course, extremely complex. A brief evolutionary perspective may be helpful in elucidating psychophysiological connections. Selective breeding advantages take place over thousands of generations, but such Darwinian effects are unlikely to have had much effect during the hundred generations or so of recorded history. Homo sapiens is presumed to have developed from primates, living in well-organised troupes with hunter-gatherer eating habits. Food scarcity may be presumed to have been normative for all societies, excluding only advanced countries for the last century or so. Social changes of the last century include the decline in muscular requirements of work for men, increased participation in waged work for women, and the artificial control of female fertility. Culture and behaviour can affect sex hormones to some extent. For example, female athletes often cease menstruating as their proportion of muscle to fat increases. This may be because of the virilising effects of testosterone or through weight loss (Bonen, 1992). However, the adaptive biological role of the sex hormones should not be underestimated when considering health problems such as depression, heart disease, eating disorders, and cancers of reproductive tissue.

Courtship involves sympathetic-adrenal activation, a process to which we have so far only referred as subserving fight and flight. In Kinsey et al.'s (1953) report on human sexuality, 14 of 18 signs of sexual arousal were also signs of aggression, so a differentiation of threat and attempts at courtship is probably made through the social behaviour that accompanies the arousal. Successful courtship culminates in erection or vaginal engorgement, and these are mediated by the parasympathetic nervous system, thereby counteracting the fight–flight response. Many animals engage in complex courtship displays, and failure in execution of the display can lead to fighting. This is particularly true of monkeys with early deprivation histories, where attempts at courtship usually led to fights. The effects of testosterone act alongside sympathetic–adrenal effects and may provide the additional distinguishing cues for sexual behaviour.

CONCLUSION

The body is adapted to stress by two main hormonal systems: SAM for fight–flight, and HPAC for conservation and withdrawal. Many coping skills can reduce unadaptive stress, but two classes are focused on: instrumental skills that modify demand, and palliative skills that modify the self and body only. Optimum arousal of the SAM system depends on demands: moderate arousal is appropriate for work and many social activities, low arousal for rest and relaxation, and high arousal for rare emergencies. Low arousal can be achieved by relaxation and moderate arousal through the appropriate use of skills such as assertion, time management.

REFERENCES

Blanchard, E.B., & Andrasik, F. (1985). *Management of chronic headache: A psychological approach*. London: Pergamon.

Blanchard, E.B., Martin, J.E., & Dubbert, P.M. (1988). *Non-drug treatments for essential hypertension*. London: Pergamon.

Bonen, A. (1992). Recreational exercise does not impair menstrual cycles: A prospective study. *International Journal of Sports Medicine, 13*, 110–120.

Brady, J.V, Porter, R.W., Conrad, D.G., & Mason, J.W. (1958). Avoidance behaviour and the development of gastroduodenal ulcers. *Journal of the Experimental Analysis of Behaviour, 1*, 69–72.

Bruehl, S., McCubbin, J., Wilson, J., Montgomery, T., Ibarra, P., & Carlson, C. (1994). Coping styles, opioid blockade, and cardiovascular response to stress. *Journal of Behavioral Medicine, 17* (1), 25–40.

Chrousos, G.P., & Gold, P.W. (1992). The concepts of stress and stress system disorders. *Journal of the American Medical Association, 267* (9), 1244–1252.

Dickson, D.A., Hargie, O., & Morrow, N.C. (1991). *Communication skills training for health professionals*. London: Chapman & Hall.

Drucker (1982). *Management by objectives*. Cited by D. Fontana, *Managing time*. Leicester: The British Psychological Society, 1993.

Eakins, B.W., & Eakins, R.G. (1978). *Sex differences in human communication*. Boston, MA: Houghton Mifflin.

Eysenck, H.J. (1990). Personality, stress, and cancer: Prediction and prophylaxis. *British Journal of Medical Psychology, 61*, 57–75.

Fontana, D. (1993). *Managing time*. Leicester: The British Psychological Society.

Gilbert, P., & Allan, S. (1994). Assertiveness, submissive behaviour and social comparison. *British Journal of Clinical Psychology, 33* (3), 295–306.

Hebb, D.O. (1955). Drives and the conceptual nervous system. *Psychological Review, 62*, 243.

Holmes, T.H., & Rahe, R.H. (1967). The social readjustment rating scale. *Journal of Psychosomatic Research, 11*, 213–218.

Jacobsen, E.J. (1938). *Progressive relaxation.* Chicago, IL: University of Chicago Press.

Jacobson, N. (1982). Communication skills training for married couples. In J.P. Curran & P.M. Monti (Eds.), *Social skills training.* London: Guilford.

Kinsey, A.C., Pomeroy, W.B., Martin, C.E., & Gebhard, P.H. (1953). *Sexual behavior in the human female.* Philadelphia, PA: Saunders.

Kumar, P.J., & Clark, M.L. (1990). *Clinical medicine* (2nd ed.). London: Baillière Tindall.

Lagercrantz, H., & Slotkin, T.A. (1986). The "stress" of being born. *Scientific American, 254* (4), 92–103.

Lakein, A. (1974). *How to get control of your time and your life.* New York: Signet.

Lazarus, R.S. (1966). *Psychological stress and the coping process.* New York: McGraw-Hill.

Marmot, M.G. (1989). General approaches to migrant studies: the relation between disease, social class, and ethnic origin. In: J.K Cruickshank & D.G. Beevers (Eds.), *Ethnic factors in health and disease.* London: Butterworth.

Matheny, K.B., Aycock, D., Pugh, J.L, Curlette, W.L., & Silva Cannella, K.A. (1986). Stress coping: A qualitative and quantitative synthesis. *The Counselling Psychologist, 14* (4), 499–549. ——

Meichenbaum, D. (1985). *Stress inoculation training.* New York: Pergamon.

Miller, N.E., Barber, T.X., DiCara, L., Kamiya, J., Shapiro, D., & Stoyva, J. (Eds.) (1974). *Biofeedback and self-control.* Chicago, IL: Aldine.

Mitchell, L. (1977). *Simple relaxation.* London: John Murray.

O'Leary, A. (1990). Stress, emotion, and human immune function. *Psychological Bulletin, 108* (3), 363–382.

Raynor, J. (1977). *Anatomy and physiology.* London: Harper.

Rotter, J.B. (1966). Generalized expectancies for internal versus external control of reinforcement. *Psychological Monographs, 80* (1, whole no. 609).

Selye, H. (1956). *The stress of life.* New York: McGraw-Hill.

Shapiro, D. (1977). A monologue on biofeedback in psychophysiology. *Psychophysiology, 14*, 213–227.

Steptoe, A. & Appels, S. (1989). *Stress, personal control and health.* Chichester: Wiley.

Tarler-Benlolo, L. (1978). The role of relaxation in biofeedback training. *Psychological Bulletin, 85*, 727–755.

Wallston, K.A. , & Wallston, B.S. (1982). Who is responsible for your health? The construct of health locus of control. In G.S. Sanders & J. Suls (Eds.). *Social psychology of health and illness.* Hillsdale, NJ: Lawrence Erlbaum Associates, Inc.

Weiss, J.M. (1972). Influence of psychological variables on stress-induced pathology. In Porter, R. & Knight, J. (Eds.). *Physiology, emotion, and psychosomatic illness* (CIBA Foundation Symposium 8). New York: American Elsevier.

Whitehead, W.E. (1992). Behavioral medicine approaches to gastrointestinal disorders. *Journal of Consulting and Clinical Psychology, 60* (4), 605–612.

3

Coping with Life Events

This chapter discusses adaptation to long-term stresses, such as divorce, unemployment, or caring for an infirm parent. While the SAM system is important in regulating arousal over minutes or hours, a second stress hormonal system, the Hypothalamic–Pituitary–Adrenocortical (HPAC) system, becomes more important during protracted stresses. Instrumental coping skills may be less effective in such situations, and palliative coping skills may be more useful. Social support, constructive expression of emotion, and seeking comfort are strategies that make long-term difficulties more bearable. A general relationship between stress hormonal systems and cognitive–behavioural processes has been described (Figure 2.1), in which palliative coping was tentatively linked with HPAC activation. The principal palliative skills to be discussed are:

3.1 expresses necessary distress, anger, and other feelings in constructive ways

3.2 maintains self-esteem to prevent anger

3.3 achieves social support during bereavement and other traumas

3.4 achieves respite from sustained stress by distraction and perspective-taking

3.5 makes life transitions with appropriate awareness, and adjusts goals and relationships appropriately

THE HYPOTHALAMIC–PITUITARY–ADRENOCORTICALSYSTEM

The HPAC system prepares the body for conservation and withdrawal. When activated, it inhibits reproductive activity, the growth and thyroid subsystem, and immune function. The functions of the medulla of the adrenal ("on-kidney") glands were described in chapter 2 in terms mainly of fight or flight. The outer layer, or cortex, of the same gland secretes hormones with a quite different adaptive purpose. The pituitary gland is located under the brain, in close proximity to, and richly innervated by, the hypothalamus. This system is also known as the CRH system because of the mediating role of Corticotrophin-Releasing Hormone (CRH). The HPAC system may be represented schematically as in Table 3.1.

Mechanisms other than HPAC for conservation and withdrawal exist. Fever is an adaptive mechanism for combating infection. During an acute infection or infestation, there is a marked increase in body temperature and white cell proliferation, accompanied by behavioural lethargy. These changes increase the likelihood that the sick animal will maximise the immune response against the infection. Dantzer (1993) has provided evidence that activated immune cells produce cytokines, which act as informational messengers to the brain's temperature control and motivational systems to produce these adaptations.

Table 3.1 The hypothalamic–pituitary–adrenocortical system

adaptive function	conservation–withdrawal; (activated during shock, e.g. injury, hypothermia)
anatomy	pituitary is in close proximity to paraventricular nucleus of hypothalamus in brain; ACTH may be initiated here or at many brain sites; adrenal cortex (rind) produces corticosteroids
digestive subsystem	stimulates liver to produce glucose; breaks down protein, e.g. in bone to produce amino acids
reproduction	sexual functions suppressed, e.g. inhibition of luteinising hormone
growth	inhibition of thyroid and growth hormones
elimination	fluid retention
immunity	suppresses cytokines and inflammation, hence T cells and NK cells

PALLIATIVE COPING
AS BIOLOGICAL ADAPTATION

Meichenbaum's (1985) distinction between palliative and instrumental skills was introduced in chapter 2. While instrumental skills such as assertion may modify the stimulus, palliative (or emotion-focused skills) mainly affect the individual's response. An analogy will be drawn at this point between palliative coping in human behaviour and conservation–withdrawal in animal physiology. Properly speaking, this should be treated as a metaphor rather than a strict reduction from cognitions to physiology.

The value of HPAC activity after defeat in conflict has been shown in primates and rats. Social dominance behaviour in baboons was studied in serum measures by Sapolsky (1990). Wild baboons were sampled regularly by anaesthetising them with hypodermic darts fired from a crossbow. Testosterone was found to be high during struggles within the troupe. Cortisol was high in middle-dominance, but low in high-dominance baboons; in other words, those who had achieved a higher position experienced low stress, while those who had been defeated experienced sustained stress. The roles of the two stress hormone systems in relation to social rank in rat colonies have been shown by Bohus, Koolhaas, De Ruiter, and Heijnen (1991) and colleagues at Groningen University. Chronic stress was induced by colony aggregation, during which dominance struggles developed. Subordinate rats, which avoided challenging dominant males, had predominantly HPAC activity. Subdominant males that entered the open area and sometimes engaged in conflict had higher levels of adrenalin and testosterone. Some empirical data are given in chapter 14.

Palliative coping in humans becomes appropriate in various "defeat" situations, though these are more likely to be symbolic losses than physical combat. Table 3.2 shows the second part of the stress-coping profile of the individual whose instrumental skills were described in chapter 2. This person was effective in dealing with high levels of work stress, but was less able to seek support, comfort, and distraction during life events that could not be altered.

Table 3.2 Stress-coping profile: Palliative skills

relaxation ability	50%
ability to take long-term view and detach self	35%
value and use of social support during stress	50%
distracting attention during unavoidable stress	70%
appropriate outward expression of anger	75%

It should be noted that avoidance is not part of palliative coping: The tendency to inhibit anger expression has been shown to be important in heart disease, and avoidance of pain has been shown to inhibit recovery from back injuries. Such avoidance is usually accompanied by high arousal and is not an adaptive form of withdrawal and conservation.

EMOTION EXPRESSION

The inhibition of distress has been implicated in cancer, and control of anger in hypertension. Overcontrol of feeling may also be relevant to asthma, bowel problems, and hyperventilation. This is not an easy area to study, since emotion expression is bound up with culture. If the effect of inhibition were strong, disease related to inhibition of emotion should be lower in people from stereotypically more expressive cultures, such as Italians, than, say, the Chinese. However, there has been very little study of culture and illness, so such knowledge as we have comes from psychotherapy with individuals within one culture.

Psychoanalysts starting with Franz Alexander have attached great importance to repressed emotion in the causation of disease. The Chicago school spoke of "nuclear conflicts", which had fairly specific connections with particular organs. Within psychoanalysis, there has been a shift away from Freud's drive theory towards greater emphasis on interpersonal relationships. These are referred to as "object relations", meaning the relationships of the subject to his or her love objects. Nemiah and Sifneos (1970), working within this framework, studied a series of transcripts of 20 patients with classic psychoanalytic diseases and noted "a marked difficulty in verbally expressing or describing their feelings and an absence or striking diminution of fantasy". Sifneos (1973) used the term "alexithymia" (from the Greek a = lack, *lexis* = word, and *thymos* = emotion) to denote this disturbance. The main feature of alexithymia was thought to be a marked difficulty in finding appropriate words to describe feelings, associated with an absence of dreaming and fantasy. Alexithymic patients were also described as acting impulsively, preferring to be alone, and describing personal problems in terms of a list of unconnected symptoms. Two French analysts, Marty and de M'Uzan (1963), had noted the same pattern of thinking, which they called *"pensée operatoire"*.

Taylor, Ryan, and Bagby (1985) developed a self-report questionnaire for measuring alexithymia. After item-analysis, 26 questions remained to be factor-analysed. The four factors that emerged, and the percentage of variance each accounted for, were as follows:

1. *identifying and describing feelings*, and distinguishing them from bodily sensations (12.3%)

2. *ability to communicate feelings* to other people (7.0%)

3. *daydreaming* (6.4%)

4. *externally oriented thinking*, at the expense of inner experience (6.1%)

The validity of these four factors is only moderately established, as indicated by the relatively small proportion of variance accounted for, but alexithymia remains one of the most tractable approaches to emotion expression.

ANGER AND SELF-ESTEEM

The appropriate expression of anger is an important task, but one where the optimum strategy is unclear. Control of temper is a social requirement, but one that is accompanied by prolonged SAM effects such as raised blood pressure. Assertion, if effective, may prevent anger developing. Some action techniques encourage the cathartic expression of anger against symbol targets—for example, the use of padded bats in psychodrama sessions, or encouraging "primal screams". There is a strong relationship between threats to self-esteem and anger, and the maintenance of self-worth is probably the most generally useful strategy. The following strategy is used by the author with people with angina pectoris, which is aggravated by feeling angry.

Write down positive self-statements.

- I can . . . (e.g. speak a foreign language; service a car; care safely for a new baby)

- I am . . . (e.g. valued by my manager; loved by my spouse; approachable to colleagues)

Now identify threats by responding to these "button pushes"

- You are . . . (e.g. disloyal; untrustworthy; just like your father; not up to the job)

What would make this threat less painful?

- Tell the person who said it you are hurt, and ask for support
        OR
- "Cover the wound", and attend to it with a trusted partner later

The first phase must leave the person feeling positive enough to engage with the threats—sometimes called "narcissistic vulnerability"—of the button pushes. The final phase is an appraisal of ways of restoring the self from narcissistic hurt. This is essential to prevent resentful and self-defeating demands directed at the source of the threat to self, such as making angry attacks on senior colleagues in an attempt to force recognition. Colarusso and Nemiroff (1981) recommend parents confronted with challenges from teenage children to "lick narcissistic wounds in silence", rather than fight for respect, which is unlikely to be forthcoming. Here again the difference between social avoidance and withdrawal for constructive self-care must be clear. A simple model of anger expression as cathartic is not well supported. Siegman (1993) provides evidence of significant cardiovascular hyperreactivity as a consequence of full expression of anger.

SOCIAL SUPPORT

John Donne's famous saying that "no man is an island" receives surprisingly strong support in epidemiological studies of illness risk. There is a well-documented statistical relationship between social isolation and the risk of cardiac events. Berkman (1984) reviews three large studies on social networks. In the Alameda County study, Berkman and Syme (1979) devised a "Social Network Index" based on four types of social connection: marriage, contacts with extended family and close friends, church group affiliations, and other group affiliations. In 1965, 6,928 questionnaires were collected in this California county, and 682 of these were retrieved when death certificates for respondents were identified. It was found that the relative risk of death for each decrease in social connection was 2.3 for men and 2.8 for women. When other risk factors were included in multivariate analyses, the relative risk diminished to about 2.0. In Tecumseh, Michigan, marital status, attendance at any voluntary associations, spectator events, and classes were each found to be significant protective factors for men after other risk factors were statistically controlled (House, Robbins, & Metzner, 1982). In the Durham county study (Blazer, 1982), impaired perceived social support gave a relative mortality risk of 3.4 among 331 men and women over 65.

Welin et al. (1985) reported on the risk associated with "lack of activity outside home": Cohorts born in 1913 and 1923 were followed up over 9 years until 1982, and death from all causes was recorded. Multivariate analysis was used to separate the influence of classic CHD risk factors and poorer health. Social activities, especially parties at home, visiting friends, and trade-union meetings were 3 to 4 times higher in the low-mortality groups. The risk of dying was 2.5 times higher in the 60-year olds with fewer outside-home activities, especially organised sport, and in those men with a smaller number of persons in the household.

DISTRACTION AND PERSPECTIVE-TAKING

An appropriate perspective on long-term difficulties can make a considerable difference to both the arousal and conservation systems. For some illnesses, attempting to ignore the present and think some months ahead is an advantage, while for others living day by day maintains emotional equilibrium better. The acute pain of surgery and the chronic pain of arthritis illustrate this difference. It often occurs that the impairment of function created by an illness coincides with independent life transitions, and these are discussed further later on.

Distraction of attention is particularly important for pain control, and the use of hypnosis and cognitive reframing for such ends is described in chapter 13. This area has received some systematic attention, but other distraction methods are mainly a matter of clinical anecdote. Sustained high-demand situations, such as divorce proceedings or litigation, make distraction particularly important. Setting boundaries can be helpful here: Changing clothes on return from work, using an answering machine for the telephone, and confining weighty correspondence to the work environment and office hours can reduce their intrusion on home life. Deliberately using music or focusing the eyes on non-threatening stimuli such as a coal fire or fish in an aquarium can prevent the intrusion of anger and distress.

LIFE EVENTS

Major transitions in life may require substantial palliative adjustment in the person. Two approaches to the operational definition of such changes will be considered: life events and life transitions. A considerable methodological problem arises in separating the demand characteristics of life events from the perception of those events: A fire-fighter might experience the work demands of a librarian as stressful, and vice versa. The solution that has been adopted over the last two decades is to take a consensus rating. Paykel (1978) gave a list of 61 events to a large number of subjects and asked them to rate the adjustment required on a 20-point scale. The consensus rating by a British sample for "death of child" was 19.53, that for "failing important exam or course" was 14.38, and that for "wanted pregnancy" was 3.70. It was found that British and US respondents broadly agreed, but there were some minor differences: "Increased arguments with husband/wife" and "minor legal offence (e.g. parking ticket/speeding)" were ranked much higher by the British sample, while "finish full-time education" and "son enlists in armed forces" were rated higher by the US sample.

A similar approach, which has become better known, was used by Holmes and Rahe (1967). The Social Readjustment Rating Questionnaire (see Table 3.3) allows the calculation of Life Change Units (LCUs). The scale was

Table 3.3 The Social Readjustment Rating Questionnaire

Family		Personal	
Death of spouse	100	Detention in jail	63
Divorce	73	Major personal injury or illness	53
Marital separation	65	Sexual difficulties	39
Death of close family member	63	Death of a close friend	37
Marriage	50	Outstanding personal achievement	28
Marital reconciliation	45	Start or end of formal schooling	26
Major change in health of family	44	Major change in living conditions	25
Pregnancy	40	Major revision of personal habits	24
Addition of new family member	39	Changing to a new school	20
Major change in arguments with wife	35	Change in residence	20
Son or daughter leaving home	29	Major change in recreation	19
In-law troubles	29	Major change in church activities	19
Wife starting or ending work	26	Major change in sleeping habits	16
Major change in family get-togethers	15	Major change in eating habits	15
		Vacation	13
		Christmas	12
		Minor violations of the law	11

Work		Financial	
Being fired from work	47	Major change in financial state	38
Retirement from work	45		
Major business adjustment	39	Mortgage or loan over $10,000	31
Changing to different work	36		
Major change in work responsibilities	29	Mortgage foreclosure	30
Trouble with boss	23	Mortgage or loan less than $10,000	17
Major change in working conditions	20		

From Holmes & Rahe (1967). Adapted by permission.

initially presented to a large number of subjects who rated them for the degree of necessary adjustment involved, by comparison with marriage. In Rahe's first study, a large number of navy personnel were asked to complete LCU scores for a period of four years prior to testing; they were also asked to recall their illness experience during the same period. The four-year period was divided into 8 six-month intervals. Whenever an illness was reported during the four-year period, the six-month interval in which it occurred was labelled the illness period. The LCU total was found to be highest for the illness period (174 LCUs). In the six-month interval prior to the illness period, the subsequently ill subjects reported an average LCU total of 125 units, and in the six months prior to that, an average of 100 LCUs. However, as the study was retrospective, subjects' memory of their illness might have exacerbated the life changes in their memories. Later prospective studies confirmed the effect, although at a weaker level.

LIFE TRANSITIONS

While Life Change Units provide a coarse measure of the demands facing an individual, Life Transitions provide a model that may be more useful clinically. The experience of a physical disability, such as a back injury or heart attack, may coincide with distress at loss of function or relationships. In such cases, recovery from the illness is blocked by lack of progress with the unrelated emotional loss. Several approaches exist for describing life transitions. Perhaps the best-known account of life transitions is Erikson's (1970) *Eight ages of man*. Erikson proposes that the successful outcome of mature adulthood is "generativity", and a poor outcome is "stagnation"; in old age, a successful outcome is "ego-integrity", and a poor one "despair". A comprehensive approach to life transitions is used by Lifeskills International (Hopson & Scally, 1984) and can be found in their manual *Build your own rainbow*. The scheme used by the author asks clients to consider the losses and gains at particular transitions. As most physical illnesses occur in the second half of life, the transition of middle life is probably most relevant to the prevention of physical illness.

It can be seen from Table 3.4 that the transitions of middle life involve more loss than gain for most people, and many people experience distress. The transitions that often coincide in the early 40s are taken from Colarusso and Nemiroff (1981). These authors report a study on 40 males aged between 40 and 45, 80% of whom reported "great struggle". It should be noted that the biological changes of middle life—decline in strength in males, and cessation of ovulation in females—are largely independent of the psychosocial changes, although the biological changes are often viewed as the cause of

Table 3.4 Losses and gains at some Life Transitions

Transition	Loss	Gain
Marriage	other partners	security in commitment
	freedom from accountability	shared income and outgoings
Parenting	free time as a couple	commitment to heirs and the future
	disposable income	
Midlife	bodily changes, e.g. greying, stoutness, decline in libido	security and purpose
	time perspective changes to "How much is left?"	
	marital relation deteriorates, search for an ideal mate may resume	
	pleasure in children declines: leave home—"the empty nest"—or distance themselves	vicarious satisfaction with children's career or achievements
	parents decline as a source of security, through death or mental frailty	grandchildren give sense of continuity
	ascending career—tends to plateau	hobbies and voluntary activities give increased sense of purpose
Retirement	external focus for activity	self-direction of activity
	time pressure	leisure time
	friendships around work	friendships around hobbies
	income (sometimes)	

distress. For a good resolution to occur, the person suffering in mid-life needs to engage actively with the gains of later middle life.

Perspective on life transitions can be achieved by a conscious letting-go and an attempt to take hold of the gains of the next phase. The graph presented in Figure 3.1, which is redrawn from data provided by Sheehy (1983), shows life satisfaction at different times. The curves average many people's experience, and individuals may peak and trough at ages widely different from the mean. The main value of the curve is to encourage optimism about gains in subsequent phases of life.

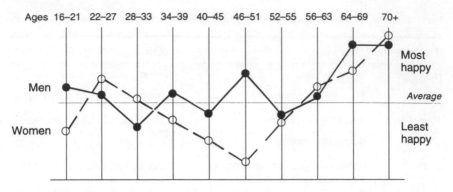

Figure 3.1 The happiest years: A comparison between men (●) and women (○)

SITUATION AND PERSONALITY

Thus far the psychological influences on physiology have been discussed in terms of "coping skills". However, much psychological literature is in terms of personality "traits" or "types".

Effective preventive strategies require identification of those individuals at risk, or those situations in which all individuals are at risk. The approach to clinical prevention used in this chapter is for the development of "coping skills", though such constructs are usually too imprecise for well-controlled scientific study. The interaction between severe life events and ineffective palliative coping has received most interest in the area of cancer-proneness. Increased incidence has been noted anecdotally after bereavement, and researchers such as Lydia Temoshok have attempted to describe a "Type-C" cancer-prone personality. We tend to anticipate human behaviour partly in terms of presumed stable dispositions of known individuals, i.e. "personality". Indeed George Kelly (1955) turned this tendency to predict by a hierarchy of constructs into a system of psychology, which he called "Personal Construct Theory". The so-called Type-A personality is a widely used categorisation for psychophysiological influences. However, "personality" turns out to be less useful than it might seem. Meehl (1954) showed that individual differences in behaviour offer less explanatory power than demand characteristics of situations. For example, the demands of work may have greater effects on arousal than does personality (see chapter 6).

The main value of type and trait approaches is in predictive research. Epidemiological researchers are obliged to use operational definitions such as traits to predict future illness. At Johns Hopkins Medical school, biological and psychological traits of medical students have been monitored since 1948 in the "precursors study". Reporting continues on these 1337 former students, now mostly physicians. Thomas and Greenstreet (1973) listed those traits emerging from a stepwise regression analysis as predictors of suicide, mental illness, heart disease, and tumours. "Habits of nervous tension" was the most predictive trait, but "closeness to parents", "father's age at subject's birth", and various Rorschach scores all emerged as predictors. Two surprises arise here: The predictors seem to be the same for very different health problems; and reports of early family influences are remarkably influential. These traits, in the form of regression variables, are fascinating, but we are obliged to put meanings on them in a theory of some kind. For example, why are males whose fathers were older more likely to suffer from hypertension?

A personality typology for prognostic studies of psychological variables on physical health is to be found in the collaboration of Hans Eysenck and Grossarth-Maticek. This personality model is complicated by Grossarth-Maticek's description of the subject in relation to his "objects of desire". For example, Grossarth-Maticek and Eysenck (1990) say of Type 1 (understimulation): "Persons of this type show a permanent tendency to regard an emotionally highly valued object as the most important condition for their own well-being and happiness. The stress produced by the continued withdrawal or absence of this object is experienced as an enormously traumatic event . . . this type shows lack of autonomy." The "Personality–Stress Inventory" is a self-report questionnaire in which questions were grouped into six putative "types". These types, with a sample question from the British version for each, are:

- *Type 1:* emotion-suppressing, conflict-avoiding, cancer-prone

  ("I am always ready to give way to people who are emotionally important to me.")

- *Type 2:* hostile, overaroused, isolated, heart-disease-prone

  ("I have tried in vain for years to distance myself from people who upset me.")

- *Type 3:* psychopathic, physically healthy, likely to abuse drugs

  ("I believe in saying: What's in it for me?")

- *Type 4:* healthy autonomous type

  ("I am emotionally a very balanced sort of person.")

- *Type 5:* anti-emotional, prone to cancer and depression

  ("I organise my life exclusively on rational principles and oppose unreasonable rules and regulations.")

- *Type 6:* antisocial, criminal, prone to drug addiction

  ("I can only be really satisfied by stepping outside the usual rules and regulations.")

The potential value of this typology is its ability to identify characteristics in apparently healthy people which might later lead to illness. In a validation study (Eysenck, 1988) they located 36 extreme scorers for each type; subjects had to have a perfect score for that type, and no more than two on any other type. These 216 people were followed up over 13 years. The occurrence of diagnoses in several typologies was much above chance level. For example, there were 11 with cancer among the Type 1s, 4 with cancer among the Type 5s, and 7 in the remaining four typologies. This study is making very strong claims for psychological influence, but has been strongly criticised on scientific grounds. Writers such as Fox (1991) criticise the unlikely numbers in some of Grossarth-Maticek's studies, and these are discussed in detail in chapter 14.

The current state of health psychology involves a great variety of trait descriptors. Some internal dysphoric states, notably trait anxiety, have a wide consensus, but generally the operational definitions of each trait or type have to be examined in each piece of research, and no general consensus exists about the most useful trait descriptors. It would be useful for treatment purposes if trait descriptors could simply be rephrased as deficits of particular palliative skills, e.g. "people with low levels of support-seeking and affect expression are more vulnerable to immune deficits". This remains largely intuitive at present.

CONCLUSION

The HPAC axis adapts us for conservation and withdrawal. There are some analogies between the cognitive–behavioural concept of palliative coping, and the physiological concept of conservation–withdrawal. Discrete life events require adaptation, even if they are favourable. Major transitions occur when becoming a parent or retiring, and difficulty in adjusting may exacerbate health problems. Emotion expression, social support, and the ability to distract and find comfort are important during unalterable stressors. Psychological theories of personality offer many alternative ways of construing the relation between mental events and illness.

REFERENCES

Berkman, L.F. (1984). Assessing the physical health effects of social networks and social support. *Annual Review of Public Health, 5*, 413–432.

Berkman, L., & Syme, S.L. (1979). Social networks, host resistance, and mortality:

A nine-year follow-up of Alameda County Residents. *American Journal of Epidemiology, 109,* 186–204.

Blazer, D. (1982). Social support and mortality in an elderly community population. *American Journal of Epidemiology, 115,* 684–694.

Bohus, B., Koolhaas, J.M., De Ruiter, A.J.H., & Heijnen, C.J. (1991). Stress and differential alterations in immune system functions: Conclusions from social stress studies in animals. *Netherlands Journal of Medicine, 39,* 306–315.

Colarusso, C.A., & Nemiroff, R.A. (1981). *Adult development.* New York: Plenum.

Dantzer, R. (1993). Stress and disease: Where do we stand? *Proceedings of the Seventh Conference of the European Health Psychology Society,* Brussels (September).

Erikson, E. (1970). *Eight ages of man.* Harmondsworth: Penguin.

Eysenck, H.J. (1988). Personality, stress and cancer: Prediction and prophylaxis. *British Journal of Medical Psychology, 61,* 57–75.

Fox, B.H. (1991). Quandaries created by unlikely numbers in some of Grossarth-Maticek's studies. *Psychological Inquiry, 2* (3), 242–246.

Grossarth-Maticek, R., & Eysenck, H.J. (1990). Personality, stress and disease: Description and validation of a new inventory. *Psychological Reports, 66,* 355–373.

Holmes, T.H., & Rahe, R.H. (1967). The social readjustment rating scale. *Journal of Psychosomatic Research, 11,* 213–218.

Hopson, B., & Scally, M. (1984). *Build your own rainbow.* Otley, West Yorkshire: Lifeskills International.

House, J., Robbins, C., & Metzner, H. (1982). The association of social relationships and activities with mortality: Prospective evidence from the Tecumseh Community Health Study. *American Journal of Epidemiology, 116,* 123–40.

Kelly, G. (1955). *The psychology of personal constructs.* London: Nelson.

Marty, P., & de M'Uzan, M. (1963). La pensée opératoire. *Revue fr. psychoanal. suppl. 27,* 1345–1356.

Meehl, P. (1954). *Clinical versus statistical prediction.* Minneapolis, MN: University of Minnesota Press.

Meichenbaum, D. (1985). *Stress inoculation training.* Oxford: Pergamon.

Nemiah, J.C., & Sifneos, P.E. (1970). Psychosomatic illness: A problem of communication. *Psychotherapy and Psychosomatics, 18,* 154–160.

Paykel, E.S. (1978). Contribution of life events to causation of psychiatric illness. *Psychological Medicine, 8,* 245–253.

Sapolsky, R.M. (1990). Stress in the wild. *Scientific American, 262* (1), 106–113.

Sheehy, G. (1983). *Pathfinders.* London: Sidgwick & Jackson.

Siegman, A.W. (1993). Cardiovascular consequences of expressing, experiencing, and repressing anger. *Journal of Behavioral Medicine, 16* (6), 539–570.

Sifneos, P.E. (1973). The prevalence of alexithymic characteristics in psychosomatic patients. *Psychotherapy Psychosomatics, 22,* 255–262.

Taylor, G.J., Ryan, D., & Bagby, R.M. (1985). Toward the development of a new self-report alexithymia scale. *Psychotherapy and Psychosomatics, 44,* 191–199.

Thomas, C.B., & Greenstreet, R.L. (1973). Psychobiological characteristics in youth as predictors of five disease states: Suicide, mental illness, hypertension, coronary heart disease, and tumor. *Johns Hopkins Medical Journal, 132,* 16–43.

Welin, L., Tibblin, G., Svardsudd, K., Tibblin, B., Ander-Perciva, S., & Larsson, B. (1985). Prospective study of social influences on mortality. The study of men born in 1913 and 1923. *The Lancet, 8434* (April 20), 915–918.

4

Psychosomatic Issues

Chapters 2 and 3 have put forward models of instrumental and palliative coping, which influence physiological events. However, clinical medicine provides an alternative conceptual system, and many of its discoveries cannot be simply encompassed in terms of psychological processes such as demand, arousal, and withdrawal. The term "psychosomatic" has been used historically to describe physical illnesses with a psychogenic component. Psychosomatic illness has been described mainly in terms of conflicting motives, and it is not simple to translate formulations based on conflicting drives into a model based on skills. Psychologists are interested in modelling the motives and cognitions behind problems such as conversion, dissociation, and hypochondriasis. This chapter is mainly theoretical and reviews different models for mind–body connections.

MEDICINE AND PSYCHOLOGY

The approach used thus far to describe connections between psyche and soma derives mainly from the academic disciplines of psychology and physiology: Normal processes such as arousal and cognition are described in controlled experiments and then applied to particular health problems. Medicine has developed historically along quite different paths. Clinicians who are confronted by patterns of symptoms and signs in patients try to fit these into accepted illness syndromes. Occasionally the fit is poor. If a series of patients is seen who show symptoms similar to each other but different from known illnesses, the clinician may be tempted to report a new pattern. If other clinicians agree that such a pattern is real, a new syndrome is defined, and a search for the pathological cause starts. Eventually, these diseases become subject to medical treatment—very often by stumbling across some remedy rather than through the deliberate planning of pharmacological treatments. Clinical medicine and therapies allied to medicine tend to progress mainly by lucky guesses that turn out to be useful, rather than through theoretically derived innovations.

The discovery of Legionnaire's Disease provides a good illustration of the success of the clinical medical approach. The illness was initially seen as a form of pneumonia, but with several unusual features: The infection was particularly severe and sometimes fatal; the usual antibiotics were often ineffective; and an epidemic had occurred, which appeared to be linked with attendance at an American Legion gathering. The pattern was sufficiently distinctive that a new syndrome was accepted, and a long and initially fruitless search for a causal organism ensued. Eventually a new bacterium was detected by an unusual staining technique, and this was subsequently called Legionella. This bacterium was found to be present in the soil, but also in the cooling towers of central-heating systems in some large buildings. This identification allowed both effective public health preventive measures and effective clinical treatments to be applied.

The success of the clinical approach for infectious diseases has not been matched in the case of illnesses involving psychological factors, where the identification of syndromes and presumed pathological agents is considerably more muddled. Nonetheless, the diverse national traditions of medicine brought together by the World Health Organisation have been able to agree a categorisation, which is enshrined in the International Classification of Diseases (ICD). In the United States, a classification used by psychiatrists has been worked out in great detail, so this will be described at some length.

DSM-III-R CLASSIFICATION

The American Psychiatric Association's (APA) classification system in its first and second versions referred to "psychosomatic illness". The definition of psychosomatic illness by Lachman (1972) was "physiological dysfunctions and structural aberrations that result primarily from psychological processes rather than immediate physical agents like those involved in the organic disorders". Half a century ago it was possible to feel confident in categorising illnesses as physical, psychiatric, and psychosomatic. Kaplan and Sadock (1985) use a psychiatric framework to describe illnesses that could be regarded as psychosomatic, and their list is presented below with some additions.

The multifactorial nature of all illnesses is now generally recognised. "Psychiatric" conditions such as depression turn out to involve hormonal changes similar to "physical" illnesses. Most illnesses actually have multiple causes, including heredity, infection, and degeneration, and it would be hard to specify a purely psychological cause for any physical illness, or any illness that has no psychological component. Even accidental fractures are more likely during "driven" behaviour. The APA later used the term "psychophysiologic disorders", and the third revision of its Diagnostic and Statistical Manual now refers to "psychological factors affecting physical condition". The classification distinguishes the following groups of problems that present as physical illnesses:

- *Psychological factors affecting physical condition.* Many; the term "psychosomatic illness" is widely misused, often as a synonym for hypochondriasis or even malingering.

- *Somatoform disorders.* These include:

  psychogenic pain disorder—pain in the absence of clear lesions; a problematic concept (see chapter 13)

  conversion reactions—conversion of an emotion into a physical experience; involves voluntary motor responses or somatosensory changes

  hypochondriasis—the anxious interpretation of benign bodily changes as symptoms of serious illness, along with suggestibility and monitoring of these changes.

- *Dissociative reactions* involve some separation of mental functions, such as:

  psychogenic amnesia—painful events, such as traumatic injury or abuse, are forgotten

  fugue—a severe but rare form of psychogenic amnesia when identity is forgotten

  depersonalisation disorder—in which the person feels unreal

  multiple personality disorder—severe dissociation between roles or subselves

- *Malingering:* The deliberate simulation of an illness, to avoid some obligation

PHYSICAL CONDITIONS
AFFECTED BY PSYCHOLOGICAL FACTORS

The following list is expanded from that presented by Kaplan and Sadock (1985) as "psychosomatic disorders". The list has been expanded to include diabetes mellitus, rheumatoid arthritis, epilepsy, multiple sclerosis, and some cancers, each of which may have a psychophysiological influence.

- *Cardiovascular*

  hypertension—persistent abnormal elevation of the blood pressure (see chapter 9)

  paroxysmal tachycardia—sudden attacks of abnormally rapid heartbeat

  arrhythmia—irregular heartbeat (see chapter 9)

  migraine—severe one-sided headache, sometimes with nausea and disturbed vision

  angina pectoris—spasmodic pain in the chest, often accompanied by feeling of suffocation and impending death (see chapter 9)

- *Respiratory*

  bronchial asthma—spasmodic contractions of air passages in the lungs and difficulty in breathing (see chapter 10)

  hyperventilation—overbreathing, causing drop in blood CO_2; symptoms include faintness, light-headedness, tingling in the limbs, feeling unable to get sufficient air (see chapter 10)

- *Gastro-intestinal*

  peptic ulcers—found in mucous membranes of stomach (see chapter 11)

  duodenal ulcers—in the small intestine; also caused by acidic action of gastric juice (see chapter 11)

  gastritis—inflammation of the stomach

  colitis—inflammation of the colon (see chapter 11)

  micturition abnormalities—e.g. painful or frequent urination

  pylorospasm—spasm of the pyloric portion of the stomach, an opening through which stomach contents are emptied into the duodenum

  anorexia nervosa—severe decrease in food intake (see chapter 11)

- *Endocrine*

  hyperthyroidism—symptoms include over-activity

  diabetes mellitus—glucose metabolism disorder (see chapter 11)

- *Skin*

  neurodermatitis—chronic inflammation and discharge of fluid

  pruritis—chronic itching

- *Musculo-skeletal*

  chronic backache (see chapter 12)

  muscle cramps

  headache—the frontalis and occipitalis muscles are prone to tension

- *Immune*

  cancer—uncontrolled proliferation of cells (see chapter 14)

  rheumatoid arthritis—widespread destruction of synovial joints (see chapter 14)

  multiple sclerosis—demyelination, causing various sensory and motor symptoms (see chapter 14)

- *Brain*

  epilepsy—synchronous firing of brain cells; may be triggered by hyperventilation (see chapter 10)

NUCLEAR CONFLICT THEORY

The concept of psychosomatic illness was formulated in terms of psychoanalytic theory, especially the conflict between different motives. For example, one may feel an obligation to care for an elderly relative, but at the same time wish to be free of such demands. Ideally, these conflicting motives can be resolved by discussion and some compromise. Without such resolution, a physical complaint that satisfies both motives may develop. Freud's psychoanalytic view was developed by Franz Alexander and the Chicago school of psychiatry, and is called "nuclear-conflict theory", because it proposes a specific nuclear conflict for each illness. The Chicago school largely defined the field of psychosomatic medicine, and most modern discussions of psychophysiological disorders are anticipated in their writings. This approach has been more important in psychiatry than in clinical psychology, and is often referred to now as "liaison psychiatry". The classic text on psychosomatic medicine was recently reprinted (Alexander, 1987). Seven conditions that were traditionally regarded as psychosomatic (in North America at least), and the postulated nuclear conflict underlying them, are listed below.

1. *Bronchial asthma:* excessive unresolved dependence on the mother

2. *Eczema:* showing the body in order to obtain attention, love and favour (exhibitionism)

3. *Rheumatoid arthritis:* repression of rebellious tendencies

4. *Ulcerative colitis:* frustrated hope of carrying out an obligation and frustrated hope in accomplishing some task

5. *Duodenal ulcer:* frustration of dependency needs

6. *Essential hypertension:* conflict over expressing aggressive impulses

7. *Hyperthyroidism:* fear of death, development of phobias related to this fear

Part of specificity theory is a postulated difference between two autonomic mechanisms. The first is preparation for fight and flight, which is not then consummated and therefore persists. Alexander believed this to account for hypertension and poor control of diabetes mellitus. The concept of arousal has been used in chapter 2 to describe the same clinical observation. Alexander's second mechanism is emotional withdrawal from action into a dependent state, when concentrated self-assertive behaviour would be more appropriate. An example of this "vegetative retreat" is the man who develops diarrhoea when faced with danger instead of confronting it—he "has no guts". Alexander sees most gastrointestinal disturbance as involving this vegetative retreat. The evidence for this as a major factor in ulcerative conditions is not strong, but avoidance is important in Irritable Bowel Syndrome (see chapter 11).

There is a weak relation between specific conflicts and specific diseases, and the following study is typical of psychosomatic disease research. Alexander, French, and Pollack (1968) published a study designed to test their theory that there is a specific type of emotional conflict for each type of illness. Interviews with 83 patients were used, so that each condition was represented by at least five patients of each sex. Recordings of clinical interviews were edited to remove references to the underlying disease and were then submitted to psychoanalysts familiar with nuclear conflict theory. The analysts were able to diagnose the specific diseases from personality alone at better-than-chance level (1 in 7, or 14%), but the percentages correct were generally below 50%. Some patients manifest the pathological personality traits, others do not; moreover, some people with the traits did not have the illness. Emotions and personality traits involving resentment, frustration, depression, anxiety, and helplessness are the most frequently reported antecedents, regardless of the disorder (Luborsky, Docherty, & Penick, 1973).

Some specificity effects have received research support, but the conceptual framework of nuclear conflict theory has limited explanatory value. Patients with eczema-like skin inflammations, which are nowadays more likely to be described as atopic dermatitis, were found to be more excitable and to cope less well than a control group of bronchitic patients (Scheich et al., 1993). Their level of immunoglobulin E (see chapter 14) was proportional to the level of such traits. Dermatitis patients were also more paranoid, but this appeared to be related to the experience of being stared at. There has been some research support for specific conflicts in hyperthyroidism, and for dependency and gastric ulcers (see chapter 11). There is much evidence connecting anger and hypertension (see chapter 8), though the exact nature of the "conflicts about expressing aggressive impulses" is problematic (Siegman, 1993). Bronchial asthma is not currently thought of as a strongly psychosomatic disease, and a specific conflict over dependency and inhibition of crying is doubtful (see chapter 10). Evidence for dependency and inhibition of emotion in rheumatoid arthritis was reported by Solomon (see chapter 14). The possibility of psychosomatic aspects of ulcerative colitis is uncertain (see chapter 11) and hinges on the credibility of concepts of concealed anxiety and defence, to be discussed shortly.

Alexander's bold and comprehensive view of specificity can now be seen as overstated, but the conflict approach remains challenging. Clinical observation unsupported by controlled research also leads to an underestimation of socio-economic factors. For example, Alexander says, ". . . the frequency of coronary accidents among patients in such professional groups as physicians, priests, lawyers, and persons who carry great responsibilities is well-known among clinicians". Recent epidemiology shows a higher rate of coronary events in people of lower social class, so Alexander's observation probably arose from selective referral of higher-class patients.

Alexithymia has been proposed as a modern framework for psychosomatics but has been only partially validated. It was defined in chapter 3 by Taylor's four components of alexithymia (identifying feelings, communicating feelings, daydreaming, and operational thinking), especially during major long-term stressors. The theoretical framework is of "object relations", meaning the relationships of the subject to his or her love objects. Developments in psychoanalysis since Alexander have involved a shift away from Freud's drive theory towards this greater emphasis on interpersonal relationships. One Italian study (Rubino et al., 1992) found that neurotics were actually less expressive than were psychosomatic patients, contrary to Taylor's basic dichotomy. Perception of emotion was equally good in 20 male alexithymics (McDonald & Prkachin, 1990), though they were much less likely to show spontaneously facial expressions of anger and happiness. Constructs in terms of conflicting motives are difficult to integrate with cognitive psychol-

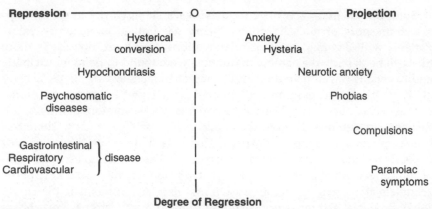

Figure 4.1 Defence mechanisms and vulnerability to physical illness
(after Bahnson)

ogy, but the clinical observations within this framework are important. Despite these conceptual problems, the implications of describing alexithymia as a contributor to a physical health problem are simple: Finding a listening environment and seeking to put obscure feelings into words are likely to be beneficial.

The psychoanalytic concept of defence mechanisms was used in an interesting dimensional approach by Bahnson (1979). This view notes that increasing somatic symptoms accompany decreasing psychological complaints and postulates an underlying dimension from "repression" to "projection" (see Figure 4.1). The more severe mental health problems are at the extreme of projection, and problems involving anxiety are at the centre. Physical illnesses with a psychological component are presumed to involve somatisation of those psychological problems, and cancer is seen as the most extreme on this dimension of repression or somatisation. A second axis indicates the degree of regression or severity of the disturbance, and this is shown as the vertical axis in Figure 4.1.

CONVERSION REACTIONS

The formal definition of conversion involves the translation of emotion into loss of sensory or motor function. This has also been called hysteria—another term that is used incorrectly more often than correctly. Conversion reactions have been thought to involve processes at a cortical level only, by contrast with psychosomatic disorders, which usually involve changes in organ systems innervated by the autonomic nervous system. Conversion reactions are distinguished diagnostically from neurological disorders such as strokes by the following features:

- *Anatomical inconsistency,* e.g. glove or stocking anaesthesia, which is incompatible with the dermotomal distribution in the brain
- *Absence of atrophy* of the muscles
- *Fluctuation* of the place of the paralysis
- *La belle indifférence:* the patient's lack of worry over the loss of function

This diagnostic term, more than any other, shows a theoretical division between the two shores of the Atlantic Ocean. One New York neurologist (Weintraub, 1993) estimates that hysterical conversion reaction (HCR) is the most frequent condition in his clinic, and he lists some 80 symptoms that can be part of HCR. In Britain, by contrast, the psychiatrist Eliot Slater (1965) has argued that the diagnosis of hysteria should not be used. He followed up cases diagnosed as hysteric and often found that some other condition, usually neurological, became manifest. Sensory anomalies, such as glove anaesthesia, may arise though carpal tunnel syndrome. Despite these objections to the concept of conversion, the relationship between emotion and unusual experience of the body has not gone away, and unusual features may variously be described as hysteria, conversion, or functional overlay.

Occasionally, a fairly clear case of classical conversion is seen. The following case referred to the author with a diagnosis of hysterical paralysis illustrates a motor conversion reaction:

Mr W, aged 39, was shopping with his wife when his left arm started to feel numb, and this sensation rapidly spread to the left leg and trunk. He was taken by ambulance to hospital with a suspected stroke and remained paralysed down the left side for the next four days. A neurologist was called and administered various pin-prick and passive manipulation tests. The area of anaesthesia moved somewhat; sensation started to return during the examination and continued to return over the next two days with no medical treatment. Full use was restored, with no difference in strength from that of the other arm. A diagnosis of hysterical hemiparesis was made. Referral was made to a clinical psychologist to identify disposing factors and prevent recurrence. The main observation was of excessive work demand—the patient's work as a security supervisor meant 60 hours on site, as well as being on call most of the remaining days and nights. Mr W had not thought this particularly unusual till it was suggested to him, indicating some lack of awareness of his own needs. In fact, he did not seem able to describe aspirations, values, or daydreams at all. His childhood had been in a stable but strict Catholic family, which placed great emphasis on honesty and hard work and very little on affection. This combination of excessive demand, lack of emotional outlet, and little use of imaginary solutions has been reported as common in conversion reactions. With discussion he was able to moderate his work demands, pay more attention to support needs, and find time for pleasurable hobbies. No return of symptoms was reported over the next year.

This case is different from a psychosomatic disorder in that no changes in tissue were observable, and muscle use returned rapidly, without any atrophy, in the supportive context of the medical examination. A further feature of the conversion reaction is the apparent secondary gain in the symptom, which does not apply to psychosomatic disorders: Mr W's symptoms meant that he could not go to work, and he received care and consideration, but there was no indication that he was intentionally creating this, i.e. "malingering". Miller (1987) considers whether cases such as this may adequately be described in terms of an illness behaviour/sick role model. This views such symptoms in terms of release from obligations, and clearly there was considerable gain in removal from a highly demanding situation for Mr W. However, "illness behaviour" may be simply be a tautology, and it is not possible at present to dispense entirely with the concepts of conversion or hysteria.

FATE AND MAGIC

Belief in harmful influences may sometimes result in those harmful effects occurring. Curses, spells, black magic, or taboos can exert powerful influences on thinking, and in some undefined way on vulnerability to illness. This is sometimes referred to as the "Nocebo effect" ("I will harm"), by analogy with the Placebo effect. Frank (1973) has described anthropological evidence for many cases in which belief systems can have a profound effect in the creation of illness. Most of these examples were in hunter–gatherer communities, such as Australian aborigines or North American Indians. Shamans were believed to be able to afflict or remove afflictions by exorcism-like rituals. A more modern example will be given next.

Traditional Chinese astrology postulates that certain combinations of birth year and disease are particularly hazardous. Phillips (1993) has provided evidence that adverse combinations of astrological signs actually predict premature deaths. Examination of 28,172 death certificates revealed that premature death was statistically linked with combinations of birth years and disease that are viewed as unfavourable in Chinese astrology. For example, Chinese females who are born in "Earth years" and suffer from malignant neoplasms die 2.29 years earlier than those born in "Fire" and "Metal" years. Chinese females born in "Metal" years and suffering from bronchitis, emphysema, or asthma die 4.02 years earlier than Chinese females with the same disease but born in non-metal years. This relationship applied to each of the major types of cancer and also for 12 of the 15 major causes of death studied. The effect was stronger for females, and the size of the effect was proportional to the person's adherence to traditional Chinese culture. Phillips interprets these findings in terms of "helplessness/hopelessness" and "stoicism", which is discussed further in chapter 14.

DISSOCIATIVE REACTIONS

Some dissociation of mental processes is observed in hypnosis, amnesia after trauma, and even in stage performances. A degree of dissociation is frequently observed in patients who had to deal with very unpleasant events. The initial numbness of bereavement may be seen as dissociation, as may the "denial" reaction observed in a minority of survivors of heart attacks. Diagnostic problems are obviously important for the doctor working in a casualty department, where very occasionally the diagnosis of "fugue" might be made. Apart from these rare and dramatic examples, "dissociative reaction" as a diagnosis is uncommon in Britain.

Dissociation was classically described by Freud using a "vertical split" model of the mind, with the unconscious mind lying beneath the conscious. An alternative approach, proposed by Hilgard (1977), is in terms of a "horizontal split", with a "hidden observer" behind a barrier. Zamansky and Bartis (1985) provide a relatively sophisticated experimental variant of the hidden-observer paradigm. Their subjects were given a hypnotic suggestion that they would neither detect an odour, nor be able to read anything written on a piece of paper. These stimuli were then presented, and those who showed no recognition went on to receive a further suggestion that "a hidden part of them would reach conscious awareness". Most subjects then recalled the smell of ammonia and the number on the paper. It is not strictly necessary to postulate an unconscious mind to explain such phenomena, and exaggerated compliance with demands may be all that is needed. Aldridge-Morris (1989) presents a view of exaggerated role-playing to account for multiple personality—the most dramatic form of dissociation. He goes on to propose that supposed multiple personalities are actually the creation of therapists. The intentional faking of multiple personality is also possible, according to the reports of Orne (1984) and other psychologists and psychiatrists who examined Kenneth Bianchi, the so-called "Hillside Strangler". Bianchi apparently faked multiple personality to avoid the consequences of a multiple murder trial, according to Orne, though Watkins discussing the same case offered evidence of genuine multiple personality.

HYPOCHONDRIASIS

Hypochondriasis is another diagnostic term that is probably better described in terms of normal processes of anxiety and body monitoring. Warwick and Salkovskis (1990) have provided a descriptive model in terms of three systems: cognition, behaviour, and physiology. Illness fear can lead to heightened awareness of normal kinaesthetic sensations and become part of a belief system about illness. Gain, in the form of medical attention, is another powerful influence. This is seen in the most dramatic way in Munchausen's syndrome, in which people injure themselves or simulate illness, sometimes to the extent of receiving exploratory surgery. A more disturbing variation, in which an adult injures a child, is known as Munchausen by proxy syndrome. Meadow (1993) reports a series of false allegations of abuse and Munchausen by proxy syndrome. These 14 cases in a Leeds hospital did not involve disputes over custody or divorce settlements and appeared to be only for the gain of medical attention. Schreier and Libow (1993) have described several such cases and draw attention to the powerful need for attention by healthcare staff, which can lead to such bizarre acts.

One implication of viewing illness as the consequence of health behaviours is the removal of the protection of the sick role. Heart attacks and cancer might come to be seen as self-inflicted disease, in the same way that parasuicide, overdosing on heroin, or Munchausen injuries were not seen as "free from blame". The implications of this have yet to be worked out, but a "professional partnership" approach, in which the client delegates some responsibility to professional health advisors, is described in chapter 7.

CONCLUSION

Organic disorders that have a partly psychophysiological basis were previously called psychosomatic disorders. The classical view was of a symptom that allowed a compromise between conflicting motives. Alexithymia theory is a modern psychoanalytic approach to the same problem, which views psychosomatic problems as communication failures. Awareness of conflicting needs is likely to be helpful. Most illnesses are now seen to have a psychogenic aspect, so the term "psychosomatic" is unhelpful. Conversion reactions involve the voluntary nervous system, but the extent of their incidence is very controversial. Dissociation may occur under hypnosis and fear, and it may be viewed variously in terms of splits in mental processes or exaggerated role-playing. Psychological models are developing as alternatives to diagnostic concepts, but medical constructs have continuing value for treatment.

REFERENCES

Aldridge-Morris, R. (1989). *Multiple personality: An exercise in deception*. Hove: Lawrence Erlbaum Associates Ltd.

Alexander, F. (1987). *Psychosomatic medicine*. London: Norton.

Alexander, F., French, T.M., & Pollack, G.H. (Eds.) (1968). *Psychosomatic specificity, Vol. 1*. Chicago, IL: University of Illinois Press.

Bahnson, C.B. (1979). Das Krebsproblem in psychosomatischer Dimension [The psychosomatic dimension of cancer]. Cited by P. Netter, Types and models in understanding and describing diseases. In L.R. Schmidt, P. Schwenkmezger, J. Weinman, & S. Maes, *Theoretical and applied aspects of health psychology* (pp. 29–50). London: Harwood, 1990.

Frank, J.D. (1973). *Persuasion and healing*. Baltimore, MD: Johns Hopkins University Press.

Hilgard, E. (1977). *Divided consciousness*. New York: Wiley.

Kaplan, R.T., & Sadock, V. (1985). *Modern synopsis of comprehensive textbook of psychiatry* (4th ed.). Baltimore, MD: Williams & Wilkins.

Lachman (1972). Definition of psychosomatic illness. Cited in D. Bakal, *Psychology and medicine*. London: Tavistock, 1979.

Luborsky, L., Docherty, J.P., & Penick, S. (1973). Onset conditions for psychosomatic symptoms: A comparative review of immediate observation with retrospective research. *Psychosomatic Medicine, 35*, 187–203.

McDonald, P.W., & Prkachin, K.M. (1990). The expression and perception of facial emotion in alexithymia: A pilot study. *Psychosomatic Medicine, 52*, 199–210.

Meadow, R. (1993). False allegations of abuse and Munchausen's syndrome by proxy. *Archives of Disease in Childhood, 68* (4), 444–447.

Miller, E. (1987). Hysteria: Its nature and explanation. *British Journal of Clinical Psychology, 26*, 163–173.

Orne, M. (1984). On the differential diagnosis of multiple personality in the forensic context. *International Journal of Clinical and Experimental Hypnosis, 32*, (2), 118–169.

Phillips, D.P. (1993). A reduction in life span associated with negative psychosocial intervention. *Proceedings of Seventh Conference of the European Health Psychology Society*, Brussels (September).

Rubino, I.A., Grasso, S., Sonnino, A., & Pezzarossa, B. (1992). Is alexithymia a non-neurotic personality dimension? *British Journal of Medical Psychology, 64*, 385–391.

Scheich, G., Florin, I., Rudolph, R., & Wilhelm, S. (1993). Personality characteristics and serum IgE level in patients with atopic dermatitis. *Journal of Psychosomatic Research, 37* (6), 637–642.

Schmidt, L.R., Schwenkmezger, P., Weinman, J., & Maes, S. (1990). *Theoretical and applied aspects of health psychology*. London: Harwood.

Schreier, H.A., & Libow, J.A. (1993). *Hurting for love: Munchausen by proxy syndrome*. New York: Guilford Press.

Siegman, A.W. (1993). Cardiovascular consequences of expressing, experiencing, and repressing anger. *Journal of Behavioral Medicine, 16* (6), 539–570.

Slater, E.T.O. (1965). Diagnosis of "hysteria". *British Medical Journal, 1*, 1395–1399.

Warwick, H., & Salkovskis, P. (1990). Hypochondriasis. *Behaviour Research and Therapy, 28* (2), 105–117.

Weintraub, M.I. (1993). *Hysterical conversion reactions*. USA: PMA Publishing.

Zamansky, H., & Bartis, S. (1985). The dissociation of experience: The hidden observer observed. *Journal of Abnormal Psychology, 94*, 243–248.

5

Food, Drink, and Drugs

Substances we take in from the environment make a substantial contribution to the maintenance of positive health. In many parts of the world and for most of human history, the central problem has been the achievement of adequate nutrition. While it is still possible to have problems such as folic acid deficiency in Europe, deficiency diseases are less important than health problems associated with the abuse of foods and drugs. The term "drugs" here mainly refers to self-administered substances such as alcohol and tobacco, rather than to controlled substances prescribed by a medical practitioner. It is necessary to discuss each substance from both biological and psychological standpoints. The following hypotheses will be presented as skills of the fit person:

5.1 eats food with about the right calorific content, low in total fats, high in fibre, and with adequate vitamins, oils, etc.

5.2 eats in social contexts with pleasure, relaxation, and social exchange

5.3 abstains from tobacco smoking

5.4 drinks alcohol in moderation or abstains, and enjoys social contexts

5.5 uses recreational drugs, if at all, in moderation and with knowledge of their effects

FOOD AS NUTRITION

Energy and nutrients

Humans need oxygen, enough food energy (calories), water, 8 to 10 essential amino acids in proteins, essential fatty acids (e.g. linoleic acid), a small amount of carbohydrate, 13 vitamins, and 18 elements scattered across the upper half of the periodic table (in addition to hydrogen, carbon, nitrogen, and oxygen). Together, they add up to over 40 nutrients, and many are normally taken for granted: The minor nutrients are present in sufficient amounts in a mixed diet of foods. The quantity of each vitamin needed is about the size of one grain of sugar a day, and the evidence for larger doses of vitamins giving benefit is not strong.

Problems of excess mainly occur in relation to fats and total calories. Generous intakes of saturated fat raise the plasma cholesterol concentration and contribute to coronary heart disease. People with high salt intakes may have more hypertension. Too much food energy leads to obesity. Table 5.1 shows the recommended daily amounts of various nutrients. The table of RDAs is taken from one of a useful series of articles on nutrition by the British Medical Journal Publishing Group (Truswell, 1986). UK DoH 1981 recommendations are quoted where available, but US and Australian RDAs are used for most of the minerals. The RDAs are for sedentary males aged 18–34. Figures for women are generally about 80% of those for younger men, but are higher for iron and during pregnancy and lactation. Figures are higher for energy if they are active; for older people, figures are generally smaller. Figures for children may be interpolated between infants and adults. Some recommendations for infants differ between breast-fed and formula-fed infants, and most increase during the four quarters of the first year of life.

Fats

Fats warrant special mention, as they are strongly implicated in heart disease, cancer, and diabetes. Energy can be derived from sugars, starches, fats, and even protein, if necessary. Fats are concentrated energy sources, and this may explain the appeal of bacon and eggs to labourers, or chocolate to mountaineers. Atherogenesis is strongly related to the level of fat consumption, and this evidence is reviewed in chapter 8. There are marked differences between countries in the incidence of cancers, which correlate with the per capita consumption of fat. Wynder (1976) estimates that one half of cancers in women and one-third in men are associated with diet, and fat intake is the principal route. The correlations for 40 countries in Table 5.2 are adapted from Carroll and Khor (1975).

The amount of fat consumed seems to increase risk of hormone-related cancers, but to reduce risk at the gastrointestinal sites of absorption. Such

Table 5.1 Representative RDAs

Nutrient	Units	Young men	Infants	
Energy	kcal	2500	530–980	
Protein	g	63	13–25	
Thiamine	mg	1.0	0.3	
Riboflavin	mg	1.6	0.4	
Niacin	mg	18	5	(equivalent mg)
Vitamin B_6	mg	2.2	0.3	
Folate	µg	200	50–70	(total µg)
Vitamin B_{12}	µg	3.0	0.5–1.5	
Vitamin C	mg	30	20	
Vitamin A	µg	750	450	(RE = retinol equivalents)
Vitamin D	µg	only if housebound	7.5	
Vitamin E	mg	10	3–4	
Calcium	mg	600	600	
Iron	mg	12	6	
Magnesium	mg	350	50	
Zinc	mg	15	3	
Iodine	µg	150	40	
Sodium	mmol	40–100	6–25	
Potassium	mmol	50–140	10–35	

From Truswell (1986). Reproduced by permission.

Table 5.2 Correlations between national fat consumption
and cancer at various sites

Site	Female		Male	
hormone-related	breast	+0.935	prostate	+0.892
	ovaries	+0.726		
intestine (exc. rectum)		+0.911		+0.928
rectum		+0.786		+0.834
skin		+0.550		+0.634
stomach		−0.112		+0.010
liver and bile duct		−0.487		−0.676

epidemiological findings may be misleading, however, because of the earlier death rate from other causes in less-nourished countries, and because of the correlation between the intake of fats and sugars, carcinogens, etc. Creasey (1985) reviews evidence from animal and cancer patient studies and concludes that fat levels do play a causal role in carcinogenesis. The effect on reproductive tissue may be via oestrogen and obesity, while the protective effect on the digestive system may be through the ability of fats to dissolve and transport carcinogens away from the gut. The proportion of calories as fat in traditional British diet is over 40%, so current medical recommendations are to reduce this to 30% or lower. The Lifestyle Heart programme (see chapter 9) recommended only 10% fat. Preference for high-fat foods seems to develop early. Men born in the 1920s in Hertfordshire who had been breast-fed and not weaned by the age of 1 year had higher Standard Mortality Ratios than those weaned earlier or bottle-fed (Fall et al., 1992). Prolonged consumption of high-fat breast milk may lead to a preference for high-fat foods.

Water and fibre

The second level of analysis of food is as water and packing. All foods contain water; in many it is more than half the weight. The percentage of water is higher in some fruits and vegetables than in milk. The more water a food contains, the fewer the calories. A sedentary adult needs about 1000 ml or grams per day, but this increases greatly if body-cooling requirements increase. The "packing" of plant foods—that is, dietary fibre—is not all inert. While the lignins are not broken down by gut action, pectins, gums, and other polysaccharides are absorbed in the human gut. The inert substances nonetheless have marked physiological effects: Hemicelluloses of wheat increase faecal bulk and speed colonic transit, and they may bind nutrients so that they are excreted; pectins slow absorption of lipids and carbohydrate. Burkitt and Trowell (1975) argued that fibre confers protection by increasing transit times, though this has not been well supported. Fibre binds bile acids and some carcinogens strongly, and this adsorption effect is the probable reason for the protective effect of fibre, according to Creasey (1985). Fibre also causes the intestinal wall to grow more thickly, which, in principle, might contribute to colon cancer, but the balance of evidence seems to point to protective effects.

All the rest and toxins

All the many other substances in foods are non-nutritive. They produce most of the flavour, colour, and other sensory qualities. In most natural foods, there are inherent substances that are potentially toxic but usually present in small amounts—for example, solanine in potatoes, nitrates and oxalates in spinach, thyroid antagonists in brassica vegetables, cyanide-producing glycosides in cassava and apricot stones, etc. Then there are substances to which only some people are sensitive—for example, in some people wheat causes gluten enteropathy, broad beans favism, and cheese a tyramine effect in patients taking monoamine oxidase inhibitors. Other toxins get into foods when their environment is unusual—for example, shellfish may be polluted with industrial contaminants, such as methyl mercury, PCB, etc. Microbiological infection can produce very potent toxins, such as botulism and aflatoxin. Minute quantities of toxins need not be a cause for health worry.

FOOD AND SOCIAL LIFE

The problems associated with food nowadays are more to do with the symbolic significance of food than with its nutritional content. Beliefs in selective dietary intake may include garlic to prevent heart disease, evening primrose oil to prevent premenstrual syndrome, or camomile to achieve relaxation. However, the effects of belief are generally stronger than the pharmacological effects, so food symbolism needs to be examined. The discussion is influenced by Orford (1985). Food has at least the following symbolic functions:

- *Body image.* Ideal weight from the point of view of physical health is that associated with highest life expectancy, as measured by the actuaries for life-insurance companies. Ideal weight is proportional to height, and to a smaller extent to bone size. Quetelet's Index (weight in kilogrammes divided by square of height in metres) is a common way of estimating this; indices in the range between 20 and 25 are regarded as ideal. Average weight is somewhat higher than ideal weight. However, body image for women is more influenced by concepts of beauty and fashion than by health, and the two criteria are often different. Perhaps the most troublesome aspect of idealised body image is that it is virtually unachievable, so that most women have a sense most of the time of having failed to reach the shape they want. Fashion photographs are commonly taken of very tall models, over 1.80 metres, and the same garments achieve different proportions on a woman of average height.

- *Comfort.* Eating is a source of pleasure that can continue when more complex satisfactions such as career or sexual relationships are suffering. In Maslow's hierarchy, this satisfaction is low in the hierarchy of needs. This is likely to be important in obesity and bulimia nervosa, and a recent discussion of this is provided by Ogden and Wardle (1991). Heatherton and Banmeister (1991) suggest that binge eating is an escape from uncomfortably high self-awareness, associated with overly high standards and expectations. Comfort eating is likely to increase when other satisfactions are low, but appetite drops during more serious depression.

- *Control through refusal or gorging.* Anorexia nervosa constitutes the most extreme form of refusal to eat. The American family therapist Salvador Minuchin views the refusal to eat as a way of maintaining autonomy in excessively "enmeshed" families. He gives examples of families in which a girl in her early teens is not able to achieve privacy and separation from parents. Minuchin spoke of "cross-generational bonding" as a symbolic process, but more recently writers such as Waller et al. (1993) have suggested that unwanted sexual experience has occurred in a high proportion of women with eating disorders. Exerting control over one's body through the refusal to eat constitutes a way of separating oneself from the body, which is seen as under the control of others, or as a retreat from femininity.

- *Relaxation pauses.* Digestion involves increased peristalsis and secretion of bile, saliva, and other digestive juices under the action of the parasympathetic nervous system. A main meal will therefore normally be followed by lowered arousal and a feeling of drowsiness. Prolonged rest or sleep will increase the amount of food absorbed—this principle is used in the body building of sumo wrestlers. Rapid eating without a digestive interval is likely to involve curtailment of the parasympathetic effects, which may have implications for those with a tendency to ulcers. Rest also increases the relaxing effect of parasysmpathetic activity, so taking time over dinner is likely to contribute to stress management. Many smokers feel the need to smoke after eating, and this may interact with short eating times: The desired mood (though also the weight gain) would follow to some extent after a slower meal, without the additional effects of nicotine.

- *Context for social gatherings.* Some cultures, especially those around the Mediterranean, place considerable importance on the evening meal as a feast for the extended family. This is likely to be the main focus for family communication and the resolution of conflict. Conversely, fast food is a relatively solitary activity. Heart disease is lower in Mediterranean than in North European countries, a trend that is usually attributed to the relative proportion of dietary fat. However, it may also reflect the role of communal eating in tension reduction.

- *Wholesomeness.* Food preferences can acquire strong emotional connotations. In childhood, a single bout of nausea can lead to a long-term aversion to the food that preceded the sickness, by a process of classical conditioning. The food preferences of other cultures can seem deeply repugnant—for example, horse-meat in France, dog in Korea, or grubs eaten by Australian aborigines. However, such aesthetic sensibilities are based mainly on habit rather than valid nutritional considerations. During periods of illness, a desire for "good" or "wholesome" food can develop. For example, patients with cancer may feel that the bad thing inside them is related to eating "unnatural" foods and turn, for example, to organically grown vegetables. However, feelings about foods being "natural" or "artificial" are often not well founded in terms of their constituents. The widely held view that E-numbers describe synthetic substances is an example and is discussed next.

Additives

Food production now involves a great variety of treatments to enhance colour, flavour, or shelf-life. Most such additives are edible substances of vegetable origin, as can be seen in Table 5.3. Concern about additives has

Table 5.3 Additives

Additive	E-number	Occurring in:
antioxidants	E300 (L-ascorbic acid)	fruit drinks and bread dough
	E307 (synthetic alpha-tocopherol)	cereal-based baby foods
colours	E100 (curcumin)	flour confectionery, margarine
	E153 (vegetable carbon black)	liquorice
	E160(b) (annatto)	crisps
emulsifiers and stabilisers	E400 (alginic acid)	ice-cream, soft cheese
	E412 (guar gum)	packet soups, meringue mixes
	E464 (hydroxypropyl-methylcellulose)	edible ices
preservatives	E200 (sorbic acid)	soft drinks, fruit yoghurt
	E220 (sulphur dioxide)	
	E252 (potassium nitrate)	cured meats, including bacon, corned beef
sweeteners	E420 (sorbitol bulk sweetener, e.g. jams for diabetics)	
others	E290 (carbon dioxide)	fizzy drinks
	E503 (ammonium carbonate)	buffer and aeration in biscuits
	E502 (sodium hydroxide)	base for cocoa, jams, and sweets

generalised from the effects of a few, such as E102 tartrazine. E-numbers merely indicate that a substance has been approved for use in foods and has been given an EEC code; these substances are not more "natural" or "artificial" than food substances without an E-number (Ministry of Agriculture Fisheries and Food, 1987).

NON-PRESCRIBED DRUGS

Apart from food, a number of substances are used recreationally to achieve feelings of well-being. The ability to achieve desired levels of arousal and feelings of intimacy and personal worth are central health behaviours. Most people rely on pharmacological agents to some extent, even if only alcohol or caffeine, so ability to use recreational drugs is an important skill.

Alcohol and tobacco are legal in most countries, while most of the others listed in Table 5.4 are illegal. From a pharmacological standpoint, dangerousness and legal status are largely historical accident. The Canadian Government Commission of Enquiry (1971) undertook a comprehensive review of recreational drugs before altering legislation, and this is summarised here. Alcohol is a fairly dangerous drug in terms of disease and accidents, but it has a long history of legal use in most cultures other than Islamic countries. On the other hand, cannabis is illegal in many, even though it has not been shown to have markedly harmful effects. The commonly used legal drugs—alcohol, tobacco, and caffeine—are analysed here in more detail. The others mentioned are important for physical health mainly in cases of overdose, self-neglect, or cross-infection, and are not otherwise highly significant for the achievement of health behaviours. Heroin and morphine are discussed further in the chapter on pain. A detailed account of brain sites of action of psychoactive drugs is given by Hollandsworth (1990). The social context of consumption in determining mood is important. It is entirely possible to become "drunk" on water, if the social influences are favourable, while the taking of an illegal drug is surrounded by a particular sense of excitement and mystique.

SMOKING

Tobacco is the most widely used drug that results in addiction, and the leading cause of preventable illness. Its psychoactive effects are mainly through nicotine, with some effect from carbon monoxide. The psychological

Table 5.4

Substance	Mechanism of action	Valued effect	Unwanted effects/ hazards
alcohol	depression of synaptic transmission in CNS, esp. reticular system	arousal reduction after work; loss of social inhibition	accidents; violence; toxic effects on liver; learning impairment
benzodia-zepines	muscle relaxation	anxiety reduction without disinhibition	dependency
barbiturates	block gamma-aminobutyric acid receptors	similar to alcohol: loss of inhibition; excitabil-ity, then mellowness	dependency
cannabis	non-specific depres-sant action on the CNS	pleasant lethargy; reduction of nausea	lower achievement motivation
heroin, opiates	stimulation of opioid mureceptors in limbic system	analgesia; warmth; contentment; ecstasy	coma in overdose
solvents	possibly similar to alcohol	disinhibition at low dose; stupor, analge-sia at high dose	asphyxiation
tobacco	stimulation of nicotinic acetylcho-line receptors	user-controlled alertness, or pain and anxiety reduction	airway obstruction; clotting, athero-genesis; carcinogens
amphetamines	adrenalin-like	rush of alertness; suppression of appetite; lack of fatigue	aggression, psycho-sis (?); weight loss; ulcers; delayed sleep needs
caffeine	increase turnover of monoamines	alertness	agitation
cocaine	noradrenalin increase	pleasurable "rush"	nasal damage
LSD	decrease in serotonin	altered perception, e.g. enhanced colour	psychosis (?)

habit of smoking serves to reduce subjective arousal ("calm one's nerves"), to control weight, and to give the appearance of maturity. The effects are similar to those of emotional arousal, so ambiguity exists about whether the cardio-vascular damage associated with smoking may be in a consequence of overarousal. Tobacco's other harmful effects are through coal-tar products in the airways.

Nicotine

Inhaled puffs of smoke produce intermittent, highly concentrated boli of nicotine in the blood. This means that the smoker can control the dose rate of nicotine he or she is delivering to the brain. By varying factors such as the size of puff and depth of inhalation, a smoker can obtain predominantly inhibitory or predominantly excitatory effects, or a mixture of both, from one cigarette. This ability to control the psychoactive effects of nicotine is probably the best explanation of why the smoking habit is so popular. The acetylcholine receptor agonistic effect of nicotine results in a dose-dependent two-way stimulant/depressant action. Small to moderate levels of the drug stimulate cholinergic activity. At higher doses or over long periods of time, nicotine may persist in these receptor sites and thus block further responding. This produces the depressant effect of nicotine at high dosages. Lethal dosages are possible, in which synaptic transmission is blocked completely.

The pleasurable effects of smoking on the cerebral cortex probably involve stimulation of the reticular system and hippocampus, although its mechanism may also involve nicotine-stimulated release of acetylcholine from the cortex. The CNS effects of nicotine induce pleasurable feelings in 90% of chronic smokers, although they do not produce a "high" comparable to that of many other drugs that induce dependence. In addition, nicotine appears to reduce pain and relieve anxiety in stressful situations; this may be due to its ability to promote the release of noradrenalin and dopamine from limbic areas and the hypothalamus. It is also possible that nicotine interacts with the opioid reward systems, as well as increasing plasma concentrations of beta-endorphin precursor (beta-endorphin-beta-lipotropin) in humans. Its psychoactive effects occur in the reward centres of the brain, while at higher dosages it seems likely that nicotine may reduce activity in the punishment centres of the brain, possibly through a depressant effect at cholinergic synapses in the periventricular system.

The properties of this volatile colourless liquid are described in detail by Hollandsworth (1990). It turns brown upon exposure to air and emits an aroma characteristic of tobacco. This plant alkaloid is structurally related to acetylcholine and acts as a direct agonist on the nicotinic cholinergic receptors throughout the body. Nicotinic receptors are found between the pre- and post-ganglionic neurons of both sympathetic and parasympathetic branches of the autonomic nervous system, as well as in the membranes of skeletal muscle at the neuromuscular junction. This explains some of nicotine's peripheral effects, which include tachycardia, vasoconstriction, and a rise in blood pressure. Thus, although smoking is often used to "calm the nerves", it actually increases the peripheral effects of emotional arousal while reducing subjective awareness of them. Nicotine is lipid-soluble, and thus it readily crosses cell membranes and, in the form of cigarette smoke, is absorbed swiftly and efficiently from the lungs. It is also rapidly absorbed from the nasal mucosa when taken as snuff and from the buccal mucosa when delivered in the form of chewing-tobacco. It exerts little effect when swallowed, because it undergoes a first-pass metabolism in the liver. Nicotine has a half-life of approximately 30 to 60 minutes. It also increases the rate of metabolism of several other drugs, through hepatic enzyme induction. Once in the blood, nicotine is quickly distributed throughout the body, reaching the brain in 7 to 8 seconds.

The presumed role of nicotine in the suppression of appetite is fairly well supported: It is known that a single cigarette inhibits hunger contractions of the stomach for 15 to 60 minutes, and its usual effect on the gastrointestinal tract is to increase tone and motor activity. In addition, nicotine appears to elevate fasting levels of blood sugar for a period of a half-hour or more. It has an antidiuretic effect on the kidneys, with non-smokers being more susceptible than smokers to this effect of reducing the flow of urine. Perkins (1992) presents evidence from cross-sectional studies that despite their lower body weights, smokers do not eat less than non-smokers or ex-smokers; in fact, they tend to eat slightly more. Similarly, laboratory studies show no acute effects of smoking or nicotine intake via other means on caloric intake in smokers, although intake of non-smokers may be reduced after nicotine. Nausea can occur, since low dosages of nicotine stimulate the medullar respiratory centre and can induce nausea and/or vomiting via stimulation of the medullary chemoreceptor zone.

Carbon monoxide and tar

Cigarette burning releases a number of volatile substances other than nicotine, including tar and benzopyrene. Tar has a cumulative effect in destroying the cilia of the airways and obstructing the alveoli of the lungs. Benzo (alpha) pyrene is the most hazardous of the substances that collect in the lungs and irritate cells, which can become cancerous. Carbon monoxide is a partial oxidation product, to which haemoglobin binds in preference to oxygen. This lowers the oxygen-transporting ability of the blood by up to 15%, but this appears to be associated with a pleasurable feeling of a light-headed "rush" for smokers.

Prevalence of smoking

Smoking has declined in Britain, partly as a result of intense publicity of its health hazards. However, this decline has been greater among white-collar workers than manual workers, greater in people in middle life than in adolescence, and more in men than in women. The proportion of people smoking remains high in Eastern European countries. Davis, Monaco, and Romero (1991) report on US smoking-cessation progress since the 1964 report of the Surgeon General described the health hazards of smoking. The prevalence of smoking in adults decreased from about 40% in 1964 to 29% in 1987. An estimated 35 million Americans who would otherwise have been smokers were non-smokers in 1985. Health knowledge alone is not a major reason for not smoking, as indicated by the high proportion of nurses who smoke. Waalkens et al. (1992) surveyed the smoking habits and attitudes towards smoking of medical students (n = 725), house officers (n = 126), and consultants (n = 236) at the University Hospital of Groningen in Holland. Of the medical students, 27% were current smokers, as were 28% of the house officers and 34% of the consultants. Smoking prevalence was highest among psychiatrists and lowest among paediatricians.

Starting to smoke in adolescence

The period of puberty is critical for the smoking habit. Children between 9 and 11 usually express a highly moralistic opposition to cigarettes. While smoking in general has declined, the rate of smoking among adolescent girls has actually increased, and about one in three teenage girls smoked in the early 1990s. Smoking appears to connote independence and perceived maturity for many teenagers, and the long-term health hazards are less significant than the strong psychosexual pressures of adolescence. Bauman (1989) studied the level of testosterone in the saliva of 14-year olds. This hormone mediates sexual arousal, and assertive behaviour generally, in both males and females. Being a current smoker, carbon monoxide in the breath, and smoking intensity were all significantly related to salivary testosterone in both boys and girls.

Initial deterrence is important, since once a smoking habit is established, quitting is extremely difficult: The relapse rate for smokers of more than 20 cigarettes a day who try to stop is about 80%.

Refusal skills have been the target of a number of interventions with early teenagers, such as that of Sallis et al. (1990). This San Diego project was called SHOUT (Students Helping Others Understand Tobacco) and consisted of eight one-hour lessons during the academic year. Types of refusal scored included:

Simple direct no: "No, that's O.K."

Broken record: "No thanks, I don't smoke; No thanks, I don't smoke."

Reason: "It can cause cancer."

Supportive: "You go ahead, none for me."

Withdrawal: "Come on, let's go dance."

Aggressive: "Only creeps smoke."

Accepts: "Sure, thanks."

Students who had received the training programme gave more simple, direct, and fewer withdrawal responses than control students exposed to the same offers of cigarettes or smokeless tobacco. This was in accord with the authors' expectation, who used their own judgement about what constituted "good" or "poor" refusal. Some external validity was found from smoking rates in the schools: Intervention students stayed at about the same level of smoking (6%), while control students increased their smoking during the seven months of intervention.

Social influences through the peer group have been seen as the key strategy in preventing adolescent smoking uptake, and reviews such as that of Flay (1985) are optimistic about the social influences model. However, a study by Murray et al. (1988) gave equivocal results for the efficacy of this approach. The major focus was on teaching and practising resistance to social pressures to smoke. Efforts were made to solicit public commitments not to smoke and to correct expectations of smoking as normative. Programmes took place in seventh-grade classrooms (12-year-olds), and most activities were pupil-led. In 1985, four or five years after the intervention, 6,135 school students were traced and agreed to a follow-up. No programme emerged as statistically superior in smoking prevention, though programmes using videotapes and those under adult leadership had marginally poorer outcomes. Among those who had experienced the peer-led social influences programme who had never smoked at the time, 8.3% now smoked on a weekly basis. Of those who had ever smoked at the time of the programme, 30.3% were now "weekly" smokers and 25.2% were "daily" smokers. The abstention rate was slightly better than among those who had had no programme at all—15.2% of those who had never smoked in the seventh grade now did so, and 41.9% of those who had smoked continued to do so.

Quitting decisions

Part of the difficulty in abstention from tobacco is that quitting and resumption are both extremely easy. Part of the solution is to make the quitting decision more strategic and preceded by a long period of reflection. This has been codified as a "Stages of Change" model (Prochaska & DiClemente, 1992). The five stages of change are: precontemplation, contemplation, preparation, action, and maintenance. About half of smokers are in the *precontemplation* stage and do not intend to quit in the next six months, while those in *contemplation* are seriously thinking about quitting in the next 6 months. The *preparation* stage implies seriously intending to quit in the next month, and having tried to do so in the last year; 10%–20% of smokers are in the preparation stage. The *action* stage is defined as 6 months after overt stopping, and *maintenance* from 6 months until smoking is no longer seen as a problem. Prochaska (1994) studied decisions across 12 health behaviours and identified only two factors in decision-making: pros and cons. Progression from precontemplation to action was a function of a one-standard-deviation increase in the pros of a behaviour change. Changes in the cons, or objections to behaviour change, were less important.

Many factors exert an influence on quitting decisions, but none is particularly strong. Physician advice, relaxation training, exposure to campaign material, experience of smoking-related illness, and environmental bans each exert small effects. Viswesvaran and Schmidt (1992) undertook a meta-analysis to cumulate the results from 633 studies of smoking cessation, involving 71,806 subjects, that reported the proportion of successful quits. Cumulation of quit rates from all available control groups indicated that, on average, 6.4% of the smokers could be expected to quit smoking without any intervention. Self-care methods did not appear to be as effective as formal intervention methods. Instructional programmes involving physicians were not more effective than other instructional programmes. Conditioning-based techniques such as aversive methods had success rates similar to those of instructional methods, and among the instructional methods, those incorporating social norms and values were more successful than those relying solely on didactic approaches.

Physician advice. This is a modest factor in quitting, but more intensive input does not seem to improve abstinence. Gilbert et al. (1992) compared a two-visit smoking cessation intervention by family physicians with the same intervention supplemented by additional follow-ups; 41 Ontario physicians and 647 patients were involved, and no statistically significant difference was found in one-year, biochemically validated, sustained cessation rates between the group offered the long-term follow-up visits (12.5%) and the group given the brief intervention (10.2%).

Relaxation. Some smokers need to complete a meal with a cigarette, and it may be that the meal has been eaten too quickly, so that the parasympathetic effects of digestion have not had time to occur. Smoking after sexual intercourse may also indicate the absence of the relaxation that follows sex in the context of emotional intimacy. Relaxation strategies alone have a small effect on achieving abstinence. Imagery for reducing stress and prolonging abstinence in adult ex-smokers was investigated by Wynd (1992). Volunteer subjects ($n = 76$) were solicited after completing a local smoking cessation programme, and participants were randomly assigned to an experimental imagery group ($n = 39$) or to a control group ($n = 37$). Both groups met for a 3-month period, and experimental group members received instruction in imagery techniques. Enhanced imagery effectiveness, reduced stress, and greater abstinence for the group receiving imagery training was demonstrated. Additionally, discriminant analysis revealed that higher stress and lower imagery effectiveness were prevalent in smoking recidivists.

Public campaigns. Smoking has been heavily promoted historically, so campaigns against smoking often seek to ban such advertising. Studies in Norway, Finland, Canada, and New Zealand have suggested that tobacco consumption could be reduced by between 3% and 7.5% by banning advertising. There are very strong financial objections to such bans, because of revenues from tobacco. Most health-promotion strategies advocating smoking abstinence operate through a one-way channel, such as television or posters, and the addition of a reverse channel seems to improve their effect considerably. Kviz et al. (1992) surveyed registrants for a smoking cessation programme on the evening television news in the Chicago metropolitan area, compared with other smokers in the population. Telephone interviews were conducted before the intervention with random samples of 641 registrants and 2,398 smokers who regularly viewed the evening news. Registration was associated with a smoker's cognitive appraisal of the quitting process, with registrants distinguished by the following: recognition of a need to act (perceived severity of and susceptibility to lung cancer); high outcome expectancies for quitting as an effective means for health promotion; realistic expectations about the effort required to quit; concern about the burden of lung cancer on significant others and related social influence factors; and motivation to quit smoking.

The work environment. Many cues for smoking are particular to the work environment, including the need to concentrate, to control anger, and to achieve separation from unpleasant work involving waste products. Employers are gradually exercising more restriction on smoking at work, and this is likely to increase with the success of claims for damage from passive smoking. Wewers and Ahijevych (1991) report that "uncertainty or ambiguity about what is expected of the worker on the job is a consistent predictor of relapse during the first year postcessation". In addition, workers who perceived a heavier load at 3, 6, and 12 months post-cessation were likely to have resumed smoking.

Stave and Jackson (1991) report on the introduction of a "smoke-free" policy at the Duke University Medical Center, but not on the adjacent University campus. Three months after the smoking prohibition went into effect, a cross-sectional telephone survey was conducted, using randomly selected groups of 400 employees from each campus. Of employees at the Medical Center, 23.6% had been smokers, compared with 20.3% on the University campus. Mean cigarette consumption during work hours declined over this same period from 8.1 to 4.3 at the Medical Center but showed little change on the University campus. A follow-up survey of the cohort of current or recent ex-smokers identified on the initial survey was conducted 6 months later. This survey revealed a smoking cessation rate of 22.5% at the Medical Center and 6.9% on the University campus.

Education in the workplace was compared with financial incentives for smoking abstinence in a study by Windsor, Lowe, and Bartlett (1988), in which 387 smokers were recruited, out of an estimated 2000 smokers at the work-site, and smoking status was validated by thiocyanate from saliva. All were given a standardised self-help cessation manual and maintenance manual before randomisation to one of four conditions. Those receiving the multicomponent health education and skill training were most successful in quitting; the monetary incentive appeared to have no effect on quit rate.

The social environment. Another set of cues for smoking is to be found in pubs, restaurants, the smoking sections of public transport, and so on. Many countries have opted for bans on smoking in public transport, as early as the 1970s in the former East Germany, and in Britain in the 1990s. The French ban on smoking in restaurants and bars was introduced in late 1992. An interesting alternative approach to bans is the use of positive incentives for clean air. Exeter Health Authority ran a "CHEERS" campaign, in which public houses were given a star rating and publicity in proportion to their smoke freedom and various food and drink criteria.

Impact of illness. The experience of major smoking-related illness may be a deterrent to future tobacco use, though this seems to be true more of heart attacks than cancers. Smoking cessation was studied in 1178 female and 1506 male cigarette smokers enrolled in the Framingham Heart Study by Freund et al. (1992). Recent hospitalisation and development of coronary heart disease were predictive of smoking cessation, while diagnosis of cancer or changes in pulmonary function were not. The impact of knowledge about smoking is illuminated by a study of 230 Norwegian smokers who had had heart attacks (Havik & Maeland, 1988). Six months after the MI, 40.6% had resumed smoking, and at a follow-up of around 43 months, 49.4% were smoking. Relapse in the first six months was associated with marital conflicts, anxiety, and depression, a less severe MI, and lower cardiac knowledge. Those who relapsed later had declined in their understanding of smoking as a risk factor. Although the early relapse is disappointing, half of the smokers had quit as a result of MI rehabilitation, which is much higher than the average rate of quitting.

Heart attack survivors seen by the present author during the three months after MI report interesting deliberate use of thoughts to control the urge to smoke. One cognition concerns "loyalty to the coronary care staff"; these patients felt they would be betraying the care shown them by nurses if they returned to smoking. The other effective cognition is a kind of covert sensitisation, in which the patient craving a smoke immediately thought of the pain of the heart attack and of a video image of a lung dissection. The rate of abstention reported in a postal questionnaire seven months after discharge from coronary care was at least 70%; this encouraging result is discussed further in chapter 9.

Weight control. Most people who smoke are aware of the health hazards, but positive reasons for continuing to smoke include stress management and weight control. However, evidence is hard to find for efficacy of a simultaneous focus on weight control and smoking abstinence. French et al. (1992) found no evidence that weight concerns interfered with smoking cessation efforts in 459 women screened for participation in a smoking cessation treatment programme. Hall et al. (1992) compared a sample of 158 smokers who completed a 2-week weight gain prevention intervention with both a nonspecific treatment and standard treatment. A disturbing, unexpected finding was that subjects in both the innovative and nonspecific conditions had a higher risk of smoking relapse than did standard treatment subjects. Both active interventions may have been so complicated that they detracted from nonsmoking. Also, caloric restriction may have increased the reinforcing value of nicotine, thereby increasing smoking relapse risk.

Pirie et al. (1992) conducted a randomised trial of 417 women smokers to test the addition of two weight control strategies to a smoking cessation programme. Participants received the standard smoking cessation programme, the programme plus nicotine gum, the programme plus behavioural weight control, or the programme plus both nicotine gum and behavioural weight control. Weight and smoking status were measured at the end of treatment and at 6 and 12 months post-treatment. Smoking cessation rates were highest in the group receiving the smoking cessation programme plus nicotine gum. Weight gain did not vary by treatment condition, and there was no significant relationship between weight gained and relapse in individuals. The added behavioural weight control programme was attractive to the participants and did not reduce smoking cessation rates.

Nicotine substitutes. The physical withdrawal effects of nicotine dependence can be strong, and provision of nicotine substitutes reduces the airway
hazards, if not the cardiovascular hazards of smoking. Sachs and Leischow
(1991) argue that nicotine activates the brain's "pleasure centre" (mesolimbic
system), and that the only agent with clear scientific evidence for treatment
efficacy is nicotine itself. The use of gum or transdermal patches that release
nicotine is a possible way of reducing the withdrawal symptoms during
smoking cessation. Nicorette is a transmucosally delivered ion-exchange
resin as nicotine polacrilex. Nicotine administered this way still creates the
taste and craved-for effects of smoking, but not the tar or carbon monoxide.
Several recent controlled studies seem to indicate that cessation is more likely
if proprietary nicotine products are used during withdrawal.

Nicotine substitutes seem to maintain smoking abstinence in proportion
to the dose, and patches seem to be more effective than gum. The Transdermal Nicotine Study Group (1991) randomly assigned 935 volunteers who
wanted to quit to a nicotine-patch system delivering nicotine at rates of 21 or
14 mg over 24 hours, or to a placebo. Group counselling sessions were provided to all participants. Cessation rates during the last 4 weeks of the two 6-
week trials were 61%, 48%, and 27% for 21- and 14-mg transdermal nicotine
and placebo, respectively. Six-month abstinence rates for 21-mg transdermal
nicotine and placebo were 26% and 12%, respectively.

Nicotine chewing gum and group sessions ($n = 37$) were compared with a
placebo group ($n = 38$) with an identical intervention by Quilez Garcia et al.
(1989) . The success rate was 35.1% in the gum and group subjects, and 13.2%
in the subjects without gum. A third group, called the "consulting room
group" ($n = 31$), was treated with nicotine chewing gum and followed up in
the programme's usual consulting room. The rate of success in this group
was 25.8%. Freedom from Smoking clinics were offered by the American
Lung Association, with or without prescription of nicotine gum (McGovern
& Lando, 1992). Abstinence outcomes at one week favoured the nicotine
gum conditions (86.3% of nicotine gum subjects were abstinent, as opposed
to 70.9% of comparison subjects). Effects for gum were no longer significant
at later follow-ups of 273 people, although there was no placebo gum condition.

A behavioural self-assessment
for gaining control of smoking

Behavioural A-B-C principles are of considerable use in quitting, and may
be applied through the checklist presented in Table 5.5. The principles are
applicable to control of any substance use and are therefore described in
greater detail in the section on alcohol.

Table 5.5 A behavioural self-assessment for gaining control of smoking

---

- **Controlling the cues for smoking (A)**

Tobacco smoking is partly maintained by a physical dependence on nicotine. More important are the habits and social situations that maintain smoking.

Look at the following list and tick those cues that apply to your smoking behaviour.

availability of matches, ashtrays, cigarettes ___

need to concentrate on a task ___

relaxing after a meal ___

drinking coffee or tea ___

drinking alcohol in social situations ___

people passing cigarettes around ___

not wanting to lose temper ___

feeling lonely or unloved ___

driving a car ___

something to do with my hands ___

too much happening at once ___

something else _____ ___

- **New behaviour (B)**

Having recognised the cues, make sure you can control them. In the case of availability, make sure smoking materials are removed from easy use.

New behaviour to develop for each cue can include:

progressive muscle relaxation ___

chewing, e.g. carrots, apples, sugarless gum ___

running (when fit enough) ___

something else _____ ___

For each of the cues you ticked, write what you will try to do in that context in future.

_____

- **Rewards (C)**

Saving the cost of smoking:

  Write down how much you spend a week on tobacco: _____

  Now write down what you can do with the money you save:

_____

Being less likely to have a heart attack ___

Better insurance premiums ___

Increasing life expectancy by six years on average ___

Feeling more able to climb stairs and so on ___

Being able to smell things ___

Not smelling unpleasant to others ___

Something else _____ ___

Passive smoking

About 85% of the smoke in a cigarette is released as "sidestream" smoke. The evidence that environmental tobacco smoke has harmful effects comes mainly from non-smokers who live or work in close proximity to smokers. Nicotine is rapidly broken down into cotinine, which can be detected in the blood, urine, or saliva. Wald et al. (1984) showed that cotinine levels were three times higher in non-smokers with spouses who smoked than in those whose partners did not. The 20% of non-smokers with the highest exposure to environmental smoke had ten times as much cotinine in their urine compared with the group with least exposure. Diseases related to passive smoking include "glue ear" and asthma in the children of smokers, and lung cancer in adults. Most lung cancer deaths occur to smokers (136,000 a year in the United States, or 40,000 in the United Kingdom). Of the 12,000 lung cancer deaths in US non-smokers, the National Research Council estimated that 2,500 may be attributed to passive smoking.

CAFFEINE

Caffeine is a very widely used legal stimulant, found in tea, coffee, and cola. Caffeine and the chemically related xanthines, theophyline and theobromine, are potent CNS stimulants that have a number of peripheral effects as well. Among the CNS effects are the improvement of cognitive performance and the alleviation of drowsiness and fatigue. Some of the peripheral effects include increased heart rate, increased vascular resistance, and diuresis. Blood pressure is increased slightly by caffeine.

Coffee contains twice as much caffeine as tea per cup on average and three times as much as a standard cola. Some of the central effects of caffeine include increased alertness, increased capacity for sustained intellectual performance, and decreased reaction time. Although it enhances motor skills at low dosages (e.g. less than 200 mg or about two cups of coffee), tasks requiring fine motor coordination may be adversely affected. At higher dosages, persons sensitive to caffeine may experience anxiety, restlessness, insomnia, tremor, and hyperaesthesia (excessive sensitivity of the senses). Dosages that exceed 500 mg may induce muscle twitches, rambling thoughts, speech disturbances, and flushing. The two sites in the brain thought to be most affected by the administration of caffeine are the reticular system and medullary respiratory centre. It is thought that caffeine's stimulant effect is due to its ability to increase the turnover of monoamines in the brain.

ALCOHOL

Alcohol is the most widely used and clinically important of the drugs that cause dependence, and it is important in social rituals in most human communities. By contrast with tobacco, its harmful effects are through excessive doses. Moderate drinking may be relatively neutral with respect to health, although this view remains controversial. Some fermentation products may have positive effects, as has been argued for red wine inhibiting the oxidation of oils to fats. The short-term hazards of excessive alcohol use are in terms of accidents (on the road or with machines), through burns, or through violence. The hazards of regular high doses of alcohol are in terms of brain and liver damage. Moderate doses of this drug are relatively neutral in terms of its cardiovascular and digestive effects, though posing some hazards to those with a tendency to ulceration. Except in Islamic communities, most preventive approaches view alcohol use as a normal behaviour that can become excessive (Robertson et al., 1984), and seek to train control, such as the Health Education Council's *That's the limit* booklet, based on an alcohol education programme in Tyne Tees area.

Units. The effects of alcoholic drinks are inversely proportional to the body mass through which they are distributed, and proportional to the percentage of pure ethyl alcohol to water. One unit or "standard drink" is the equivalent in pure alcohol of half a pint of ordinary beer, a standard glass of wine, or an English standard measure (sixth of a gill) of spirits. Stronger beer, such as Dutch or German lagers, may contain twice the alcohol units, and wines such as sherry, which are fortified with distilled alcohol, are about twice as strong as table wine. The recommended limit in the United Kingdom is currently 21 units for men and 14 for women. Alcohol seems to have a greater effect on women, partly because men have a higher mass and a higher proportion of water in body mass than do women; in addition, the liver seems to be more vulnerable to cirrhosis in women. It takes one hour on average for the liver to eliminate one unit of alcohol. After drinking six pints of beer by 11.00 p.m., an average drinker might still have four units in the blood when driving to work at 7.00 the following morning.

Brain changes. Alcohol is a general CNS depressant that produces a dose-dependent decrease in arousal similar to that obtained from general anaesthetics. At small doses, there may be the appearance of a slight stimulant effect due to disinhibition. Larger doses, however, are associated with a deterioration of judgement, concentration, and attention, as well as impairment of psychomotor and sexual performance. Higher doses are accompanied by ataxia (uncoordinated motor movements) and slurred speech. Very high doses may induce stupor, deep anaesthesia, and even coma. At high blood concentrations, respiratory response to carbon dioxide becomes depressed, which may have lethal consequences. The extended use of alcohol coupled with vitamin deficiencies associated with chronic alcoholism may lead to degenerative changes in brain cells. Wernicke's encephalopathy and Korsakoff's psychosis are two disorders resulting from excessive alcohol consumption over a period of time. The impurities in alcohol, such as the aldehydes that give sherry its characteristic smell, are more toxic than ethyl alcohol itself, so purer alcohol such as vodka is less likely to result in a hangover.

Mood. The effects of alcohol on mood are complex and partly depend on disinhibitory effects on previous mood, and contextual cues during drinking. One memorable aphorism is that "the conscience is the only human organ that is soluble in alcohol". People in a humorous and relaxed environment who believe they are drinking alcohol often imitate others' disinhibited states, even if they are in fact drinking alcohol-free beverages. Small doses of alcohol may produce a mild euphoria and a pleasant sense of relaxation. With increasing dosage, alcohol may precipitate aggressive behaviour or a sense of increased poignancy or sentimentality. Paradoxical effects often follow some hours later: Sleepiness may be followed by an inability to sleep. Robertson et al. (1984) view this as part of an "opponent process". This theory postulates an adaptive change in the nervous system, which opposes the drug effect. The relaxation response of alcohol is opposed by higher arousal, which persists after the alcohol is eliminated.

Circulation and digestion. As a food, ethyl alcohol provides energy only, while destroying some vitamins. A pint of average beer delivers about 180 calories. Alcohol at concentrations greater than the electrolyte concentration in the body cells causes dehydration, which contributes to waking in the night. This can be prevented if wine and spirits are accompanied by water to maintain the isotonic balance. Alcohol is also a diuretic, partly because of its ability to suppress the pituitary antidiuretic hormone. As far as the cardiovascular system is concerned, alcohol increases myocardial excitability and may induce hypertension in some subjects. On the other hand, the daily ingestion of alcohol in moderate amounts may increase the concentration of high-density lipoproteins and thus provide some protection against coronary heart disease. Peripherally, alcohol causes vasodilation in the skin and sweating. This gives the sense of warming, while in reality increasing heat loss, so the traditional remedy of giving brandy after shock or injury can actually aggravate hypothermia of the body core. Alcohol also increases gastric secretions and thus may contribute to gastritis and peptic ulceration. Other conditions related to chronic alcohol abuse include pancreatitis and hepatic cirrhosis. In pregnancy, foetal alcohol syndrome is found in as many as a third to one-half of babies of mothers who are chronic alcoholics.

Heredity. Genetic factors in alcoholism may be most important in determining whether an individual is capable of becoming alcohol-dependent. In a 1971 study, Vesell, Page, and Passananti (cited in Hollandsworth, 1990) administered a single oral dose of 1 ml per kilogram of body weight of 95% ethanol to 14 sets of non-medicated, non-hospitalised healthy twins. Half of the twin pairs were monozygotic and half were dizygotic. The rates of elimination were more similar between monozygotic than dizygotic twins, which suggested that individual differences in ethanol elimination were genetically controlled and that "environmental factors played a negligible role". In fact, elimination rates were identical for 5 of the 7 monozygotic twin pairs, whereas only 1 of the 7 dizygotic pairs exhibited exactly the same rate of elimination. Elimination studies raise the possibility that some individuals have a genetic intolerance of alcohol that protects them from developing alcoholism. The view of alcoholism as a disease put forward by Jellinek (1952) was once widely accepted, not least by chronic alcohol abusers. However, problem drinkers can exert more control than this theory implies. Mello and Mendelson (1971) found that problem drinkers given the opportunity to work for alcohol remained abstinent for a whole day's work in order to accumulate enough alcohol for the next binge.

Functional analysis of alcohol use

A behavioural approach is particularly useful for modifying habit disorders. The principles will be elaborated here for alcohol, and a self-assessment for smoking is given in Table 5.5, on p. 79. Alcohol is a central feature of social life in most European cultures, and any account of its use must be essentially psychosocial, despite the physiological adaptations that also occur. One useful framework, derived from operant conditioning theory, is "functional analysis" (Sobell & Sobell, 1981). Functional analysis distinguishes setting events (or "Antecedents", so that the acronym is an A–B–C sequence), Behaviour, and Consequences.

- *Setting events*

   In the functional analysis model, the term "setting events" is used to connote a complex of factors that, taken as a whole, set the stage for a possible drinking decision:

   distal individual: genetic endowment, early drug learning

distal social: peer group's alcohol use, family climate, parental drug use

proximal individual: beliefs or expectations about drinking, response tendencies, prevailing mood state

proximal situation-specific: physical setting, presence of specific others, licensing laws, cost, ease of access to alcohol.

The individual may or may not be aware of the various components of the setting events complex. Enough assessment information is needed to be relatively confident that most of the major setting events have been identified, without spending an undue amount of effort elucidating trivial components. Any simple functional approach—such as "alcohol abusers drink to reduce anxiety"—is likely to ignore important aspects of drinking decisions.

• *Behavioural options*

Drinking may be in association with:

avoidance learning: forgetting unpleasantness

approach learning: getting up courage to speak to others

Behaviour can be specified by:

Q: *quantity* per sitting

F: *frequency* of drinking occasions

V: *variability* between occasions

Drinking intentions may be:

to drink heavily, with the avowed intention of becoming clearly intoxicated, or

to drink in a limited manner, to achieve pro- or antisocial effects

Some options for control of alcohol use involve drinking, and others do not. The response-consequence contingency defines whether or not a given behaviour is a problem, rather than any reference to a "disease" or "alcoholism".

• *Consequences*

The payoff matrix for alcohol use includes many factors, with different valencies:

immediate positive consequences: change in mood state, avoidance of something aversive, social approval; the immediate positive consequences are hypothesised to be the most important influences on behaviour because of their close temporal contiguity with the drinking

primarily negative but delayed consequences: hangover, declining self-perception, health deterioration, legal difficulties, money shortage, psychosocial problems (e.g. embarrassment at having to deal with problems created for oneself while drinking), etc.; delayed aversive consequences of drinking may go unnoticed by the drinker—for example, some drinkers may not be aware that other people have started to avoid opportunities to socialise with them in drinking situations

Functional analysis will enable many problem drinkers to achieve better control. Where professional intervention is needed, other forms of behavioural management may be appropriate, such as aversive conditioning in addition to the contingency management described above. Emotional dependency is a substantial factor in alcohol use, so dynamic psychotherapy focusing on dependency needs is also valuable.

CONCLUSION

Food can have substantial adverse effects on health if particular nutrients are taken in excess; the proportion of fats is the most important factor. The requirements of low fat and high fibre intake suggest the value of green vegetables, cereals, and fruit. Nutritionally, some fish and white meat is acceptable; milk products and red meat need to form a relatively small proportion of intake. Deficiency problems are now uncommon in industrialised countries, but vitamin deficiencies still occur in some restricted diets. Arguments for dietary supplements and specialised patterns of eating are generally less well supported, at least in terms of their impact on physical health. Aesthetic, religious, and other values may argue for more restrictive diets. Eating also has important pro-social functions, including comfort, relaxation pauses, and social participation. Selective eating may also be used to achieve personal control or feelings of wholesomeness. Various recreational drugs may also be used to achieve a sense of well-being, and users need to be well-informed about their benefits and hazards. Tobacco smoking is very hazardous to the cardiovascular and respiratory systems, and abstinence is discussed in detail. Alcohol is hazardous mainly in excess, so control strategies are analysed.

REFERENCES

Bauman, K.E. (1989). Testosterone and cigarette smoking in adolescents. *Journal of Behavioral Medicine, 12* (5), 425–434.

Burkitt, D.P., & Trowell, H.C. (Eds.) (1975). *Refined carbohydrate foods and disease: Some implications of dietary fibre.* London: Academic Press.

Canadian Government Commission of Enquiry (1971). *The non-medical use of drugs.* London: Penguin.

Carroll, K.K., & Khor, H.T. (1975). Dietary fat in relation to tumorigenesis. *Progr. Biochem. Pharmacol., 10,* 308–353.

Creasey, W.A. (1985). *Diet and cancer.* Philadelphia, PA: Lea & Febiger.

Davis, R.H., Monaco, K., & Romero, R.M. (1991). National program for smoking cessation. *Clinics in Chest Medicine, 12* (4), 819–833.

Fall, C.H., Barker, D.J., Osmond, C., Winter, P.D., Clark, P.M., & Hales, C.N. (1992). Relation of infant feeding to adult serum cholesterol concentration and death from ischaemic heart disease. *British Medical Journal, 302,* 801–805.

Flay, B.R. (1985). Psychosocial approaches to smoking prevention: A review of findings. *Health Psychology, 4,* 449–488.

French, S.A., Jeffery, R.W., Pirie, P.L., & McBride, C.M. (1992). Do weight concerns hinder smoking cessation efforts? *Addictive Behaviors, 17* (3), 219–226.

Freund, K.M., D'Agostino, R.B., Belanger, A.J., Kannel, W.B., & Stokes, J., III (1992). Predictors of smoking cessation: The Framingham Study. *American Journal of Epidemiology, 135* (9), 957–64.

Gilbert, J.R., Wilson, D.M., Singer, J., Lindsay, E.A., Willms, D.G., Best, J.A., & Taylor, D.W. (1992). A family physician smoking cessation program: An evaluation of the role of follow-up visits. *American Journal of Preventive Medicine, 8* (2), 91–95.

Hall, S.M., Tunstall, C.D., Vila, K.L., & Duffy, J. (1992). Weight gain prevention and smoking cessation: Cautionary findings. *American Journal of Public Health. 82* (6), 799–803.

Havik, O.E., & Maeland, J.G. (1988). Changes in smoking behaviour after a myocardial infarction. *Health Psychology, 7* (5), 403–420.

Health Education Authority (1991). *Smoking: The facts.* London: Health Education Authority.

Heatherton, T.F., & Banmeister, R.F. (1991). Binge eating as escape from self-awareness. *Psychological Bulletin, 110* (1), 86–108.

Hollandsworth, J.G. (1990). *The physiology of psychological disorders: Schizophrenia, depression, anxiety, and substance abuse.* London: Plenum.

Jellinek, E.M. (1952). Phases of alcohol addiction. *Quarterly Journal of Studies on Alcohol, 13,* 673–684.

Kviz, F.J., Crittenden, K.S., Belzer, L.J., & Warnecke, R.B. (1991). Psychosocial factors and enrolment in a televised smoking cessation program. *Health Education Quarterly, 18* (4), 445–61.

McGovern, P.G., & Lando, H.A. (1992). An assessment of nicotine gum as an adjunct to freedom from smoking cessation clinics. *Addictive Behaviors, 17* (2), 137–147.

Mello, N.K., & Mendelson, J.H. (1971). Drinking patterns during work contingent and non-contingent on alcohol acquisition. In N.K. Mello & J.H. Mendelson (Eds.), *Recent advances in alcoholism*. Washington, DC: National Institute of Mental Health.

Ministry of Agriculture Fisheries and Food (1987). *Food additives* (leaflet). London: HMSO.

Murray, D.M., Davis-Hearn, M., Goldman, A.I., Pirie, P., & Luepker, R.V. (1988). Four- and five-year follow-up results from four seventh-grade smoking prevention strategies. *Journal of Behavioral Medicine, 11* (4).

Ogden, J., & Wardle, J. (1991). Cognitive and emotional responses to food. *International Journal of Eating Disorders, 10* (3), 297–311.

Orford, J. (1985). *Excessive appetites: A psychological view of addictions*. London: John Wiley.

Ornish, D., Brown, S.E., Schwerwitz, L.W., Billings, J., Armstrong, W., Ports, T., McLanahan, S., Kirkeeide, R., Brand, R., & Gould, K. (1990). Can lifestyle changes reverse coronary heart disease? The Lifestyle Heart Trial. *The Lancet, 336*, 129–133.

Perkins, K.A. (1992). Effects of tobacco smoking on caloric intake. *British Journal of Addiction, 87* (2), 193–205.

Pirie, P.L., McBride, C.M., Hellerstedt, W., Jeffery, R.W., Hatsukami, D., Allen, S., & Lando H. (1992). Smoking cessation in women concerned about weight. *American Journal of Public Health, 82* (9), 1238–43.

Prochaska, J.O. (1994). Strong and weak principles for progressing from precontemplation to action on the basis of twelve problem behaviors. *Health Psychology, 13* (1), 47–51.

Prochaska, J.O., & DiClemente, C.C. (1992). Stages of change in the modification of problem behaviors. In M. Hersen, R.M. Eisler, & P.M. Miller (Eds.), *Progress in behavior modification*. Sycamore, IL: Sycamore Press.

Quilez Garcia, C., Hernando Arizaleta, L., Rubio Diaz, A., Granero Fernandez, E.J., Vila Coll M.A., & Estruch Riba, J. (1989). Double-blind study of the efficacy of nicotine chewing gum for smoking cessation in the primary care setting [Spanish]. *Atencion Primaria, 6* (10), 719–726.

Robertson, I., Hodgson, R., Orford, J., & McKechnie, R. (1984). *Psychology and problem drinking*. Leicester: British Psychological Society.

Sachs, D.P., & Leischow, S.J. (1991). Pharmacologic approaches to smoking cessation. *Clinics in Chest Medicine, 12* (4), 769–791.

Sallis, J.F., Elder, J.P., Wildey, M.B., de Moor, C, Young, R..L., Shalkin, J.J., & Helme, J.M. (1990). Assessing skills for refusing cigarettes and smokeless tobacco. *Journal of Behavioral Medicine, 13* (5), 489–503.

Sobell, M., & Sobell, L. (1981). A functional analysis model of drinking decisions. In: C.K. Prokop (Ed.), *Medical psychology—Contributions to behavioural medicine*. London: Academic Press.

Stave, G.M., & Jackson, G.W. (1991). Effect of a total work-site smoking ban on employee smoking and attitudes. *Journal of Occupational Medicine, 33* (8), 884–890.

Transdermal Nicotine Study Group (1991). Transdermal nicotine for smoking cessation. Six-month results from two multicenter controlled clinical trials. *Journal of the American Medical Association, 266* (22), 3133–8.

Truswell, A.S. (1986). *ABC of nutrition*. London: British Medical Association.

Viswesvaran, C., & Schmidt, F.L. (1992). A meta-analytic comparison of the effectiveness of smoking cessation methods. *Journal of Applied Psychology, 77* (4), 554–561.

Waalkens, H.J., Cohen Schotanus, J., Adriaanse, H., & Knol, K. (1992). Smoking habits in medical students and physicians in Groningen, The Netherlands. *European Respiratory Journal, 5* (1), 49–52.

Wald, N.J., Boreham, J., Bailey, A., Ritchie, C., Haddow, J.E., & Knight, G. (1984). Urinary cotinine as a marker of breathing other people's tobacco smoke. *Lancet, i*, 230–231.

Waller, G., Hamilton, K., Rose, N., Sumra, J., & Baldwin, G. (1993). Sexual abuse and body-image distortion in the eating disorders. *British Journal of Clinical Psychology, 32* (3), 350–352.

Wewers, M.E., & Ahijevych, K.L. (1991). Work stress after smoking cessation. *Aaohn Journal, 39* (12), 547–551.

Williams, H. (1983). *Facts about smoking for young and old* (leaflet). London: The Chest, Heart, & Stroke Association, Tavistock Square, WC1H 9JE.

Windsor, R.A., Lowe, J.B., & Bartlett, E.E. (1988). The effectiveness of a worksite self-help smoking cessation program: A randomized trial. *Journal of Behavioral Medicine, 11* (4).

Wynd, C.A. (1992). Relaxation imagery used for stress reduction in the prevention of smoking relapse. *Journal of Advanced Nursing, 17* (3), 294–302.

Wynder, E.L. (1976). Nutrition and cancer. *Federal Proceedings, 35* (21 July), 1309–1315.

6

Work and Play

Apart from eating and drinking and psychophysiology, a number of other aspects of lifestyle within the control of the individual can make a substantial contribution to preventive health. The topics to be considered here are exercise, paid work, and sexual relationships. Paid work occupies a major portion of the adult life-span, and its effects on health both positively and negatively are enormous. Many of the parameters of work are determined by market pressures and even national traditions, and the scope of the individual is relatively small. Public health and occupational health are fields that can have the greatest impact on healthy working, but most such issues are beyond the scope of this book. Sex is considered mainly in terms of behaviour that reduces risk of sexually transmitted disease.

EXERCISE

The following account is simplified; a more comprehensive treatment can be found in Bouchard et al. (1990). Any muscle will increase its strength in proportion to the demand placed on it. Regular exercise can therefore have the effect of strengthening muscle, particularly before the age of 50. Overload is required, which means that the muscle is required to do more than it has been accustomed to. Reversibility of improvements is the rule, so activity levels need to be maintained. There are three purposes of exercise:

- *stamina*: activities involving the thighs and other large muscles, which make demands on the cardiac muscle

- *strength:* weight-lifting or similar activities, which make demands on particular skeletal muscles

- *suppleness:* stretching exercises, which increase range of movement

The distinction between strength and stamina training involves the duration and intensity of exertion. Muscles supplied with plenty of oxygen make adenosine triphosphate (ATP) by completely breaking down stored carbohydrate, in the form of glycogen, and fat. Under moderate demand conditions, these reactions can produce ATP for hours—long enough to run a marathon. They come to a halt only when glycogen stores are depleted. When the demand exceeds the capacity of the aerobic system, the muscles rely on biochemical pathways that are anaerobic (occur without oxygen), mainly in "fast-twitch" fibres. Anaerobic metabolism comes into play when weight-lifters, shot putters, and sprinters make brief but massive efforts, or when a long-distance runner sprints to the finish. At such times, glycogen is only partially broken down without oxygen to lactate. This type of metabolism produces the maximum power output and can happen immediately, without the heart increasing the supply of oxygen to muscles. Lactate soon builds up in the muscles and leads to aching and fatigue and, ultimately, exhaustion. Anaerobic training—lifting weights and the like—causes the muscles to grow stronger, partly by increasing contractile protein and the concentrations of enzymes in the "fast-twitch" muscle fibre that specialises in anaerobic glycolysis. Strength training does not give much benefit to the cardiovascular system.

Aerobic exercise, on the other hand, causes physiological changes in the body that seem to be linked with cardiovascular health. Aerobics is about exercising in such a way as to enhance the ability of "slow-twitch" muscles to use oxygen to make the energy-rich compound ATP, which fuels contractions. Training for aerobic fitness leads to improvements in the efficiency of the circulation, mainly through increases in peripheral muscles. Muscles trained for endurance rather than anaerobic strength also oxidise more fat and less carbohydrate, and they can work harder and longer before reaching "anaerobic threshold"—the point at which aerobic metabolism becomes inadequate and the muscle begins producing lactate. Endurance improves after regular exercise, largely because the muscle fibres that specialise in aerobic metabolism, the slow-twitch fibres, synthesise more oxidative enzymes and more mitochondria, the mediators of aerobic respiration in the cell.

Exercise may be prescribed for particular purposes, usually stamina increase or weight loss. As much as 50% of the muscle's energy can come from fat, so a prescription of 300 kilocalories per session might be prescribed for weight reduction. The duration of exertion required to build stamina might involve running fast enough to elevate the heart rate substantially for at least

10 minutes, or brisk walking for 30 to 40 minutes. Frequency of exercise sessions needs to be fairly high, and three such episodes a week are often recommended. The following activities have associated energy expenditure for a man of average weight, and would be lower in proportion for a woman of average weight.

Energy expenditure of selected activities (after Astrand & Rodahl, 1986)

- *sleeping*:   1 kcal/min

- *walking* at 3 m.p.h.:   3–5 kcal/min

- *running* at 10 m.p.h.:   19 kcal/min

- *cycling* at 13 m.p.h.:   5–11 kcal/min

- *swimming* (the crawl):   5–11 kcal/min

There are substantial psychological benefits of exercise, but it is unclear how these are derived. Vigorous physical activity leads to increased levels of catecholamines being released from the brain, the sympathetic nerve endings, and the adrenal medulla. "Jolts" of adrenalin and noradrenalin activate the hypothalamus and may give rise to a pleasurable sensation; this is discussed further in the context of pain control (see chapter 13). Naturally occurring peptides with opium-like qualities have been isolated from brain and other tissue. One of these substances, beta endorphin, has been reported to increase significantly in the plasma after bouts of severe exercise (a 100-mile run). It has been suggested that the so-called physical "high" experienced by the runner, as well as the post-workout feeling of relaxation and physical gratification, is due to endogenous opioid release. The effect of belief on the sense of well-being that accompanies exercise is also strong. Desharnais et al. (1993) gave 24 healthy young adults a suggestion that an exercise programme would enhance both well-being and aerobic capacity. A second group were given the expectation of aerobic increase, but not of well-being, and engaged in a similar 10-week programme. Self-esteem improved significantly in those given the placebo expectation, but not in the control group.

Suppleness

There are a number of methods of training posture to achieve relaxation or suppleness, and these are usually embedded in some philosophical tradition. Yoga is perhaps the best known; its benefits are mainly for breathing, and hence arousal reduction. Yoga disciplines can also improve musculoskeletal suppleness, but they have little or no effect on stamina. Suppleness is important in preventing strain injuries during sport and exercise rehabilitation (see chapter 9), and in maintaining full-range movement in spite of ageing (see chapter 12). Many types of pain and disability can be reduced by understanding the normal function of muscles and connective tissue. Voluntary muscles tend to be grouped in antagonist pairs, such as the biceps and triceps in the upper arm, with additional muscles called synergists and fixators used to prevent movement in another dimension. Overuse of an agonistic muscle will lead to fatigue in the short term, but longer-term muscle building; the antagonist muscle may not strengthen in proportion. One example of this is the overuse injury of the wrists experienced by some regular users of word-processors (see chapter 12). Some knowledge of normal function can prevent such problems developing or recurring.

The disciplines of Yoga and the Alexander Technique have respiratory advantages, in maintaining air flow and preventing panic. Pranayama yoga breathing involves the slowing of breathing and an inspiration-to-expiration–duration ratio of 1:2. Singh et al. (1990) asked 18 patients with mild asthma to practise slow deep breathing of the pranayama type for 15 minutes twice a day. Expiratory flow rate and volume, as well as symptom score and inhaler use, all improved more than with the placebo device, but the differences were not significant. There was a statistically significant increase in the dose of histamine needed to provoke a 20% reduction in forced expiratory volume, which indicates a lowered tendency to bronchospasm.

The Alexander Technique (AT) is a postural training method, designed by an actor to overcome problems of voice and posture on stage. As described by Leibowitz and Connington (1990), it may be considered as proprioceptive musculoskeletal education, in that it increases awareness and voluntary inhibition of personal habitual patterns of rigid musculoskeletal constriction. Austin and Ausubel (1992) reported a subjective sense of enhanced ease of breathing after instruction in the Alexander Technique. They investigated the effects of AT instruction on respiratory function in 10 healthy adult volunteers who received 20 private AT lessons at weekly intervals. These showed a 9% increase in peak flow, and small increases in other upper-respiratory-tract measures; 10 healthy controls showed no significant changes.

Work as exercise

Work in the sense of productive activity for which one earns a payment also involves work in the biological sense of muscle activity and energy expenditure. Before the nineteenth century, most work involved considerable muscular activity, whereas in the late twentieth century the degree of automation means that most jobs involve relatively small energy expenditure.

Traditionally strenuous work, such as that of the trawler-man, lumberjack, or foundry-man, are now principally machine-supervision tasks. The following energy expenditures are also taken from Astrand and Rodahl (1986):

- *postman climbing stairs:* 10–14 kcal/min
- *shovelling:* 6–10 kcal/min
- *hewing coal:* 3–10 kcal/min
- *tree-felling with saw:* 9–12 kcal/min
- *washing clothes:* 3–5 kcal/min
- *heavy engineering:* 4–6 kcal/min
- *driving a car:* 1–3 kcal/min
- *making beds:* 4–5 kcal/min

Even where considerable exertion is required—for example, in shovelling coal into a furnace—the activity can be done in bursts of a few minutes, so that the worker rarely reaches aerobic levels of sustained activity. It can be seen that domestic work can have moderately high energy demands, but activities such as making beds are usually of short duration. Consequently, housework does not bring about good stamina, even though it involves long hours of activity. Work that involves long periods of sitting and short bursts of strenuous activity, such as driving a lorry, seem to be particularly unhealthy.

Jobs that involve much walking or climbing stairs, such as delivering milk or letters, seem to develop stamina. In the 1950s, Professor Jerry Morris examined the rate of heart attacks in London Transport staff. It was found that bus drivers were much more likely to have heart attacks than were conductors. The latter are much more active, though they may also have suffered lower emotional stress than drivers. Paffenberger observed a similar trend in American dockers. The men whose jobs regularly required high energy expenditures (5.2–7.5 kcal/min) were half as likely to die of heart attack as those whose jobs required lower energy output (2.5–5.0 kcal/min). Strenuous work is now uncommon, so both these researchers have gone on to advocate leisure-time aerobic activity as a preventive measure against heart disease (Morris et al., 1980; Paffenberger et al., 1984).

Work and arousal

For many adults, paid work occupies the major part of waking life and has major consequences for SAM arousal. The extent to which an individual can exert control over the work process is limited, and the organisation of work is beyond the scope a book on individual behaviour. Our interest will be on those aspects that can be brought under personal control or compensated. Work stress is strongly associated with the sense of being under external control, and this sense may reflect a lack of assertiveness or time management (see chapter 2). Physical harm may arise from the direct psychophysiological effects of arousal, or from the use of recreational drugs to reduce arousal. There are also well-known hazards of exposure to harmful substances at work, including: dust and paint vapour on asthma and COAD; benzene, asbestos and similar mineral fibres on cancer; and solvents such as toluene on brain function. These hazards are subject to public health influences rather than individual health behaviour, so the following illnesses are of greater interest as occupational influences:

- *myocardial infarction:* overarousal through high reactivity; low-exertion occupations, e.g. driving; smoking (active and passive) (see chapter 8)

- *gastric ulcers:* overarousal; high-fat meals, inadequate digestion time (see chapter 11)

- *back and neck injuries:* lifting of unbalanced loads; sustained use of a stooped or otherwise asymmetric posture, or of the forearms (see chapter 12)

- *accidents:* disturbed sleep through shift work; intrusive imagery in occupations handling trauma, e.g. police, ambulance

Before describing hazards of work, some account of the rewards of paid work is necessary. Satisfaction with work is dominated by two theories, according to Cox (1982): Maslow's (1954) "hierarchy of needs" (see Figure 6.1), and Herzberg's (1966) "motivation-hygiene" theory. The hierarchy approach proposes that less potent needs (esteem, self-actualisation) do not come to govern behaviour until the more potent (food, safety) are fulfilled. The needs for self-esteem and self-actualisation are the dominant motives in work behaviour. Herzberg proposes that job satisfaction depends on motivator factors, whereas dissatisfaction relates to the absence of hygiene factors. Motivator factors relate to the job itself and include achievement, recognition, responsibility, and advancement. Hygiene factors include pay, working conditions, security, and interpersonal relations. According to Herzberg, improving hygiene factors will reduce dissatisfaction, but not increase motivation. One surprising implication is that increasing pay will not increase motivation. Herzberg based his theory on a study of 200 engineers in Pittsburgh. The critical-incident technique he used forces individuals to make dichotomous choices, and studies that have used this method tend to confirm Herzberg's theory, while other research fails to support it.

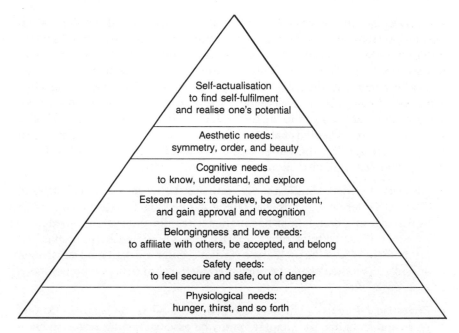

Figure 6.1 A hierarchy of human needs (after Maslow)

Arousal is likely to be excessive where satisfaction is lowest, in a very general sense. External demands of the work situation have attracted most attention during wartime, when hours are long and conditions severe. Factors associated with "work neurosis" according to Lader (1975) include *overload* (75 or more hours of industrial work in a week) and *high attention/low discretion*, as discussed later on. However, opposite demand characteristics were also associated with work neurosis: *boring* and disliked work, *very light* or sedentary work, and *repetition*. *Skill mismatch* (having to work at too high a level of skill, or vice versa) and *domestic pressures* (inadequate diet, restricted time for leisure contacts, low recreational time, widowhood or separation, family illness, finance, housing, excessive travel) also contributed. Specific factors that have been shown to have adverse effects in maintaining excessively high arousal, include:

- *Reactivity.* Occupations where demand fluctuates in an unpredictable way are likely to lead to excessive arousal and cardiovascular reactivity in employees. This hypothesis was advanced by Marmot in relation to messengers in the civil service (see chapter 8), but it also applies to other service providers including ambulance or maintenance personnel. Predictable high demand seems to be more acceptable than variation between high and low demand.

- *Low decision latitude* was identified by Karasek et al. (1981) on the basis of the American Quality of Employment Surveys. Factor analyses disclosed two closely related components—"skill discretion" and "authority over decisions", which have usually been combined subsequently. Swedish working-men who described their job as demanding and possessing a low level of decision latitude were more likely than others to develop cardiovascular symptoms and to die from CHD during follow-up. Using similar questionnaires, Theorell et al. (1987) interviewed men who had developed MIs before age 45 within three months of disease onset. The MI sufferers described less skill discretion than those without MI.

- *Job monotony* was a significant discriminator between MIs and controls in Theorell's interviews. Knox et al. (1985) showed that Swedish men aged 28 in non-learning occupations had higher adrenalin and systolic blood pressure than those with learning opportunities. Olsen and Kristensen (1991) estimate that 6% of the premature cardiovascular mortality in Danish men and 14% in women would be prevented by the elimination of monotonous high-paced work.

- *Recreational drug use.* The well-documented association between manual work and smoking (see chapter 5) may be associated with restoring emotional equilibrium in relatively unpleasant work environments. The use of alcohol to reduce tension after work by air-traffic controllers is associated with above-average rates of hypertension and ulceration in this group (see chapter 11). Smoking by nurses may reflect the need to restore a sense of balance during short meal breaks.

- *Shift work* has major implications for health, mainly through reduction in sleep quality. Where a morning shift requires the worker to wake around 4 a.m.—at the lowest point in the circadian rhythm—fatigue will persist through the working shift. It seems to be difficult to achieve compensatory changes in earlier induction of sleep. Rotating shifts have been reported to entail a higher proportion of accidents and mistakes in police personnel, so the Lexington police department moved to permanent shift assignments (Phillips et al., 1991). Absenteeism rates fell during the six months following the change, and reported sleep quality and psychological well-being also improved.

- *Bus and lorry driving.* Professional drivers seem to have an increased risk of heart disease, as noted by Morris et al. (1980). While unfitness combined with sudden exertion may be contributing factors, the sustained attentional demands are also important. The relative risk of CHD death among 2,000 Danish bus drivers was 1.6 times higher in those working in a high-traffic-intensity area during a 10-year follow-up (Netterstrom &

Suadicani, 1993). This was in line with other reports, but satisfaction with the work was associated with a six-fold increase in risk. Those who reported never experiencing mental exhaustion after work, that their job was very varied, that their job was something special, and those who reported that they would choose the same job again, had an excess risk.

• *Unwanted unemployment.* While work may be hazardous, its absence also has major adverse effects on health. These are often described as a reduction in "scope", and include decline in intellectual efficiency and mood. There is an epidemiological association between economic recession and admissions to mental hospital, and a rise in cardiovascular mortality about two to three years after redundancy (Brenner, 1971). Having some paid work outside the home was reported as a protective factor against depression in women by Brown and Harris (1978).

Occupational stress may manifest itself in various ways, including increased sickness and absence, excessive use of alcohol, and poor performance. Although work has strong demand characteristics, some variation in pacing and arousal at work can be achieved by the individual. Driven behaviour and heart disease (see chapter 8) can be reduced by improved self-esteem. The careful use of meal breaks can reduce arousal, and this is particularly true for reactive occupations such as ambulance personnel. Setting up boundaries from work—by changing clothes, or keeping papers, tools, and work-related telephone conversations out of the home—can achieve some distancing. Debriefing after particularly unpleasant and disturbing work, such as handling of bodies after a major accident, can reduce later intrusive imagery and accidents. Where a major illness such as infarction or perforated ulcer has been heavily influenced by the work environment, a worker may achieve most control by moving within or between employment, or in some cases by retiring from paid employment.

SEX

Of all the areas of personal behaviour that can promote health or incur illness, sex is probably the greatest. Sexual activity is one of the greatest human pleasures, which can protect from stress and the effects of ageing, and it provides the most intimate human contacts. From a strictly biological viewpoint, it is both a strenuous physical activity and also the opportunity for many infectious hazards. It is appropriate to consider HIV prevention in the context of "work and play", since the behaviours concerned are pleasurable activities that are not viewed as connected with health. This disconnection between behaviour and its health risks is discussed in chapter 7 in terms of the "health belief model".

Sexually transmitted disease (STD)

Intercourse has always been a prime route for transmission of infection. In nineteenth-century China, for example, the majority of the population suffered from at least one STD—either gonorrhoea or syphilis. Concern about STD was high in the early twentieth century, when about 60,000 people a year died from syphilis in Britain, and during the Second World War, when STDs became widespread. Concern declined considerably after the war, partly because of reliable drug treatments for syphilis. The rise in genital herpes, which is not easily curable, reawakened concern, but the identification of AIDS in the early 1980s has dominated lay thinking about the hazards of sex since then. The world-wide incidence figures for sexually transmitted diseases given in Table 6.1 give some indication of the relative risk of contracting each STD (WHO, 1990). Some of the more serious hazards of each STD are indicated.

Human Immunodeficiency Virus (HIV) is not a robust virus, so infection is only likely through blood-to-blood contact. Infection through exchange of semen or vaginal fluid can occur, but mainly in association with ulcers, gonorrhoea, or other genital conditions associated with bleeding. Anal intercourse, involving exchange of semen and perhaps blood, carries a relatively

Table 6.1 Some infections transmitted during sexual intercourse

Infection	Yearly increase (in millions)	Effects
chlamydia	50	non-specific urethritis/cervicitis; may cause infertility/arthritis
genital herpes simplex	20	recurring illness with painful itching; see chapter 14
human papilloma virus	30	causes genital warts, which can lead to cancer of the cervix
gonorrhoea	25	may cause infertility
syphilis	3.6	may cause damage to brain, heart etc., persists for decades
hepatitis B	2	causes liver damage, can be fatal
HIV	1.6	fatal; see below and chapter 14

high risk of infection. There is no definite evidence that HIV can be transmitted through saliva or sweat, so activities such as kissing, oral–genital sex, and mouth-to-mouth resuscitation are thought to be largely safe. Infection between lesbians is rare but has been reported in connection with practices causing bleeding. Public awareness of the modes of transmission of HIV rose rapidly in the 1980s, so that most people can now identify penetrative sex and procedures involving blood as the risky behaviours, and are less concerned about superficial contact such as handshakes. However, there is a large discrepancy between knowledge of STD and risky sexual behaviour.

Sex between men

AIDS was first identified in homosexual men, and initially thought to be unique to that community. Education about the mode of transmission was rapidly taken up by gay organisations, and their efforts have been fairly effective in informing men who are part of a gay support network. The experience of the San Francisco gay community, by comparison with that of New York, is salutary. This community of 150,000 was well-organised and vocal, and was able to organise secondary prevention education and buddying systems for infected persons. This openness contrasted with that of New York, where gay men were less organised, and early public reactions such as closing public bath houses had the effect of driving sexual activity and drug use further underground. Unfortunately, many of the San Francisco gay population were probably infected by the time the risk was identified, but the lessons for effective prevention have to be learned at the expense of this community.

More cautious sexual behaviour was found in 80% of over 2,000 homosexual men surveyed by McKirnan and Peterson (1989). Caution was not principally a move towards monogamy, since the proportion of stable couple relationships was unchanged from that found 16 years earlier. While the average number of sexual partners reported by gay men had declined, 19% were still reporting two or more new partners a month. The sexual lifestyles of gay and bisexual men were investigated by Project SIGMA (1992). One in seven gay men had never participated in anal intercourse, and nearly half had not recently done so. Most of those who practised anal sex did so both actively and passively. Condom use was usual where the partnership was seen as casual or part of an "open" relationship. However, in stable couples it was often seen as a sign of mutual trust not to use a condom. This link between romantic love and unsafe sex is unfortunate, since the average lifespan of gay partnerships is about four years, while the incubation period for HIV can be up to ten years.

In the early 1990s, the relative abstinence of the late 1980s was replaced by some increase in the frequency of unsafe sex among gay men. Gold et al.

(1991) studied the thought processes associated with unsafe encounters through a postal questionnaire of 219 gay men in Melbourne; 35.7% reported desire for unprotected anal intercourse in advance of the encounter, rather than being overtaken by unplanned desire. Nearly all respondents had known of the AIDS hazard of anal intercourse, and ejaculation had occurred in 48% of cases. Unavailability of condoms was not a substantial reason for unsafe practice, as 56.6% reported that they could have obtained one. Self-justifications included thoughts that the other person was too attractive or too healthy-looking to be infected, or could be a long-term lover. Positive thoughts that the partner's attractiveness implies health are common justifications for unsafe sex.

Nitrites are sometimes used by gay men to enhance sexual potency, and the inhalation of nitrites was identified as a risk factor for AIDS and Kaposi's sarcoma in the early 1980s. This class of drugs is prescribed to treat angina, and as liquid incense. Research interest in nitrites declined once HIV was identified as the causal organism. Seage et al. (1992) report a strong relationship between using nitrite inhalants during unprotected receptive anal intercourse and the risk of HIV infection. These drugs increase blood flow and may increase vascular permeability to the virus.

Recent preventive education by organisations such as the Terence Higgins Trust has focused on the eroticisation of safer sex. Erotic fantasy may include masturbation while speaking to one's lover on the telephone. While sex drive may disappear entirely after a diagnosis of HIV status has been received, sexual feelings often return later. Communication of erotic feeling may be preferable to attempting to achieve total abstention, with the risk that this will break down in reckless sexual behaviour.

Syringe sharing

Procedures involving blood in medical contexts are very unlikely to cause the spread of HIV and are fairly unlikely to spread the more infectious Hepatitis B. Procedures for sterilising blood appear to have stopped the spread to haemophiliacs, and strict adherence to aseptic surgery is now usual in hospitals. Several thousand patients treated by HIV-positive dentists and surgeons were traced following concern over several patients infected by one Florida dentist, and no evidence of infection was found in any other case (JAMA Editorial, 1993), though the reasons in that case remain a puzzle.

By contrast, syringes used for recreational drug use are often not aseptic, and syringe-sharing has led to further epidemic spread in cities such as Edinburgh. In an Edinburgh sample interviewed by Morrison (1991), injecting of substances less associated with the stereotype of recreational drugs use were reported, including prescribed tranquillisers and pain-killers such as DF118. In an Australian sample, Loxley, Marsh, and Lo (1991) report that amphetamines were the most common injected drug in the under-23s, while heroin was more common in older injectors. Another reason for syringe-sharing is the use of anabolic steroids by body-builders: The loan of a syringe to a new member at a gym may be seen by body-builders as a friendly induction procedure and unconnected with "drug use".

Many health authorities now support needle-exchange schemes to reduce the risk of contaminated materials being shared. The use of household bleach as an emergency sterilisation procedure is recommended in some areas. Morrison (1991) and Klee et al. (1991) both report a considerable reduction in syringe-sharing after appropriate counselling. There was greater avoidance of using others' equipment, but injecting partners and close friends continued to share. Both studies report little increase in condom use among these clients.

Sex for money

Commercial sex constitutes a potential focus for epidemic spread of HIV, particularly since offering sex for money is often undertaken to finance injecting drug use. Ashton and Seymour (1990) provide evidence on HIV prevalence among prostitutes. The vast majority of prostitutes in central African countries are seropositive, but only a small percentage of sex-industry workers in Western Europe carry the virus. In 1985–86, among 400 prostitutes in Nuremburg none was seropositive; 101 were in Denmark, 84 in Amsterdam, and 56 in Paris. Of 200 registered prostitutes in Greece, 6% were found to be seropositive, and 12% of 53 Amsterdam prostitutes carried HIV in 1983–84. Recent prevalence is reported by the European Working Group on HIV Infection in Female Prostitutes (1993). In various countries, 866 prostitutes provided blood, or saliva in some cases, for HIV testing. The prevalence of HIV overall was 5.3%, but most of the positives were among intravenous drug users, where prevalence was 31.8%. The use of petroleum-based lubricants emerged as an additional risk factor, probably because they cause the latex rubber of condoms to perish. Condom use is usual among regular prostitutes who are part of a support group, but less so among women who occasionally offer themselves for money. Unsafe sex is also associated with lack of opportunity for the prostitute to assess a client, who might be coercive.

Male prostitution is a higher-risk though less common activity. Bloor et al. (1992) argue that the male prostitute is often unable to be proactive in achieving safer sex because control is with the client. These researchers managed to contact 32 male prostitutes in Glasgow at the pubs, parks, and lavatories where they worked. Most offered masturbation, oral sex, or spanking, but 10 reported that they at least occasionally accepted anal intercourse. Factors that reduced the male prostitute's control included illegality, low income, and rape in some cases, but the notable common feature was the lack of verbal communication about the act. Contact might be initiated simply by gaze or showing an erection, and there was often no discussion of the type of act, or even if money was to be paid. Unsafe acts that occurred thus did so usually at the client's insistence.

Outreach

Syringe-sharing and commercial sex together provide a major route for epidemic spread. Unfortunately, these behaviours are covert and associated with illegality and shame or guilt. Effective epidemic prevention strategies must therefore take services to people engaged in these risky behaviours, rather than hoping that they will use statutory health services.

The Liverpool outreach scheme (Ashton & Seymour, 1990) started with a survey of 34 prostitutes, who claimed to be providing services to an average of 8 clients a day. Although 70% claimed always to carry condoms, 36% admitted to being prepared to have intercourse without a condom, usually at the insistence of the client; 41% were using injectable drugs; 56% had used the STD clinic of the university hospital, but 24% had never had an STD check. This level of high-risk behaviour was accompanied by a high level of avoidance of health services. Reasons for avoiding services centred on the risk of losing a child to social services care, followed by unfriendliness and lack of confidentiality. Services that were considered more acceptable were a free condom service (88% said they would visit), breast cancer screening (75% acceptable), and HIV or STD screening (75%).

The Maryland outreach centre was located at the edge of the street prostitution area of Liverpool and aimed to provide treatment services including antibiotics, syringe exchange, free condoms, an STD clinic, and other primary screening services. The activities of legal agencies were revealed as a possible aggravating factor: Intensive policing could prompt prostitutes to make rapid pickups, reducing their ability to prepare for safer sex and avoid aggression; large fines by courts might be payable only by further acts of prostitution; dependency on illegal drugs increased the need for money, and hence the risk of unsafe sex. A history of having been in care was shared by 65% of the women, and the same percentage had been in prison. Local authority care may thus be seen as another point of vulnerability for becoming a prostitute and abusing drugs, and hence a point of contact for outreach.

The first wave of HIV cases in each country has been mainly among homosexual men, but transmission by this means tended to slow as AIDS awareness increased. Sharing of contaminated needles is the route for the second wave of infections. An outreach campaign in the King's Cross area of Sydney is often cited as an example of success in preventing the secondary epidemic of HIV transmission by intravenous drug users. New cases of AIDS will only appear several years after infection, but the indications are that the epidemic spread in this community has been slower than predicted.

Sex between men and women

HIV is also spread by heterosexual intercourse, but this knowledge has not greatly affected heterosexual behaviour as yet. Behaviours that reduce the risk of transmission are abstention and "safer sex"—the latter mainly involves the use of condoms or femidoms during intercourse, or masturbation and other methods that do not involve exchange of body fluids. The probability of infection during heterosexual intercourse is not high, as indicated by the low rates of infection among wives of haemophiliac men; on the other hand, some unlucky people have become infected during their first act of sexual love.

In Africa the picture is very different, and it is estimated that 80% of transmission is through heterosexual intercourse. The difference is thought to arise through prevalence of genital lesions and circumcision practices, and in Zimbabwe through the use of drying herbs in the vagina to increase erotic pleasure. Anal intercourse is also practised by some heterosexual couples. Reliable data on this is difficult to find, as the activity is stigmatised and illegal, but it is likely that more heterosexual women than homosexual men have participated in anal sex at some time.

Agreement to use condoms during sex requires good communication, which makes their use more likely between regular couples than between new partners. Phillips and White (1991) found that 70% of the adolescents they surveyed reported themselves to be sexually active, but only 15% had changed their behaviour as a result of the threat of AIDS. Only 24% of sexually active New Jersey college students reported consistently using condoms (O'Leary et al., 1991). By contrast, condom use usually becomes regular in married couples where one partner is seropositive, once HIV status has been disclosed and sensitive counselling has occurred (Kamenga et al., 1991). At an 18-month follow-up, 77% were still using condoms consistently.

Early health-promotion campaigns used mainly aversive imagery. The UK government campaign on AIDS prevention was launched in 1986 and involved giving information about HIV transmission, along with visual images of mortality. The Australian campaign launched in 1987 was still more aversive, starting with a television commercial of "The Grim Reaper". This skeletal figure cut down with a scythe the "pins" in a bowling alley, which assumed the form of men, women, and children. Rigby et al. (1989) interviewed 525 Adelaide residents shortly after the campaign, of whom 94% recalled the television advertisements. There was no significant increase in concern about AIDS, and older viewers actually reported less concern following the campaign. Among the 29% who most approved of the campaign, knowledge about AIDS was no greater than in those who approved less, although concern was heightened. Hardly any research has found knowledge of HIV risk by itself a predictive factor in condom use.

The contrast between aversive approaches and those that eroticise safe sex has been seen in previous STD prevention campaigns. During the Second World War, pragmatic approaches to prevention of syphilis and gonorrhoea in troops were evolved by medical officers in the British and other armies. In the early part of the war, medical officers would give highly aversive demonstrations of the effects of syphilis, which reportedly led to many soldiers fainting. However, there was no evidence that this reduced the likelihood of unprotected intercourse. Later on, a more "two-sided" approach was taken, in which the attractions of sex were stated along with reminders about the risk to regular partners on returning home and the value of condoms. Comparisons of one-sided and two-sided messages have found that the educational level of the audience plays a significant role: Less-educated subjects are more likely to comply with a message that did not state the opposite case, while more-educated subjects were more likely to comply if the counter-case was stated.

The probability of safer sex in a new liaison is lower if the relationship is appraised as love, or the partner as attractive and therefore healthy. Most people appraise their personal risk as low, and not sufficient to modify the tense and exciting process of sexual courtship. One response to the lack of effect of AIDS campaigns would be to increase the aversive nature of the message, but this is likely to create "two-stage coping" (see chapter 7): The viewer needs to cope with the anxiety created by the message, separately from the behaviour that entails infection risk. Personal acquaintance with an AIDS sufferer is likely to constitute a strong reminder, but unfortunately the long delay between exposure and symptoms is likely to mean that many people will have been exposed to the virus by the time their health beliefs become powerful enough to achieve effective prevention. The probability of contracting an infection is clearly much higher for STDs such as chlamydia than for HIV, so the experience of the rapid development of soreness from more common infections may act as a deterrent in future sexual encounters.

The perception of low personal risk makes HIV prevention among heterosexuals particularly difficult, and there is not yet a clear strategy for promoting safer sexual practices. The misleading connection between trust and unsafe sex is a further obstacle: Either partner may feel that suggesting condom use may imply one's own promiscuity. Good communication in the context of courtship can overcome some of these barriers to safer sex practices. Some of the models for homosexual courtship combine physical explicit discussion with humour, and these models may be valuable for heterosexuals.

CONCLUSION

Exercise can make a substantial contribution to preventive health. Stamina is particularly important in the prevention of heart disease, while suppleness can prevent musculoskeletal and some respiratory problems. Exercise and arousal aspects of work have been described in this chapter, and some implications for individual compensatory behaviours presented. Sexual behaviour is a major influence on well-being and illness, and the achievement of safer sexual practices requires good communication in courtship situations.

REFERENCES

Ashton, J., & Seymour, H. (1990). *The new public health*. Milton Keynes: Open University.

Astrand, P.O., & Rodahl, K. (1986). *Textbook of work physiology* (3rd ed.). Singapore: McGraw Hill.

Austin, J.H., & Ausubel, P. (1992). Alexander Technique. *Chest, 102* (2), 486–490.

Bloor, M.J., McKeganey, N.P., Finlay, A., & Barnard, M.A. (1992). The inappropriateness of psycho-social models for understanding HIV-related risk practices among Glasgow male prostitutes. *AIDS Care, 4* (2), 131–137.

Bouchard, C., Shephard, R.J., Stephens, T., Sutton, J.R., & McPherson, B.D. (Eds.) (1990). *Exercise, fitness, and health: A consensus of current knowledge*. Leeds: Human Kinetics Publishers.

Brenner, M.H. (1971). Economic changes and heart disease mortality. *American Journal of Public Health, 61* (3), 606–611.

Brown, G.W., & Harris, T. (1978). *Social origins of depression: A study of psychiatric disorder in women*. London: Tavistock.

Cox, T. (1982). *Stress*. London: Macmillan.

Desharnais, R., Jobin, J., Coté, C., Lévesque, & Godin, G. (1993). Aerobic exercise and the placebo effect: A controlled study. *Psychological Medicine, 55*, 149–154.

European Working Group on HIV Infection in Female Prostitutes (1993). HIV infection in European female sex workers: Epidemiological link with use of petroleum-based lubricants. *AIDS, 7*, 401–408.

Gold, R., Skinner, M., Grant, P., & Plummer, D. (1991). Situational factors and thought processes associated with unprotected intercourse in gay men. *Psychology and Health, 5*, 259–278.

Herzberg, F. (1966). *Work and the nature of man*. London: Staples.

JAMA Editorial (1993). HIV-infected surgeons and dentists. *Journal of the American Medical Association, 269* (14), 1843–1844.

Kamenga, M., Ryder, R.W., Jingu, M., Mbuyi, N., Mbu, L., Behets, F., Brown, C., & Heyward, W. (1991). Evidence of marked sexual behavior change associated with low HIV-1 seroconversion in 149 married couples with discordant HIV-1 status: Experience at an HIV counselling centre in Zaire. *AIDS, 5*, 61–67.

Karasek, R., Baker, D., Marxer, F., & Ahlbom, A. (1981). Job decision latitude, job demands and cardiovascular disease: A prospective study of Swedish men. *American Journal of Public Health, 71*, 694–705.

Klee, H., Faugier, J., Hayes, C., & Morris, J. (1991). Risk reduction among injecting drug users: Changes in the sharing of injecting equipment and condom use. *AIDS Care, 3* (1), 63.

Knox, S., Theorell, T., Svensson, J., & Waller, D. (1985). The relation of social support and working environment to medical variables associated with elevated blood pressure in young males: A structural model. *Social Science Medicine, 21*, 525–531.

Lader, M.H. (1975). The nature of clinical anxiety in modern society. In C.D. Spielberger & I.G. Sarason (Eds.), *Stress and anxiety, Vol. 1*. New York: Halstead.

Leibowitz, J., & Connington, B. (1990). *The Alexander Technique*. Melksham, Wilts.: Redwood Press.

Loxley, W., Marsh, A., & Lo, S.K. (1991). Age and injecting drug use in Perth, Western Australia: The national AIDS and injecting drug use study. *AIDS Care, 3* (4), 193.

Maslow, A. (1954). *Motivation and personality*. New York: Harper & Row.

McKirnan, D.J., & Peterson, P.L. (1989). AIDS risk behaviour among homosexual males: The role of attitudes and substance abuse. *Psychology and Health, 3*, 161–171.

Morris, J.N., Everitt, M.G., Pollard, R., Chave, S., & Semmence, A. (1980). Vigorous exercise in leisure time: Protection against coronary heart disease. *The Lancet, 8206*, 1207–1210.

Morrison, V. (1991). The impact of HIV on injecting drug users: A longitudinal study. *AIDS Care, 3* (2), 193.

Netterstrom B., & Suadicani P. (1993). Self-assessed job satisfaction and ischaemic heart disease mortality: A 10-year follow-up of urban bus drivers. *International Journal of Epidemiology, 22* (1), 51–56.

O'Leary, A., Jemmott, L.S., Boocher-Lattimore, D., & Goodhart, F. (1991). Condom use by New Jersey college students: A social-cognitive analysis. Cited in D. Carroll, *Health psychology: Stress, behaviour, and disease*. London: The Falmer Press, 1992.

Olsen, O., & Kristensen, T.S. (1991). Impact of work environment on cardiovascular diseases in Denmark. *Journal of Epidemiology and Community Health, 45*, 4–10.

Paffenberger, R.S. Jr., Hyde, R.T., Wing, A.L., et al. (1984). A natural history of athleticism and cardiovascular health. *Journal of the American Medical Association, 252*, 491–495.

Phillips, B., Magan, L., Gerhardstein, C., & Cecil, B. (1991). Shift work, sleep quality, and worker health: A study of police officers. *Southern Medical Journal, 84* (10), 1176–84.

Phillips, K., & White, D. (1991). AIDS: Psychological, social, and political reactions to a modern epidemic. In R. Cochrane & D. Carroll (Eds.), *Psychology and social issues*. London: Falmer Press.

Project SIGMA (1992). *The sexual lifestyles of gay and bisexual men in England and Wales*. London: HMSO.

Rigby, K., Brown, M., Anagnostou, P., Ross, M.W., & Rosser, B.R.S. (1989). Shock tactics to counter AIDS: The Australian experience. *Psychology and Health, 3,* 145–159.

Seage, G.R., Mayer, K.H., Horsbrugh, C., Holmberg, S., Morn, W., & Lamb, G. (1992). The relation between nitrite inhalants, unprotected receptive anal intercourse, and the risk of human immunodeficiency virus infection. *American Journal of Epidemiology, 135* (1), 1–11.

Singh V., Wisniewski A., Britton J., & Tattersfield A. (1990). Effect of yoga breathing exercises (pranayama) on airway reactivity in subjects with asthma. *The Lancet, 335* (8702), 1381–1383.

Theorell, T., Perski, A., Akerstedt, T., Sigala, F., Ahlberg-Hulten, G., Svensson, J., & Enevoth, P. (1988). Changes in job strain in relation to changes in physiological state: A longitudinal study. *Scandinavian Journal Work Environment Health, 14* (3), 189–196.

WHO (1990). *Incidence of sexually transmitted diseases*. Geneva: World Health Organisation.

7

Medical Services

This book is based on a model of skilled behaviours that can be practised by people who want to know what to do to remain healthy, particularly after some episode of ill health. Most of the material thus far has been on methods the individual can use alone, but sometimes it is essential to seek the services of a medical practitioner. This does not entail relinquishing total control to the doctor but achieving some shared responsibility for procedures. Health beliefs are central to effective health behaviour, and competing beliefs need to be understood. Better mutual understanding, contracts, and more sensitive use of screening can improve adherence to medical regimes. The knowledge and attitudes that are most relevant to a fit person are:

7.1 has sufficient awareness of human biology to maintain personal health

7.2 consults medical and other practitioners for expert advice if this is suggested, or if personal health behaviours appear ineffective (see also 2.4)

7.3 uses prescribed drugs with knowledge of their actions

7.4 complies with surgical procedures entailing discomfort or embarrassment

CONSULTING A DOCTOR

At its simplest, traditional medical practice is somewhat similar to garage services: One person (patient) brings a problematic object (body) to another person (doctor). The second person exercises judgements about the malfunction based on a large knowledge of such objects and executes repairs to the object before returning it to its owner. In practice, the medical practitioner is usually one element in a large healthcare network, but we can ignore this for the moment. This model often works moderately well where the owner of the problematic body is unable to act at all alone to remedy the problem—for example, during a cardiac arrest, or for removal of an inflamed appendix. However, the majority of medical consultations involve the patient exercising some degree of control over the problematic body, so a somewhat different relation of the three elements becomes appropriate. The patient (or client) takes continuing responsibility for the body, but takes advice and training from the doctor in the care of it. The relationship between patient and doctor is then more analogous to that of student and teacher. The different types of doctor–patient relationship are contrasted in Table 7.1. This chapter describes a client-led approach to use of medical services.

Table 7.1 Models of doctor, client, and illness

	Doctor-led model	Client-led model
doctor's role	takes control of defective body	accepts patient's problem definition
	diagnoses deviations from ideal	diagnoses deviations from ideal
	prescribes and administers drug or surgical remedy	recommends remedy, trains use
	informs patient of required role	revises advice after hearing patient's competing health beliefs
client's role	relinquishes control	seeks advice on defined problem
	complies with prescribed remedy	accepts advice or raises incompatibilities
	remains passive until directed	agrees to practise behaviour recommended
appropriate context	medical emergencies with high immediate risk of deterioration	chronic or recurring with low risk of rapid deterioration
examples	severe asthmatic attack, cardiac arrest, perforated ulcer	routine control of asthma, angina pectoris, recurrent ulceration

ADHERENCE

The traditional model of medical practice is relatively ineffective in enlisting the patient's participation in the health-maintenance process, so the model of service delivery is critical in addressing the major problem of non-adherence. The term "adherence" refers to the extent to which the person is able to achieve optimum dosage and timing of the drug or other self-administered procedure. "Compliance" is another frequently used term and is defined by Haynes as "the extent to which a person's behavior . . . coincides with medical or health advice" (Haynes, Taylor, & Sackett, 1979). The term "compliance" has the drawback that it assumes decision-making power exclusively in the prescriber, with which health behaviour can "coincide". Health behaviour, which involves the knowledge, beliefs, and skills of the person using the drug, are of central importance for adherence to be achieved. Perhaps "compliance" is the more appropriate term when describing surgical procedures, and "adherence" when describing procedures the client undertakes alone.

Despite their importance in medicine, prescribed drugs are probably misused as often as they are used appropriately. DiMatteo (1985) estimates noncompliance to medical advice at about 40%—that is, two out of every five patients fail to adhere reasonable closely to their regimens—but he does not distinguish between misunderstanding and rejection. Comparisons of acute and long-term conditions indicate the following conclusions (Becker & Rosenstock, 1984; Sackett & Snow, 1979):

- *Acute illnesses* have average adherence rates for taking medicine with short-term treatment regimens at about 78%.

- *Chronic illnesses* with long-term regimens have adherence dropping to about 54%; 37% to 50% of tuberculosis patients ceased treatment, against medical advice (Drolet & Porter, 1949).

- *Preventive medication* use achieves average adherence rates of roughly 60% for both short-term and long-term regimens. In anti-hypertensive therapy, as many as 50% of patients drop out during the first year, most of them during the first two months of treatment (Armstrong et al., 1962; Caldwell et al., 1970).

- *Scheduled appointments* are missed 20% to 50% of the time, but attendance is much higher if the patient initiated the appointment than if the practitioner did.

- *Referral failure:* 34% of families referred to child guidance did not attend at all (Cauffman et al., 1974) (see further on).

- *Components of adherence:* Adherence among clients of a health centre serving a low-income population was reported by Svarstad (1976). About 50%

could not correctly report how long they were supposed to continue taking their medications, 26% did not know the dosage prescribed, 17% could not report the prescribed frequency for taking their medications, 16% thought that their drugs marked *"p.r.n."* were to be taken regularly, and 23% could not identify the *purpose* of each drug they were taking.

Pendleton et al. (1984) suggest a "rule of thirds" for summarising these findings—one-third use the drug as prescribed, one-third misunderstand the advice, one-third reject the medical advice. Rejection of medical advice is of particular concern. Rejection is rarely an explicit refusal to the prescribing doctor, but some implicit contrary belief. The health beliefs behind some such rejections that patients have given to the author include:

"I know I'm supposed to take that steroid spray for my asthma, but it feels like oil in my throat, so I take an extra puff of my Ventolin if I feel bad."

"I take those beta-blockers for my blood pressure, but I stop taking them when I'm on holiday so I can have a drink."

Rejection of medical advice without this being declared has led to adherence monitoring in some medical centres. There are three relatively objective approaches for assessing adherence to using medication:

- *Pill or quantity accounting*, in which the remaining medication is measured, such as by counting the number of pills left, and then compared against the quantity that should be left at that point in treatment if the patient has been following the directions correctly. This method does not reveal whether the patient used the medication at the right times, and patients who expect an accounting and want to conceal their non-compliance can discard some of the contents.

- *Medication dispensers with recording devices* (mechanical or electromechanical) that can count and record the time when the dispenser is used. Although this approach is expensive to implement, it assesses compliance accurately as long as the patient does not deliberately create a ruse. If patients know about the device and want to avoid taking the medicine, they can operate the dispenser at the right time and discard the drug.

- *Biochemical tests*, such as the patient's blood or urine. This approach can accurately assess recent medication use, but it can also be very time-consuming and expensive to implement.

Information on levels of adherence and health has only become available in the last few years. Hays et al. (1994) followed 2,125 patients with hypertension, diabetes, recent myocardial infarction, and congestive heart failure, using self-report measures of adherence. Significant benefits were found in insulin-using diabetics on measures such as social function and energy, but only 9 significant effects (7 positive, 2 negative) were found out of 72 possible. These authors recommend a return to assessing the positive, null, and negative outcomes of medical recommendations, rather than spotlighting failure to adhere to such recommendations.

HEALTH BELIEF MODEL

Strategies to increase adherence need to engage with the patient's health beliefs. Over the past few decades, a variety of models have been constructed to help explain public response to preventive programmes. Although these formulations offer different orientations and variables, most contain elements of a particular model initially developed to predict compliance with such preventive health recommendations as obtaining immunisations, screening tests, and annual check-ups. The Health Belief Model (HBM) has been one of the most influential, though other approaches such as the parallel response model have been more predictive in some situations. Niven (1989) attributes the HBM model to Hochbaum, Kegeles, Leventhal, and Rosenstock (Rosenstock, 1974), later modified by Becker (1974).

This "Health Belief Model" contains the following elements:

- *susceptibility:* the person's perception of vulnerability to the particular illness

- *severity:* perception of the physical and social impact of that disease

- *benefits:* evaluation of the feasibility and efficaciousness of the advocated health behaviour (i.e. an estimate of the action's potential benefits in reducing susceptibility and/or severity)

- *barriers:* perceived physical, financial, or psychological costs which might offset benefits.

The Health Belief Model has now been applied successfully in a large number of research efforts to explain and predict individuals' health-related behaviours in preventive situations, including: screening for cervical, breast, or other cancers; screening for tuberculosis, heart disease, Tay-Sachs disease, and for dental problems; immunisations against various illnesses; adoption of an accident-preventive device; risk-reduction actions to prevent coronary heart disease; a postpartum programme of contraception; and well-child (preventive) clinic visits. Apart from the four basic variables of the HBM, various other modifiers have been added in later developments of the theory. These include demographic, ethnic, personality, family factors, and cues to action. A cue to action must occur to trigger the appropriate health behaviour; this stimulus can be either internal (e.g. the perception of symptoms) or external (e.g. interpersonal interactions, mass media communications).

A tendency to be aroused by health-related stimuli and a general concern for health helps in explaining mothers' decisions to adhere to a ten-day penicillin regimen prescribed for their children (Becker, Drachman, & Kirscht, 1972). But, in screening situations, general concern with health did not account for people's decisions to participate in a programme to detect the Tay-Sachs trait (Becker & Maiman, 1975). It should be noted that the first of these studies concerned behaviour under conditions of diagnosed illness, whereas the second concerned behaviour to be initiated by a healthy target audience. Perhaps health consciousness helps to explain illness or sickness (compliance) behaviour, but it is less valuable in explaining preventive behaviour. While correlations among four preventive health actions studied (chest X-rays, medical and dental visits in the absence of symptoms, and tooth-brushing after meals) were positive, they were quite modest (Haefner et al., 1967). Other investigators have been unable to demonstrate the existence of a uni-dimensional preventive health orientation. Behaviours such as brushing one's teeth have health implications but are probably cued by non-health habits developed in childhood, such as preparing for bed (Haefner, 1974).

Inoculation behaviour against swine influenza will be used to illustrate how the Health Belief Model has been employed in studying preventive health behaviour (Becker & Rosenstock, 1984; Cummings et al., 1979). In 1976, swine influenza was widely believed by public health officials to threaten the population of the United States. Predictor variables for inoculation included HBM dimensions, measures of behavioural intention, physicians' advice, and other variables hypothesised to have some potential impact on the decision. The research design consisted of a telephone survey one week prior to the start of a mass campaign and a follow-up survey on a random half of the sample immediately after the campaign and the other half two months later. One adult respondent was randomly chosen from each household selected into the sample. The subject group comprised 374 adults in the initial survey and 286 adults in the follow-up survey. Each of the four main HBM variables—perceived susceptibility, severity, efficacy, and barriers—yielded a significant correlation with inoculation behaviour. Socio-economic status was the only demographic variable to have a significant relationship with vaccination behaviour, and the other traditional demographic indicators (age, sex, marital status) demonstrated weak correlations with the dependent variable. It should also be noted that for those individuals who sought the advice of a physician, the physician's recommendation had a powerful influence on their subsequent behaviour. Finally, behavioural intention was significantly associated with behavioural outcome.

THREAT MINIMISATION

Appraising a health consultation as threatening may actually prevent attendance for screening—a finding that HBM has difficulty in explaining. Invitation to attend mass cancer screening was less likely to be accepted in those who saw themselves as at risk for cancer (Seydel, Taal, & Weigman, 1990). Leventhal (1970) proposes a parallel response model, in which fear control is separated from danger control. Action to reduce danger would involve knowing the presence of a vulnerability, but actions to reduce the unpleasant effects of fear may include avoidance. The tendency to minimise threat was studied in a screening simulation by Croyle and Barger (1993). Subjects were invited to attend for screening of saliva for a hereditary trait. All subjects were then asked to estimate the seriousness and prevalence of the condition, the accuracy of the test, and the probable symptoms. Those who were told they carried the trait estimated the trait to be less serious and more prevalent, and the accuracy of the test lower, than those told they did not carry the trait. In fact, the trait and disease were entirely fictitious, and subjects were debriefed to that effect.

INCREASING ATTENDANCE AND ADHERENCE

The drop-out phenomenon has been well studied in the psychiatric area and is clearly a considerable problem in the TB and hypertension treatments described above. Why do people discontinue treatment? To begin with, the picture may not be as bleak as the drop-out rates suggest. Patient adherence decisions have been studied by Cummings, Becker, and Maile (1980), and by Baekeland and Lundwall (1975). The latter authors conclude (in a review of psychiatric literature) that not all drop-outs are lost to treatment, since many of them seek care elsewhere; moreover, some persons may drop out because their health has improved. These reviewers conclude that likelihood of dropping out is also positively related to:

- social isolation or lack of affiliation
- negative therapist attitudes and behaviour
- low personal motivation
- long waiting-time for treatment
- low socio-economic status

- young age

- female sex

- social instability

Personal contact. Features of the treatment setting and system of care are clearly involved in the problem of drop-out. Relatively simple changes in the system, such as reminders and provider continuity, have demonstrated notable effects on keeping patients in treatment for alcoholism (Baekeland & Lundwall, 1975). Similarly, modification of clinic procedures towards more personalised, convenient care has proved valuable in reducing drop-out among hypertensive patients (Finnerty, Mattie, & Finnerty, 1973). Finally, in a review of the drop-out and broken-appointment problem in general adult clinics, Deyo and Inui (1980) conclude that most successful interventions have concentrated on features of clinic organisation and on interactions between patient and provider. The following features were suggested:

- individual timed appointments systems

- specific physician assignment

- mailed prospective reminders

- access to physician by telephone

- elimination of pharmacy delays

- educational efforts aimed at conveying knowledge of disease, its therapy

- modifying health beliefs, e.g. the importance of continuing care

- eliciting and discussing reasons for previously missed appointments.

It has long been known that many clients referred by one agency for care at another never complete these referrals. For example, Levine, Scotch, and Vlasak (1969) have shown that most children referred to child guidance clinics for service fail to obtain service at those clinics. Cauffman et al. (1974) have probed this problem and emerged with some surprising findings. The overall aim of their project was to develop and implement an on-line computer system for making referrals for health care throughout the Los Angeles area, using a comprehensive health service data bank to which health workers in various agencies would be linked by terminal devices. Thirteen diverse agencies in the East Los Angeles Health District participated in a feasibility study of the system. Over the study period, data were collected on a total of 471 consumers, each with a single referral. It was found that over 40% of consumers referred for care did not receive care; some of these appeared for care but did not receive it, perhaps for good medical reasons, but 34% of the total group did not even appear at the care facility. Only two factors studied showed significant relationships to referral follow-through: whether the consumer was given the name of a person to see at the provider's office, and a time; those consumers given specific appointments and/or a named person to contact were more likely to show up than were other consumers.

These findings are reasonable, and the action implications seem obvious. Of greater theoretical importance are those factors that did not distinguish shows from no-shows. These included sex, type of health problem, convenience problems (including transportation, language, child care, parking), financial difficulties, time interval between referral and appointment, distance from care, and type of provider. Some of the "non-findings" are surprising, especially those concerning convenience problems in obtaining care. It is clear that referral failures are widespread, and it is likely that the rate of no-shows could be reduced by giving clients specific appointments with named providers.

Contracts. A relatively recent development that attempts to capitalise on (and in some ways improve) the relationship between provider and patient is the "therapeutic contract". Both parties set forth a treatment goal, the specific obligations of each party in attempting that goal, and a time limit for its achievement. Lewis and Michnich (1977) argue that, as a compliance-enhancing intervention, the contract is supposed to work by clarifying and making explicit relative responsibilities of both provider and consumer in achieving an agreed-upon goal and by transferring some power from provider to consumer. A provider–client contract increased the likelihood of patient compliance with ambulatory haemodialysis (Cummings et al., 1981).

INFORMATION AND ITS RECALL

The surprisingly low recall by patients of information given by doctors has been extensively documented by Ley (1982, 1988). The following features of the message and the audience are relevant to recall of information:

- *Primacy.* There is a strong tendency to recall information given first. In three analogue studies, subjects typically recalled 10% more of the first half (or third) of the information than in subsequent half (or thirds).

- *Medical knowledge.* Recall of medical information depends heavily on previous medical knowledge. In three analogue studies, correlations of at least +0.33 were reported.

- *Intelligence.* Only a slight effect of general education and intelligence has been reported, equivalent to a correlation of +0.20.

- *Amount of information.* Recall decreases with the number of separate pieces of information given, as we would expect from research on memory. Subjects given six statements recalled 64% in two experiments by Ley, while those receiving twelve statements recalled 41% or 52%.

- *Anxiety.* Moderate anxiety has been shown to lead to greater recall than low anxiety in four studies. The Yerkes-Dodson U-curve (see chapter 2) would lead us to expect poorer recall at very high levels of anxiety, and high anxiety is likely when serious diagnoses are being given. This has been demonstrated only in an analogue study by Ley.

- *Time elapsed.* Memory research generally tends to show considerable decay between recall immediately after presentation and some hours or days later. However, this does not seem to be the case for personally meaningful medical information.

- *Age.* No general effect of age on recall has been shown, though patients over 65 may recall slightly more poorly.

IMPROVING COMMUNICATION

- *Simplification.* The use of shorter words and sentences increases the likelihood of recall. Where written material is used, formal checks on the required reading age can be made. Videotapes achieve better attention-control than does written material.

- *Explicit categorisation.* A preliminary statement giving the categories of information (e.g. diagnosis: "What you must do for yourself . . .") is made, then each category is expanded.

- *Repetition.* Immediate recall increased from 76% to about 90% if either the patient or the physician repeated the information, in a study by Kupst et al. (1975). However, in analogue studies recall has not increased much with repetition.

- *Specific advice.* Statements such as "You must lose two stone in weight" were shown to be seen as significantly more important than "You must lose weight".

- *Reminders.* Stickers, calendars, and packages may act as prompts to memory, especially with elderly patients. Adherence using mechanical prompts tends to decline to the general level of non-adherence (Rehder et al., 1980).

- *Threat* may increase adherence in a treatment context but create avoidance in screening contexts. Mothers of obese children were randomly assigned to a high-threat communication condition, a low-threat communication condition, and a non-communication control by Becker et al. (1977). Each parent had an oral message and a booklet, then received dietary counselling and re-appointments to the clinic. The group receiving the high-threat message lost more weight than did the one receiving the low-threat version, and both lost more than the no-commmunication group.

SATISFACTION

Satisfaction with technical aspects of medical services is usually much higher than for communications with the medical practitioner. The increased emphasis on communication in medical education, and special efforts by doctors, do not seem to improve the rate of satisfaction, according to Ley (1988). That author repeated a survey at the same hospital nine years apart, and satisfaction was about 53% in both cases. In a review of studies of satisfaction with information given, Ley found the following percentages dissatisfied: hospitals 38%; G.P. and community samples 26%; psychiatric patients 39%. Korsch, Gozzi, and Francis (1968) have undertaken one of the largest studies of patient satisfaction: They studied 800 consultations in a paediatric clinic, and satisfaction was found to be related to the doctor being friendly, rather than businesslike, and seen as understanding the patient's concerns; the patient's expectations about treatment and the like being met; the doctor being perceived as a good communicator; the provision of information.

Communications have both information-giving and affective aspects. The affective dimension of satisfaction with consultations was revealed in the study of 34 consultations by Larsen and Smith (1981), who used three measures of non-verbal communication:

- *"immediacy"*:   based on touch, eye contact, and leaning forward

- *"relaxation"*:   inferred from asymmetry and leaning sideways or back, and

- *"responsiveness"*:   based mainly on speech characteristics.

Overall satisfaction was mainly related to physician immediacy, and to its touching, forward-leaning, and body orientation components. Two relaxation measures also related to satisfaction.

SCREENING

Public and preventive health programmes place considerable emphasis on early detection of problems, such as complications of pregnancy, abnormal cells of the cervix, or raised blood pressure. Such screening should enable prompt remedies if a problem is detected, and reassurance if nothing is detected; in practice, a variety of outcomes occur. Screening programmes generate errors at each level, as Marteau (1993) has shown. The outcomes of screening can be shown in terms of four possibilities (see Table 7.2), borrowing a model used in signal detection theory (Green & Swets, 1966).

A *miss*, or failure to detect the target abnormality, is of greatest concern. Some cytology screening programmes have been shown to pass doubtful smears, perhaps through technician fatigue, and information is sometimes lost through incorrect addresses and other processing errors. However, many more misses arise through failure to take up screening opportunities. Some patients avoid screening because of fear of the presumed illness. This seems particularly true of breast and cervical screening, where many women appear to believe that the purpose of screening is to find cancers rather than early deviant cells. The most disturbing situation is that revealed in a follow-up of non-attenders by Nathoo (1988): In 12 of 17 cases traced, the invitation to attend for screening was interpreted as a concealed message that cervical cancer was present, which resulted in the patient being too scared to attend.

Correct rejection may be a good outcome medically but create either unrealistic confidence or undue pessimism. The purpose of ante-natal screening is frequently misunderstood as being given a clean bill of health. Amniocentesis is intended to detect only Down's syndrome and neural tube defects, but some parents have interpreted a subsequent congenital abnormality as an indication of medical negligence after a negative result. Similar reactions are sometimes seen by the author in patients who have been in told they were in good shape after a routine check of blood pressure and urine, only to sustain a heart attack a few weeks later. Many patients who receive negative findings are not reassured and remain anxious about the illness. The screening test may alert the patient to the possibility of illness, and this anxiety does not recede on being given a negative result (Stoate, 1989).

The *False Alarm* situation arises fairly frequently, since tests do not have unambiguous cut-offs. The probability of recall after an initial cervical smear is much higher than most patients realise, though the probability that second

Table 7. 2 Outcomes of screening

	Client's health status	
Screening verdict	Abnormality present	No abnormality present
abnormality reported	**Hit** remedy administered	**False alarm** repeat screening
no abnormality reported	**Miss** illness	**Correct rejection** client reassured

and third tests will incorrectly lead to diagnosis of abnormality is still quite low.

OVERUSE OF MEDICAL SERVICES

The consultation model described at the beginning would require the patient to consult only when he or she has problems that would improve with medical treatment and exceed personal coping resources. Problems that require psychological help could be presented directly to a counsellor or psychologist of some kind, or referred onwards by a general practitioner if they required longer or more skilled consultations. Despite this, many problems are presented to doctors for which they have no constructive response. These include problems of excessive illness concern (hypochondriasis) and problems where the patient makes use of the "sick role", when more independent coping would be possible. The most extreme form of hypochondriacal concern is the Munchausen syndrome, in which a patient manages to convince medical practitioners of some serious internal illness, sometimes involving surgery.

"Sick-role" behaviour has been conceptualised in the context of social roles by Talcott Parsons, and this model has been widely quoted. In 1951 this sociologist posited the sick role as a construct to account for the rights and obligations of the sick person in the context of US values. Parsons' (1972) discussion begins with the notion that the sick person suffers a disturbance of capacity. Once the incapacity is recognised, the individual moves into the sick role; occupants of this role are *not held to be responsible* for the incapacity since it is viewed as beyond their control, and they are, therefore, *exempted from normal social role obligations*. However, continued legitimation of the sick role requires that the occupant take every reasonable action towards achieving recovery, including (where appropriate) an *obligation to seek technically competent help* and co-operate in the process of getting well. These three attributes of the sick role acount for much inappropriate use of medical services, but not those of the chronically ill patient; indeed, by definition, chronic illnesses are not "curable", and the requirement on the patient would, therefore, be more one of adjusting to the condition than of trying to get well.

KNOWLEDGE OF NORMAL BIOLOGY

Greater knowledge of normal biology would eliminate many consultations. Some body sensations are disturbing until their adaptive significance is known. Reflex pathways have adapted over millions of years for preserving life, and many sensations interpreted as symptoms of disease are actually trustworthy allies.

- *Fear.* The normal increase in heart rate and stomach tightening associated with fear-arousal are very frequently misinterpreted as signs of illness. Knowledge of the fight/flight syndrome is usually helpful. Deliberately experiencing some physical hazard such as rock-climbing makes useful fear familiar and more controllable.

- *Vomiting.* Reflex elimination of stomach contents, either by being sick or diarrhoea, is adaptive in cases of gut infection. These symptoms alone should not be prevented, since starving and taking only water will usually allow normal function to return in one or two days.

- *Fever.* Part of the response to systemic infection is a rise in body temperature and increased lethargy. These are adaptive in increasing white cell proliferation and preventing energy expenditure. "Positive reframing" of fever as a healthy struggle against an alien invader is described further in chapter 14.

- *Aching muscles.* Heavy use of a skeletal muscle creates a build-up of lactic acid and consequent aching. Recall of the previous day's carrying or bending can often put a benign meaning on disturbing sensations for the person with a back or heart problem.

CONCLUSION

Consultations with medical practitioners are necessary for patients to use preventive remedies, and a client-led, shared-care model is often appropriate. Patients' health beliefs in using such medical services are often discrepant from those of doctors, so the rate of adherence is surprisingly poor. Costs and benefits of attendance must be assessed in relation to fear-reduction. Communications are received more effectively if contact is personal, and if messages are framed carefully. Knowledge of normal adaptive reactions can prevent unnecessary worry.

REFERENCES

Armstrong, M.L., Bakke, J.L., Dodge, H., Conrad, L., Freis, F., Fremont, R., Kirkendell, W., Pilz, C., Ramirez, E., Richardson, D., & Williams, J. Jr. (1962). Double-blind control study of hypertensive agents. *Archives of Internal Medicine, 110,* 222–237.

Baekeland, F., & Lundwall, L. (1975). Dropping out of treatment: A critical review. *Psychological Bulletin, 82,* 738–783.

Becker, M.H. (Ed.) (1974). The health belief model and personal health behavior. *Health Education Monograph, 2* (4), 324–508.

Becker, M.H., Drachman, R.H., & Kirscht, J.P. (1972). Predicting mothers' compliance with pediatric medical regimens. *Journal of Pediatrics, 81* (4), 843–854.

Becker, M.H., Haefner, D.P., Kasl, S.V., Kirscht, J.P., Maiman, L.A., & Rosenstock, I.M. (1977). Selected psychosocial models and correlates of individual health-related behaviours. *Medical Care, 15,* 27–46.

Becker, M.H., & Maiman, L.A. (1975). Sociobehavioral determinants of compliance with health and medical care recommendations. *Medical Care, 13,* 10–24.

Becker, M.H., & Rosenstock, I.M. (1984). Compliance with medical advice. In A. Steptoe, & A. Mathews (Eds.), *Health care and human behaviour* (Ch. 6). London: Academic Press.

Caldwell, J., Cobb, S., Dowling, M.D., & Jongh, D.D. (1970). The dropout problem in antihypertensive therapy. *Journal of Chronic Disease, 22,* 579–592.

Cauffman, J., Lloyd, J.S., Lyons, M., Cortese, P., Beckwith, R., Petit, D., Wehrle, P., McBroom, E., & McIntire, J. (1974). A study of health referral patterns. *American Journal of Public Health, 64,* 331–356.

Croyle, R.T., & Barger, S.D. (1993). Illness cognition. In S. Maes, H. Leventhal, & M. Johnston (Eds.), *International review of health psychology* (chapter 2). Chichester: Wiley.

Cummings K.M., Becker, M.H., & Maile, M.C. (1980). Bringing the models together: An empirical approach to combining variables used to explain health actions. *Journal of Behavioral Medicine, 3,* 123–145.

Cummings, K.M., Becker, M.H., Kirscht, J.P., & Levin, N. (1981). Intervention strategies to improve compliance with medical regimens by ambulatory haemodialysis patients. *Journal of Behavioral Medicine, 4,* 111–127.

Cummings, K.M., Jette, R.P.T., Brock, J.M., & Haefner, D.P. (1979). Psychosocial determinants of immunization behavior in a swine fever campaign. *Medical Care, 17,* 639–649.

Deyo, R.A., & Inui, S. (1980). Dropouts and broken appointments: A literature review and agenda for future research. *Medical Care, 18,* 1146–1157.

DiMatteo, M.R. (1985). *The psychology of health, illness, and medical care: An individual perspective.* Belmont, CA: Brooks/Cole.

Drolet, G., & Porter, D. (1949). *Why patients in tuberculosis hospitals leave against medical advice.* New York: New York Tuberculosis and Health Association.

Finnerty, F.A., Jr., Mattie, E., & Finnerty, F.A., III (1973). Hypertension in the inner city: I. Analysis of clinic dropouts, and II. Detection and follow-up. *Circulation, 47,* 73–78.

Green, D.M., & Swets, J.A. (1966). *Signal detection theory and psychophysics.* New York: Wiley.

Haefner, D.P. (1974). The health belief model and preventive dental behaviours. *Health Education Monographs, 2,* 420–432.

Haefner, D.P., Kegeles, S.S., Kirscht, J.P., & Rosenstock, I.M. (1967). Preventive actions concerning dental disease, tuberculosis, and cancer. *Public Health Reports, 82,* 451–459.

Haynes, R.B., Taylor, D.W., & Sackett, D.L. (Eds.) (1979). *Compliance in health care.* Baltimore, MD: Johns Hopkins University Press.

Hays, R., Kravitz, R., Mazel, R., Shelbourne, C., DiMatteo, M., Rogers, W., & Greenfield, S. (1994). The impact of patient adherence on health outcomes for patients with chronic disease in the medical outcomes study. *Journal of Behavioral Medicine, 17* (4), 347–360.

Korsch, B.M., Gozzi, E.K., & Francis, V. (1968). Gaps in doctor–patient communication. *Paediatrics, 42,* 855–871.

Kupst, M.J., Dresser, K. et al. (1975). Evaluation of methods to improve communication in the physician–patient relationship. *American Journal of Orthopsychiatry, 45,* 420–429.

Larsen, K., & Smith, C.K. (1981). Assessment of non-verbal communication in the physician–patient interview. *Journal of Family Practice, 12,* 481–488.

Leventhal, H. (1970). Findings and theory in the study of fear communications. In L. Berkowitz (Ed.), *Advances in experimental social psychology.* New York: Academic Press.

Levine, S., Scotch, N.A., & Vlasak, G.J. (1969). Unravelling culture and technology in public health. *American Journal of Public Health, 59,* 237–244.

Lewis, C.E., & Michnich, M. (1977). Contracts as a means of improving patient compliance. In I. Barofsky (Ed.), *Medication compliance: A behavioral management approach* (pp. 69–75). Thorofare, NJ: Charles B. Slack.

Ley, P. (1982). Satisfaction, compliance and communication. *British Journal of Clinical Psychology, 21,* 241–254.

Ley, P. (1988). *Communicating with patients.* London: Chapman & Hall.

Marteau, T. (1993). Health-related screening: Psychological predictors of uptake and impact. In S. Maes, H. Leventhal, & M. Johnston (Eds.), *International review of health psychology.* Chichester: Wiley.

Nathoo, V. (1988). Investigation of non-responders at a cervical screening clinic in Manchester. *British Medical Journal, 296,* 1041–1042.

Niven, N. (1989). *Health psychology: An introduction for nurses and other health care professionals.* Edinburgh: Churchill Livingstone.

Parsons, T. (1972). Definitions of health and illness in the light of American values and social structure. In E.G. Jaco (Ed.), *Patients, physicians, and illness* (2nd ed., pp. 107–127). New York: Free Press.

Pendleton, D.A., Schofield, T., Tate, P., & Havelock, P. (1984). *The consultation: An approach to learning and teaching.* Oxford: Oxford University Press.

Rehder, T.L., McCoy, L.K., et al. (1980). Improving medication compliance by counselling and special prescription container. *American Journal of Hospital Pharmacy, 37,* 379–386.

Rosenstock, I.M. (1974). The health belief model and preventive health behavior. *Health Education Monographs, 2,* 354–386.

Sackett, D.L., & Snow, J.C. (1979). The magnitude of compliance and non-compliance. In R.B. Haynes, D.W. Taylor, D.L. Sackett (Eds.), *Compliance in health care.* Baltimore, MD: Johns Hopkins University Press, 1979.

Seydel, E., Taal, E., & Weigman, O. (1990). Risk-appraisal, outcome, and self-efficacy expectancies: Cognitive factors in preventive behaviour related to cancer. *Psychology and Health, 4*, 99–109.

Stoate, H. (1989). Can health screening damage your health? *Journal of the Royal College of General Practitioners, 39*, 193–195.

Svarstad, B.L (1976). Physician–patient communication and patient conformity with medical advice. In D. Mechanic (Ed.), *The growth of bureaucratic medicine* (pp. 220–238). New York: Wiley.

II

BODY SYSTEMS

8

Circulation: Maintenance

Maintenance of energy supply is the body's most critical function. Cessation of the heart action for as little as three minutes leads to death, but fortunately the heart is a highly efficient self-repairing pump. The arteries age more rapidly than do most other bodily systems, through the combined effects of plaque deposition and loss of elasticity. The processes that lead to this are predominantly in the realm of personal behaviour. Heart disease is, in principle, highly preventable, but the extent to which campaigns to reduce it have any effect remains debatable. Most scientific knowledge about maintenance of circulation is from disease epidemiology. This chapter presents research on risk factors, and inferences for positive skills are drawn in the conclusion.

PHYSIOLOGY OF CIRCULATION

The heart has the function of circulating blood, which is the transport medium for substances that need frequent changes, including oxygen, energy-releasing substances, cells of the immune system, and waste products. The following brief summary can be amplified by reference to medical textbooks—for example, Kumar and Clark (1990). Blood from the heart is distributed into the arteries; after the exchange processes in capillaries it returns under lower pressure via the veins. Control of the heart-beat involves a complex electrical "clock". Normally the heartbeat is initiated by the sino-atrial node within the heart, and the wave of depolarisation spreads through

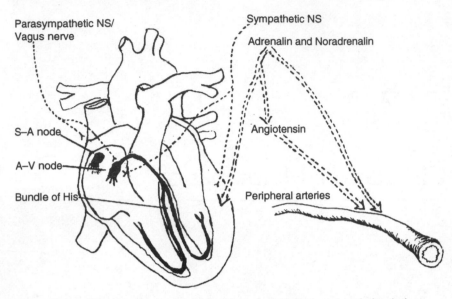

Figure 8.1 Nervous and hormonal control of the heart and circulation

the myocardium like ripples on a pond: From the atrium, the spread is slowed at the boundary with the ventricles by the atrioventricular node, and continues via the bundle of His and the left and right bundle branches (see Figure 8.1). This electrical activity can be monitored on the surface of the body by electrocardiogram (ECG): Atrial depolarisation shows as a P wave, followed by a short interval; ventricular activation shows as a QRS complex; and T is the recovery phase. The complex electrical activity of the heart means that a great variety of electrical dysfunctions can occur, and these can be monitored closely with the ECG.

The "rate of ticking" of the electrical clock is influenced by both sympathetic and parasympathetic descending pathways. Adrenergic nerves supply atrial and ventricular muscle, which have predominantly beta-receptors. Cholinergic nerves in the vagus supply the Sino-Atrial (SA) and Atrio-Ventricular (AV) nodes. Under resting conditions, parasympathetic vagal effects dominate, resulting in a slow heart rate; increased sympathetic stimulation causes the heart rate to rise. The blood vessels have walls consisting of smooth muscle, and the diameter of these vessels can be altered via their beta-receptors and the ANS according to different demands placed on the organism. Such demands include increased muscle requirements for energy during exertion, or diversion via deeper vessels during cold, but it also includes more subtle changes such as blushing during emotion. With such sophisticated nervous and behavioural control, it is hardly surprising that the heart and arteries are especially susceptible to stress-related illness.

PREVALENCE OF HEART DISEASE

The majority of our knowledge of normal circulation comes from epidemiological research on one type of illness—myocardial infarction. A myocardial infarction (MI) occurs when a clot of blood blocks a coronary artery. This will cause death of the muscle tissue supplied by that artery. This is often accompanied by great pain in the centre of the chest and sometimes in the left arm, sweating, and changes in blood pressure and heart rhythm. Death follows within one hour in approximately 40% of initial incidents. Other circulatory accidents, including stroke and sudden death, are described in chapter 9.

It is often claimed that coronary heart disease (CHD) is at epidemic proportions in Britain and other industrialised countries. Epidemiological research shows this to be largely accurate, with marked differences according to age, gender, and nationality. Leeder et al. (1983) looked at the rates of MI among 238,028 men and women during 1979 in an Australian community. The incidence rates show the dramatic increase in incidence during middle life, and the effect of gender:

- *under 39:* 4.1 per 1000 per year (men)
              0.7 per 1000 per year (women)

- *65–69:*   42.4 per 1000 per year (men)
              20.7 per 1000 per year (women)

The differences between countries are shown in the 1971 report of the US National Heart and Lung Institute (see Byrne, 1987). The trend since that time appears to be that CHD has increased in Japan but declined by about 3% a year in the 1980s in the United Kingdom. 1971 data show the death rates per 100,000 people from arteriosclerotic and degenerative heart disease in 1967 for men aged between 45 and 54 years:

- *Finland* had the highest incidence: 500

- *The United States* was also high: 370

- *Britain* was slightly lower: about 250

- *Italy and Mediterranean countries*: about 150

- *Japan* was lowest: less than 100

Many factors have been implicated as risks for CHD, but three "classic risk factors" stand out and will be discussed in detail: cholesterol, blood pressure, and tobacco smoking. These factors are influenced by eating habits, emotional arousal, and fitness, so inferences for these skills will be drawn further on.

Cholesterol and atheroma

MI and related problems such as angina and hypertension have received most research attention as possible stress-related diseases. MI is predisposed mainly by the reduction of effective arterial diameter. Loss of elasticity of the smooth muscle of the artery and sudden spasm of the muscle will reduce this diameter, but the main pathological influence is the deposition of fatty substances in the form of atheroma. Such depositions are most likely where the level of low-density lipoproteins in the serum is regularly high. Cholesterol is difficult for the body to dissipate and can only be excreted from the body in the form of bile. Being relatively insoluble, it is easily deposited as plaques to form atheroma. It is therefore plausible, though not proven, that people under chronically high stress without the releasing effect of vigorous physical activity are likely to develop atheroma.

Cholesterol is one of four forms of lipid present in plasma, the others being fatty acids, triglycerides, and phospholipids. Lipids combine with proteins in blood plasma to form lipoproteins, which are more soluble. Heredity plays a moderate role in CHD risk, and much of this seems to be via Lipoprotein A (Lawn, 1992). The level of this particle in the blood remains fairly stable throughout life, irrespective of diet. Recently it has been found that density of lipoproteins is better than cholesterol as a measure of pathology. High-density lipoprotein (HDL) is found to be beneficial, while low-density (LDL) and very low-density lipoprotein (VLDL) are found to be associated with atheroma formation. However, serum total cholesterol is still the widely used clinical measure. Cholesterol levels by country are strongly correlated with CHD risk for the same country, as can be seen in Figure 8.2.

Doyle and Kannel (1970) published the findings of the National Cooperative Pooling Project. Serum cholesterol was measured at entry to the study, in milligrams per 100 millilitres (the more usual unit is millimols per litre; 1 mmol/litre = 39 mg/100 ml). All subjects were males. Outcome figures are 10-year age-adjusted rates for first major coronary events including fatal or survived myocardial infarction:

Cholesterol	MIs/1000
<175	45
175–199	52
200–224	53
225–249	67
250–274	112
275–299	115
>300	162

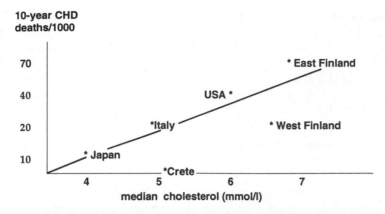

Figure 8.2 Serum cholesterol and deaths by country.
(Redrawn from Truswell, 1986)

Because of the correlations between CHD rates and cholesterol in the serum, currently recommended diets contain a low proportion of total fat, in the hope that this will reduce cholesterol. Until recently polyunsaturated fats, chiefly linoleic, found in sunflower and maize oil, were thought to be protective, but it now appears that these are oxidised in the body and may be equally harmful. Eating cholesterol sources such as eggs has less effect for most people than eating fats. Polysaturated fats such as palmitic and myristic acids appear in the serum after about 10 days. Monounsaturates, found in olive oil and fish oil, do not contribute to cholesterol but may not reduce it, while eicosopentenaenoic acid, also found in fish oil, is thought to reduce cholesterol.

It is widely known that excessive dietary cholesterol is harmful and that it is found in animal substances that store energy, such as eggs or liver. The role of endogenous cholesterol is less well known: Cholesterol from food is transported to the human liver, which is also where endogenous cholesterol is synthesised. It serves as a medium-term energy source and is therefore produced in increased quantities when muscular demands are high. Physiologists usually study lipids in static laboratory situations, so rather little is known about the relationship between cholesterol, mood, and behaviour. In the light of the findings of Carruthers (1969) and Manuck, Kaplan, and Clarkson (1983) discussed later on, it is reasonable to assume that the sympathetic-adrenal mechanisms that mediate fight or flight will also increase cholesterol production. However, preparation for fight or flight is often not followed by vigorous action in modern society, and this may be the reason why emotional stress may be associated with sustained increases in serum cholesterol.

In humans, Taggart and Carruthers (1971) demonstrated that cholesterol levels are extremely high in car drivers in demanding situations: This finding was first made on racing drivers before a major competition and repeated on inexperienced women drivers in busy traffic. Manuck et al. (1983) have reported on a series of studies of coronary atherosclerosis of cholesterol-fed, male cynomolgus monkeys (*Macaca fascicularis*). In the 1983 experiments, he subjected macaque monkeys to a moderate laboratory stressor (threat of capture) and classified the monkeys as high or low heart-rate responders to this threat. They were fed a moderately atherogenic diet for 22 months, then sacrificed. It was found that the high stress responders had nearly twice the level of arterial occlusion of the low responders. Atheroma was exacerbated among animals that exhibited the largest heart rate (HR) reactions to a standard laboratory stressor.

Behavioural influences on lipids in the serum have been implicated in other diseases, notably diabetes mellitus. The regular achievement of optimum levels of blood glucose in insulin-dependent diabetics is mainly a function of calorie intake, energy expenditure, and level of insulin. Deviations from this optimum are fairly frequent and create many long-term health hazards, including increased risk of MI. Many of these lapses arise through lack of skill in the sufferer in giving doses according to input and output, or through casual or rebellious attitudes to the drug regime. A further pathway seems to occur if the diabetic has sustained high levels of lipids associated with chronic stress. Minuchin (1977) gave a rather extraordinary demonstration of this by taking blood serum measure during therapy with a family. Two children with diabetes were involved, one with good and one with poor glucose control. As the session progressed, the second child was seen to be experiencing rejection by the family, and this was associated with rising levels of lipids in the serum.

Blood pressure and CHD risk

Pressure of the arterial blood increases with greater peripheral vascular resistance, and resistance reflects atherogenesis and ageing, but also short-term vasoconstrictive processes. Raised blood pressure increases the risk of cerebrovascular accident (stroke), but also the risk of MI, kidney disease, retinal bleeding, and numerous other diseases. Management of hypertension is therefore an important part of the general-practice doctor's role. Julian Tudor Hart (1980) is well known for his work on management of high blood pressure. As with cholesterol, risk is elevated in proportion to the elevation of the reading. Arterial blood pressure is normally measured with a sphygmomanometer outside the body, although a more accurate reading requires an arterial canula. The cuff is pressurised and stops blood flow until the cuff pressure is dropped to the peak pressure generated by the heart. This is known as the systolic pressure. As the cuff pressure drops further, the pulse disappears when the diastolic or base pressure is reached. Systolic pressure at rest is considered normal if it is around age plus 100. For example, normal pressure at age 20 is 120, and at 65 is 165.

A cut-off at 140/90 was regarded as "normal" in the American high blood-pressure education project (see chapter 9). Since BP readings fluctuate and drug treatment has side-effects, GPs use ascertainments such as Hart's recommended cut-offs for diastolic pressure:

Men and women	Drug treatment	Observation	Residual
age 40–64	>105	90–104	<90
age < 40	>100	85–99	<85

One relationship between resting blood pressure and behaviour that has proved tractable to research is the subjects' report of their usual mode of expressing hostility. Spielberger et al. (1985) asked high-school students to report on their usual way of expressing anger. His statistical analysis found two principal factors, which he labelled "anger-in" and "anger-out". Questions correlating with anger-in included "I am secretly critical of others", while items such as "I slam doors" correlated with anger-out. Spielberger measured the blood pressure of over a thousand students and found that BP was highly correlated with anger-in. While there was little relationship between anger-out scores and BP, the highest-scoring teenagers on anger-in had average systolic BP of 132, compared with 115 for the lower scorers. A comprehensive account of hostility and CHD risk is provided by Chesney and Rosenman (1985).

There is evidence that fear combines with inhibition of effective response to the threat to create high blood pressure. A study by Gentry et al. (1982) of male black Americans identified these risk factors: black/white; urban/suburban residence; and anger-in/anger-out. The percentage of the male population with hypertension was in proportion to the presence or absence of these three factors. Of black males residing in high-stress areas, who also suppressed anger, 39% were classified as hypertensive. The effect of fear on BP was also shown in a study of pregnant women in Israel (Rofé & Goldberg, 1983). Women receiving ante-natal care were classified according to the level of military activity in the region where they lived. It was found that average blood pressure was proportional to the level of military activity.

Measurement of blood pressure is normally made under clinical conditions of rest, where the level of demand is low. Resting blood pressure is not a good measure of the subject's blood pressure under stress, and some measure of the average increase in blood pressure is needed. Cardiovascular reactivity has been repeatedly associated with CHD risk (Matthews et al., 1986). One approach to measuring the reactivity of the cardiovascular system is ambulatory monitoring, in which readings can be taken repeatedly in normal environments by automatic recording devices. Another approach is to induce environmental stress artificially under clinical conditions, such as asking the subjects to perform a mentally demanding task while playing loud noise to them. Steptoe (1990) reviews studies on reactivity in humans and reports moderate reliability in that 12 out of 23 reactivity measures were unchanged on repeated testing, but fairly low correlations between ambulatory measures and reactivity.

Research on blood pressure under demand conditions such as exertion and stress include Manuck's measures described earlier implicating atheroma and reactivity. Keys et al. (1971) studied the effects of cold immersion on diastolic blood pressure. The 23-year follow-up shows that CHD was significantly related to the magnitude of the diastolic response to this cold-pressor stress. At least two other studies have confirmed this trend, while two more have failed to find prediction from cold pressor response (see Steptoe, 1990). Although behaviour has strong effects in developing high blood pressure, homeostatic control at hypertensive levels by the kidney may not be easily reversible by changes in behaviour (see chapter 9).

Smoking

Tobacco smoking is the best statistical predictor of MI, if age and sex are discounted. The cardiovascular effects of nicotine are mainly through its cholinergic effects and include tachycardia, vasoconstriction, and platelet aggregation. To these is added the effect of carbon monoxide in blocking the transport of oxygen, further increasing the pulse rate. The risk of a clot large enough to obstruct a coronary artery is much increased after cigarette smoking. Results of many studies continue to confirm the association between smoking and CHD. The US Pooling Project (Doyle & Kannel, 1970; also cited in Byrne, 1987) found that men smoking more than 20 cigarettes a day were three times more likely to die of CHD than were men who had never smoked. The following results are for first major coronary events (fatal or survived). Smoking status was at time of entry to the study and was measured in terms of "packs per day" of cigarettes; those who had given up smoking are noted as "past only", while those who smoked a pipe or cigar were aggregated.

Smoking status	Rate/1000
never	40
past	50
pipe/cigar	50
<10/day	66
20/day	83
20+/day	131

This showed a clear association between the number of cigarettes smoked and risk. However, the risk for pipe and cigar smokers was only slightly higher than for non-smokers, and this may relate to different inhalation practices. The rate for those who had given up smoking was much lower than for those who currently smoked and only slightly higher than for non-smokers. Smoking cessation has an immediate positive effect on CHD risk, but a much smaller and slower effect on risk of lung disease. Public awareness of these hazards is now high. Smoking has declined, though behaviour change has lagged far behind attitude change. In the 1985 Welsh Heart Survey, 42% of men and 33% of women were recorded as smokers (HPAW, 1990). The General Household Survey has shown a continuing fall in prevalence since then. Manual workers continue to smoke more than non-manual workers, and adolescent girls smoke more than adolescent boys. Data from the Welsh Youth Survey showed validated smoking prevalences for boys as 22%, and for girls as 31%.

The reasons for starting smoking in adolescence are an important focus for preventive health. Reported reasons for smoking rarely include pleasure; indeed, most teenagers report nausea in connection with first cigarettes. More important are toughness and independence. Peer pressure towards mature-seeming images at puberty is the most probable factor. The increase in smoking by teenage girls may be related to the increased independence and role stress of women. The problems of cessation and prevention and the use of tobacco to control arousal and substitute for intimacy are discussed in detail in chapter 5.

PSYCHOPHYSIOLOGY OF HEART DISEASE

Several physiological processes are partly under behavioural control, and most of these are increased by sympathetic–adrenal activity. The term "overarousal" is used here to describe these changes, to distinguish internal response from environmental stress factors. "Overarousal" is an umbrella term for these diverse psychological states of anger, fear, and grief. This term was used by, for example, Eysenck and Grossarth-Maticek (1990) in reporting a Yugoslav study, which also found CHD prediction. Psychophysiological processes include:

- *Heart-rate rises*, to meet the energy demands of exertion or emotion. The S–A node has adrenergic inputs and parasympathetic input via the vagus nerve, and their relative influence determines the pulse rate.

- *Vasoconstriction,* which leads to increased peripheral resistance and hence higher blood pressure; this is commonly measured by the blood pressure at rest, but reactivity of blood pressure under emotional stress is emerging as a better measure (Matthews et al., 1986; Steptoe, 1990). Some "reactive" individuals seem to experience strong vasoconstrictive effects, with consequent surges in blood pressure.

- *Serum lipids,* notably cholesterol or low-density lipoproteins, are produced in increased quantities to maintain the muscular ATP supply; recent evidence (Muldoon, Manuck, & Matthews, 1990) suggests that lowering cholesterol by drugs does not reduce CHD risk, so research on lipids in relation to behaviour seems necessary.

- *Blood-clotting time,* often measured by serum fibrinogen or platelet levels, is thought to be another part of the fight/flight response, in preparation for wounds. Platelet activation was found by Patterson et al. (1994) to be increased by mental arithmetic stress and to some extent by watching films of surgery.

- *Electrical discharge* patterns may become deviant: Schwartz et al. (1991) provide evidence that the Q–T interval lengthens with adrenalin; fibrillation and tachycardia are arrhythmias that may arise in older people if the balance is wrong.

A great variety of behavioural events can have unhealthy cardiovascular consequences, across very short or very long time scales (Conduit, 1992). Human patients with a hereditary condition called long-QT syndrome are very vulnerable to fatal arrhythmias after relatively small emotional shocks, such as loud noise. They can be protected by drugs or surgical procedures that block sympathetic activity (Schwartz et al., 1991). At the other end of the time-scale is the lifelong process of atherogenesis. Manuck et al. (1983) demonstrated that macaque monkeys subject to dominance interruptions or threats of capture show increased atheroma, particularly if their heart rates are reactive to such stresses.

Most research has focused on the search for a "coronary-prone personality", either in terms of "Type-A behaviour pattern" or in terms of various aspects of hostility. The following review starts with "trait" influences, moves on to "states" associated with MI, and finishes with environmental demands; in the case of work pressures, overarousal might either be a trait or an environmental issue. A further ambiguity to be noted at this point is the possible role of other mediating risks, such as lower exercise tolerance in the socially isolated, or more smoking during bereavement.

The coronary-prone personality

Osler (1896) described the heart-attack victim as "a keen and ambitious man, the indicator of whose engine is always set at full speed ahead". Dunbar's (1947) profile studies of various diseases included the following stereotype of the coronary patient: "A consistently striving person of great control and persistence, aiming at success and accomplishment; a long-term planner; he is often distinguished-looking; he displays the capacity for subordinating actions to long-term goals".

Type-A behaviour pattern (TABP) has dominated research on traits associated with CHD risk, and a strong association between TABP and heart attacks was popularised by Friedman and Rosenman (1974) and Price (1982). The term comes from two cardiologists, Ray Rosenman and Meyer Friedman. A memorable phrase they have used for describing the person with TABP is that "he is engaged in a chronic struggle against time and other people". More usually, a list of traits is given, such as:

• time-urgency
• job involvement
• competitiveness
• hostility

The Western Collaborative Group Study (WCGS) in 1964 involved some 3,524 men aged between 39 and 59, who were located through employers in California and were therefore mainly white middle- and upper-level executives. Upon entry, about half were classified as Type A and half as the more relaxed Type B. After 8½ years of follow-up, 257 men had developed CHD; 178 had been initially categorised as Type A, and 79 as Type B. TABP was statistically independent of smoking, cholesterol, and other risks. Briefly, apparently healthy middle-aged Type As were more than twice as likely as Type Bs to develop CHD (Rosenman et al., 1964, 1975). Worse still, the mortality rate was higher following infarction in Type As, and the risk of subsequent infarction was also higher. They were assessed by Structured Interview (SI), as well as by serum and ECG tests. The SI asks questions about time-pressure, job-involvement, etc., but behavioural observations of non-verbal leakage are also included.

Type A replications. A number of major studies have attempted to replicate the findings of the WCGS. The Framingham Study (Haynes, Feinlieb, & Kannel, 1980) also followed men over 8 years and found Type As had at least 50% higher rates of CHD. A Belgian study (Kornitzer et al., 1981) also found predictive significance of TABP. However, the MRFIT study showed no increased risk associated with Type-A status over a 7-year follow-up (Shekelle et al., 1983). Major studies in Hawaii, Belgium, France, and elsewhere failed to find any predictive value of TABP. About half the well-controlled studies find TABP predicts CHD, while the other half fail to find any prediction. Studies using the SI have usually shown greater prediction than those using questionnaires, so it is worth examining the SI in greater detail. The Bortner analogue scale has lower predictive validity than does the Jenkins Activity Survey, and both are generally poorer than the SI.

The Structured Interview with a videotaped record (VSI) was described by Friedman and Powell (1984) and remains similar to that used in the WCGS. The interview is scored for free-floating hostility and time-urgency, and some pathophysiological indicators (pigmented eyelids and excessive sweating) are also scored. Overt answers to questions about time-urgency are sought, such as "Does your wife ever tell you to slow down?" The content of the answer is noted, but the interviewer is also trying to elicit psychomotor manifestations, including:

- rapid eye blinking
- knee jiggling
- facial tautness
- head nodding when interviewer speaks
- retraction of eyelid, showing cornea round pupil
- motorisation accompanying responses, e.g. mimes shaving

Questions used to elicit hostility include admiration and respect for doctors, by comparison with the attitudes of the respondent's father and mother. Signs of hostility concurrently monitored include:

- harsh voice quality
- use of swear-words
- taut set of face and jaw
- finger-tapping
- tendency to interrupt (the interviewer deliberately stammers at times to see whether the subject would interrupt)

Psychometric aspects of TABP. The concept of two types, A and B, has passed into psychology from medicine, and Friedman and Powell (1984) regards TABP as a "diagnosis". Yet elsewhere in psychology "personality types" have been found unreliable. Moreover, Meehl (1954) demonstrated that situational determinants of behaviour usually account for more variance in outcomes than traits, i.e. presumed stable behavioural dispositions of the individual. It might be useful to re-examine "time-urgency" to see how much was a situational reaction to work pressure (as CHD patients often assert), and how much a long-term disposition in the subjects. The SI classification is into four categories, including stronger and weaker versions called A1 and A2, thereby introducing range rather than type concepts. A more substantial problem with the A/B typology is that Type Bs are quite a rare breed. The postulation of a type conveys a stereotype of a group of males who are uniformly urgent, competitive, work-involved, and suppressing anger. In the WCGS study, 50% of subjects were identified as A and 50% as B, while in later studies the split has been nearer 75:25. In one study in the Pentagon, fewer than 10% were identified as Bs! The discriminative validity of the construct fades when most of the population has it.

Age and TABP. The significance of Type A for CHD appears to decline with age. The WCGS subjects were followed up at 22 years (Ragland & Brand, 1988), at which time the men were in their 60s and 70s. Among those who had died from CHD, the ratio of As to Bs was only 119:95 at that time. TABP seems to correlate with atheroma in younger subjects, at least according to the large and careful study of Williams et al. (1988). Type-A behaviour was found to predict angiographically documented coronary atherosclerosis in 2289 patients. Other studies involving subjects of all ages, such as Krantz et al. (1981), have failed to find a relationship between atheroma during angiography and TABP.

Reduction of Type A behaviour in healthy persons. Research on attempts to prevent CHD by psychological means is rather stymied by the current state of ignorance about the relation between TABP or hostility on the one hand, and physiological risk on the other. Ethel Roskies (1987; Roskies et al., 1979) was previously a strong advocate of stress management for healthy Type As. Her colleague Seraganian used resting pulse rate, oxygen uptake, and strength of voluntary muscles as outcome measures (Seraganian et al., 1987). Comparison groups engaged in aerobics or weight training. There were small non-significant trends in the desired direction with each type of training on each of the physiological measures, and the authors report the preventive effort as a failure. However, the selection of these physiological measures as the presumed risk correlates of TABP is not well established. The authors also took a reactivity measure in the form of a 25% increase over baseline in 3 out 5 measures during the initial assessment. The proportions of subjects who fell below reactivity criterion at post-testing for heart rate were 12% in the stress management group, compared with 4% and 6% in the aerobic and weight-training conditions. There were similar trends to reduction of reactivity of both diastolic and systolic BP in each training condition, but none of these trends reached significance.

Hostility

Cardiovascular changes with anger are very quick and strong, so it is not surprising that hostility emerges most frequently in CHD research (Chesney & Rosenman, 1985). Hostility is a very global concept and may include level of anger, its expression, and social distancing.

Re-analyses of TABP studies. Recent research has tended to confirm the clinical insight about "chronic struggle" in TABP but has diminished the importance of time urgency. Thoresen and Ohman (1987) have reported several re-analyses of the WCGS data to various end-points. The speech components (harsh voice quality, etc.) of TABP were found to be a negative predictor of CHD in studies at Duke University, perhaps supporting Julius and Harburg's construct of anger-out. Matthews et al. (1977) followed up a sub-sample of the WCGS who had experienced a heart attack and compared them with a matched sub-sample of healthy controls. Among these 186 men, seven items out of 44 significantly differentiated coronary from healthy subjects, and all seven items involved anger or hostility. Time urgency did not distinguish the two groups. Spielberger followed up the same data for an additional four years and confirmed the predictive validity of the anger–hostility items. Using principal components analysis, a single factor accounting for 65% of the variance was identified, and they dubbed this the anger–hostility factor. Items related to rapid psychomotor movement (e.g. eats rapidly), a high drive level, and job involvement were not predictive. Hecker et al. (1988) re-examined 250 CHD cases and 500 controls from the Western Collaborative Group Study. Of the 12 behavioural characteristics extracted from the Structured Interview (SI), only hostility remained as a component when all 12 were included in the model.

"*Cynicism*", as measured by the Cook-Medley scale of the MMPI, was the operational definition of hostility used by Barefoot, Dahlstrom, and Williams (1983). Items included

> "People make friends because friends are likely to be useful to them."

> "I have frequently worked under people who seem to have things arranged so that they get credit for good work, but are able to pass mistakes off onto those under them."

Medical students were classified into five score ranges on hostility/cynicism, and the 255 subjects were followed up over a 25-year period. By this time,

1.5% and 3% of the low-scoring doctors had had heart attacks, while 9% and 12% of the two highest-scoring categories had had heart attacks. A non-significant finding on the Ho scale was reported by Hearn, Murray, and Luepker (1989), who undertook a telephone follow-up of 1399 men for whom Cook-Medley Ho scores from 33 years previously were available. Subjects had completed the MMPI as freshmen at a mean age of 19 years and were traced through driving licences, university records, and other means; 6% could not be traced. Missing subjects are especially critical when death rate is an outcome, and ascertainment was not as precise as in Barefoot's study; the follow-up age in this sample is over 50, by which time many of the most vulnerable subjects had died. The incidence of CHD events (death and MI) for each Ho score band was:

Ho score mean	% of CHD events
8	3.6
14	4.2
20	5.0
28	3.7

"*Anger suppression*" was the form of hostility reported by Julius et al. (1986) with 696 Michigan subjects. Anger-coping was assessed by response to the hypothetical question, "Imagine that your (husband/wife/sweetheart) yelled in anger or blew up at you for something that wasn't your fault. What would you do?" A similar kind of hypothetical unjustified attack from a policeman was presented later. Five possible responses were grouped into two "anger-in" and three "anger-out" codes. Follow-up over 12 years found that those who reported suppressing anger at spouse were twice as likely to have died, while suppression of anger at a policeman increased risk by 1.24. There was an interaction with hypertension, which in this study meant systolic pressure over 140 mm—a very mild increase. Those mildly hypertensive subjects with high total anger suppression were five times more likely to die than were those who scored low on suppressed anger. By contrast, overt irritability and impatience was found to be associated with angina and MI in men of low socioeconomic status (Mendes de Leon, 1992).

Social isolation

This CHD predictor is probably connected with hostility. The person who is wary of others may not make sufficient use of social support when under stress, and is likely to remain aroused for a longer time. The protective value of extended families has been suggested as a reason for the relatively low rates of CHD in Mediterranean countries. Traditional Italian communities in the United States have low rates of MI, despite high fat consumption, smoking, and lack of exercise. Social factors may also be relevant in Japanese culture, since ethnically Japanese citizens in the United States seem to have more heart attacks than those living in Japan. Japanese culture and work relationships are discussed later.

Berkman (1984) devised a "Social Network Index" based on four types of social connection: marriage, contacts with extended family and close friends, church group affiliations, and other group affiliations. Questionnaires from 6,928 residents in a California county were collected in 1965, and 682 of these were retrieved when death certificates for respondents were identified. It was found that the relative risk of death for each decrease in social connection was 2.3 for men and 2.8 for women. When other risk factors were included in multivariate analyses, the relative risk reduced to about 2.0. Welin et al. (1985) reported on "lack of activity outside home": Cohorts born in 1913 and 1923, with few activities, were more than twice as likely to have CHD as those with several activities; such a trend might be mediated by hostile self-isolation or by absence of aerobic exercise.

Ruberman et al. (1984) used membership of clubs or religious organisations as criteria of social integration in a study of 2,320 male survivors of MI. Those who were judged to be socially isolated and to have high levels of stress had four times the death rate of those who were low in both. Social support has also been shown to be prognostic of recovery from MI (Ruberman et al., 1984). Medalie and Goldbourt (1976) undertook a prospective study of 10,000 Israeli men. Love and support by wives emerged as a preventive factor against the emergence of new angina pectoris, even in the presence of cholesterol and hypertension.

Phobic anxiety

Anxiety is not generally regarded as a risk for heart disease, though anxious people frequently misinterpret normal rises in heart rate with emotion as signs of illness. During the Romanian uprising in December 1989, cardiovascular referrals in the Cluj district increased significantly, but among these no increase in MI or angina rates was observed (Dumitrascu, Hopulele, & Baban, 1993). Phobic anxiety was reported as a predictor of CHD death by Haines, Imeson, and Meade (1987). A score of 5 or over on the Crown-Crisp Experiential Inventory increased the relative risk of a fatal MI by a factor of 4 in 1457 men in North-West London. This result is unusual, and the implication for sudden cardiac death are explored in chapter 9. Trait anxiety may contribute to CHD if excessive and prolonged, presumably because this implies higher average levels of catecholamines.

Bereavement

Grief is a very powerful emotion, associated with restless searching, sleep disturbance, loss of appetite, and increased levels of the stress hormones. Parkes, Benjamin, and Fitzgerald's (1969) study of London widows found a 1.4 times increased risk of MI in the first six months after loss of husband, and this finding was dubbed the "broken-heart" effect. Kraus and Lilienfield (1959) reported that mortality was at least seven times greater in bereaved men and women under the age of 45 than for control groups of married people. Males had a mortality rate 10 times greater, and most of these deaths were related to Coronary Heart Disease (CHD). Helsing, Szklo, and Comstock (1981) reported the same trend: Mortality of bereaved males was consistently greater than for bereaved females, but those who remarried lived longer than those who did not. Katsouyanni, Kogevinas, and Trichopoulos (1986) reported increased CHD in an account of earthquake victims. Bennet (1970) studied victims of the 1969 Bristol flood and demonstrated an increase in morbidity and a 50% increase in mortality in the subsequent year in those who had been flooded, compared with those whose homes had been spared.

Rees and Lutkins (1967) conducted a prospective study on 903 close relatives of 371 individuals who had recently died in the Aberfan disaster. A non-bereaved control group was formed using 878 close relatives of 371 individuals from the same community, matched for age, sex, and marital status. The mortality rate for the bereaved group was seven times that of the non-bereaved group during the first year of bereavement. Rates were also higher, but not significantly so, during the second and third years.

Vital exhaustion

Grief is one emotional state with strong adverse cardiovascular effects, but the experience of demoralisation and exhaustion seems to be similar. The term "vital exhaustion" has been provisionally attached to this state by Appels (1989), who sees it as related to but not identical with depression. The Maastricht vital exhaustion questionnaire was constructed by Appels, who undertook a prospective study of 3877 male Rotterdam civil servants aged between 39 and 65 in 1979–80. During the 4.2 years of follow-up, 59 had new cardiac events. The age-adjusted relative risk for myocardial infarction associated with five complaints during 4 years of follow-up is shown in Table 8.1.

No increased risk of cancer or duodenal ulcer in association with vital exhaustion was found, so this pattern is seen as specific to CHD. The predictive value is short-term, so vital exhaustion is seen as a transient state. Later research found that Type-A trait might lead to vital exhaustion, but the two

Table 8.1 Predictions from Maastricht questionnaire items

Complaint	Year of follow-up			
	1	2	3	4
Want to be dead	7.65 **	4.32 **	3.60 **	2.90 **
Not accomplishing much	4.53**	2.80**	1.89	1.37
Easily irritated	5.88**	1.90**	1.53	1.40
Strange bodily sensations	3.30**	1.04	0.91	1.04
Shrink from work	3.01**	1.49	1.39	1.33
Relative risk of above-median score on Maastricht Form B	10.05	2.23	3.04	0.68

** = statistical significance

were statistically independent. No statistical interaction between vital exhaustion and age, BP, cholesterol, or smoking was detected. The standardised regression coefficient for vital exhaustion was found to be 0.31, lower than that for cholesterol (0.36), but higher than that for systolic blood pressure (0.26). Coefficients for age (0.63) and smoking (0.54) accounted for most of the prediction, as in most MI research.

Social class and work

The Type A stereotype and Dunbar's profiles have tended to propagate a stereotype based on white-collar or executive occupations. WCGS subjects were employees of large corporations, and this sample and those of subsequent Type A studies tend to under-represent semi-skilled and unskilled manual workers.

There are strong connections between work activity and arousal. A comprehensive review by Kristensen (1989) found many studies supporting Karasek's strain model, and some influences from shift work, noise, and temperature extremes. Standardised mortality ratios (SMR) for 1979–83 show manual workers had an SMR of 1.4, while married women had 2.4 times the SMR of their counterparts whose husbands had white-collar occupations (Marmot & McDowell, 1986). While much of the CHD risk associated with lower social class may be attributed to higher rates of smoking and other biological factors, psychological risks also increase with lower social class.

Marmot also found that CHD rates in the Whitehall civil service were highest in lowest grades, such as messengers, and lower in professional and executive grades. Particular features of jobs such as "excessive demand", "low decision latitude", and "poor possibility of learning new things" have been described by reviewers such as Marmot and Kristensen, and further details are given in chapter 6.

Russek and Russek (1973, 1976) provide extensive evidence about the demand characteristics of various occupations, although much of it is, admittedly, retrospective. They surveyed CHD rates among 25,000 men in 20 occupations and ranked specialities within various occupations against the presumed stressfulness of those specialities; for example, the CHD prevalence among G.Ps. in medicine was reported as 11.9%, compared with 3.2% for dermatologists. In earlier studies they found that 91% of 100 patients with recent MIs had had excessive occupational demand compared to 20% of controls. "Demand" was defined as holding down two or more jobs, working more than 60 hours a week, or experiencing particular frustration in relation to employment. "Overwork" may be seen as a third state that sometimes precedes MI. In a survey by the present author of 50 consecutive MI admissions, a third of those in work had been exceeding Russek's 60–hour threshold, although most of the patients were not in work.

The low rate of CHD in Japan

Particularly interesting are attempts to identify what gave the Japanese such a low rate of MI—about 100 per 100,000, compared with 300 to 500 in most advanced countries in the Pooling Project. However, Hayano et al. (1989) report a doubling of the rate of CHD in Japan in the previous decade. Apart from a diet high in seafood (but also salt), an important predictor of CHD is adherence to Japanese culture: Americanised Japanese have similar rates of MI to Americans, while those who remain culturally Japanese in the United States have low rates of MI, according to Marmot (1987). Marmot et al. (1975) have attempted to separate cultural and dietary influences by comparing CHD rates in 11,900 Japanese citizens with various degrees of assimilation to American lifestyles. Ethnically Japanese men were classified as having definite or possible CHD. In Japan the rate was 25.4 per 1000, compared with 34.7 in Hawaii, and 44.6 in Japanese living in California. Although there were also differences in cholesterol and hypertension rates, the differences were not large enough to explain the difference in incidence rates. Traditional Japanese culture requires greater group conformity, politeness, and prolonged commitment to an employer than American or British culture, and it may be that group membership and rituals for reducing hostility are important factors in preventing CHD (Marmot, 1989). Hayano et al. (1989) surveyed TABP in 1682 Japanese male employees. When the occupational level was controlled, they found that the prevalence of global A on the Jenkins questionnaire was 40%—similar to that in the WCGS. Scores on the WCGS factor H (hard-driving and competitive) were considerably lower, and scores on WCGS factor J (job-involvement) were much lower. This suggests that "hard-working" is not necessarily "hard-driving" in Japan, and continuity of employment and promotion by seniority and cooperativeness, rather than individual achievement, still apply in Japanese public utilities.

Intimacy and gender

There is a strong but unexplained effect of gender on MI risk. Heart attacks are unusual in women during the reproductive years, and the lower life expectancy of men is largely attributable to the greater risk of MI. After the menopause or surgical removal of the ovaries, the rate of MIs in women rises considerably. Patients having heart attacks at age 75 are more likely to be female than male. The protective factor has been thought to be oestrogens, and hormone replacement therapy at the time of the female menopause is thought to extend protection against CHD risk into the 50s, though the evidence is inconclusive (Findlay, Cunningham, & Dargie, 1994).

Psychosocial predictors of MI in women have only been studied in the last few years. Of females entering Dutch hospitals with a first MI, 63% met the criterion for vital exhaustion in a study by Appels, Falger, and Schouten (1993), although 39% of the women in the control group with orthopaedic problems also scored above the median. Eighty-three women enrolled in the Recurrent Coronary Prevention Program (see chapter 9) were separately analysed by Powell et al. (1993). The six who had died were more likely to be divorced and to be employed without a college degree. The factors of exhaustion, anger, and isolation seem to be similar for men and women, while the patterns of lower social class and dual roles constitute a stronger risk in women. The reasons for masculinity increasing risk were studied by Helgeson (1991), who interviewed 99 post-MI males about social support and masculine attitudes before discharge. Lack of disclosure to spouse predicted worse outcomes on re-hospitalisation, chest pain, and perceived health. Masculine attitudes predicted more severe chest pain, but not the other two factors. The small amount of research on gender suggests that lack of intimacy and sustained work demands may be part of the risk associated with gender, as much as the absence of female hormones.

EXERCISE

The value of three types of exercise was discussed in chapter 6, and the greatest benefit appears to be derived from stamina-building exercise, which maintains circulation. Jobs that involve much walking or climbing stairs, such as delivering milk or letters, seem to develop stamina and reduce the risk of CHD. Aerobic fitness entails an increase in cardiac output, which, in turn, lowers the pulse rate and reactivity (the surge of BP in response to stress and exertion).

The hazards of unfitness associated with sedentary work were discussed in chapter 6, as was the protective value of strenuous work among San Francisco dockers reported by Paffenberger. A correlation between level of fitness and risk of heart disease has been shown many times, and the argument for exercise as an independent risk factor is made by Sandvik et al. (1993). They report on physical fitness as a predictor of mortality among healthy, middle-aged Norwegian men: Through employers, 2,014 apparently healthy men were recruited, and the results of bicycle ergometer tests led to them being classified into four fitness quartiles. Over an average 16-year follow-up, 271 men had died, about half of them from CHD. The relative risk of death from any cause in the fittest quartile was 0.54 of that in the least fit quartile. The adjusted relative risk of death from cardiovascular causes in Quartile 4 in relation to the least fit quartile 1 was 0.41. The relative risk in Quartile 3 was 0.45, and in Quartile 2 in relation to Quartile 1 it was 0.59. The evidence that fitness is a graded long-term predictor of CHD mortality is therefore strong, although confounding variables that could account for risk include age, smoking, work stress, and lower social class. The mean age in Quartile 1 was 6 years older than in Quartile 4, and Quartile 1 had a higher proportion of smokers. Sandvik's risk ratios corrected for these factors, and also for systolic blood pressure, BMI, and several other biological risks. However, psychosocial risks were not assessed, so there may still be confounding factors such as isolation or overwork.

The leisure-activity levels and health of Harvard graduates has been monitored over many years by Paffenberger et al. (1986, 1993). A physical activity index was calculated from the energy used each week in stair-climbing, walking, and light and vigorous sports. Men with an index of over 2,000 kcal per week had 39% fewer MIs than those below 2,000. Among 50,000 former university students, men who had completed questionnaires between 1962 and 1966 and again in 1977 were classified according to changes in lifestyle in that interval. Beginning a moderately vigorous sports activity (at an intensity of 4.5 or more metabolic equivalents) was associated with a 23% lower risk of death; quitting smoking was associated with 41% lower risk than continuing smoking; blood pressure and BMI also affected risk. Evidence for either unfitness and emotional stress in the CHD risk of bus drivers has been offered by Morris and Netterstrom (see chapter 6). While the mediating variables are unclear, there is little doubt that an exercise habit contributes to the maintenance of circulation.

RISKS AND CAUSES

A great variety of "risk factors" have emerged in epidemiological studies of CHD. These include caffeine and salt consumption, body mass index (a measure of obesity), lack of exercise, soft drinking water, and up to 200 others. The central problem of epidemiological research is that it shows only correlations, not causes, and many factors that emerge from regression equations may be artefacts of something else. Caffeine was at one time identified as a substantial risk, but on re-analysis the correlation with tobacco consumption was identified. Caffeine is probably a minor risk factor, through its small effect on BP. Debate continues about salt, which appears to increase BP in susceptible subjects. Numerous artefacts emerge in dietary research, as regression coefficients may arise through quite spurious associations. Risk reduction has been reported in association with alcohol or milk consumption, which probably reflect relaxed aspects of lifestyle.

The reliance on epidemiological associations makes it difficult to evaluate true causes. The diagram presented in Figure 8.3 goes beyond the evidence but allows a mass of diverse research to be integrated along two main pathological routes: atherogenesis and thrombogenesis. It differs somewhat from recent medical schemata in that it gives the psychosocial factors a more central position.

PRIMARY PREVENTION

The ideal preventive situation would be for all citizens to practise the main health behaviours regularly, and considerable energy is expended by health promotion agencies towards this end. Primary prevention may take the form of mass communication through TV announcements or posters. A middle road is the "well-woman" (or -man) method, using literature, health checks, and advice in health centres. The most interventionist approach is to identify subjects in fair health, but at risk, and to engage them in face-to-face preventive dialogue.

Evaluation of such efforts remains difficult, since health promotion is the hardest area in which to evaluate the effects of intervention. The province of Karelia in Finland was the target of a major health-promotion campaign because of its extremely high rate of CHD. The inhabitants of this part of

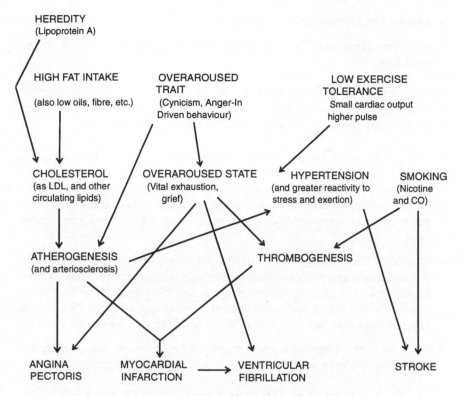

Figure 8.3 Some connections between risk factors and cardiac events

Finland made substantial changes in their diet and smoking rates, but residents of neighbouring provinces also made changes when they heard of the special campaign in Karelia. There were also population movements into urban areas and a partial return to rural areas. It is difficult to infer what impact changes in lifestyle had on CHD rates in Finland.

The Multiple Risk Factor Intervention Trial

The Multiple Risk Factor Intervention Trial Group (1982) carried out a CHD prevention programme at 28 medical centres across the United States. Out of 361,662 men examined, 12,866 were selected as being at high risk on three factors, but they were young and thus in a preventable category. At the outset, the factors were assessed as follows:

- 66% smoked cigarettes

- 66% had had hypertension early in life

- 60% were obese, and their diet contained twice the recommended cholesterol level

The subjects were randomly divided into "usual care" and "special intervention" groups. The "special intervention" group attended 10 group sessions, held at weekly intervals. They received the following programme:

- *Diet:* They were taught low-cholesterol purchasing and cooking, recorded diets, signed contracts to restrict particular foods, and were given reinforcement for achievement of dietary goals. They achieved a 42% cut in cholesterol, a 28% cut in saturated fat intake, and a 21% cut in total calories; serum cholesterol dropped by 5%–6.7% (two assay methods).

- *Smoking:* They were given health lectures from physicians; success stories from quitters; monetary rewards for savings on cigarette purchase; stimulus control—e.g. placing cigarettes in inaccessible places. After four years, half of the smokers remained abstinent, exceeding the target; 75% of light smokers had quit, but only 33% of those smoking two packs had done so.

- *Blood pressure:* They were given regular BP monitoring and prescription of antihypertensive drugs according to a stepped-care regime.

The study reported that 87% moved below the moderate hypertension threshold, and 66% achieved a specific BP goal in the normal range. Antihypertension medication had caused cholesterol to rise by 7%.

The results of this study were tallied in 1982, after nine years. The cause of any deaths was judged by three cardiologists with no knowledge of the subjects. Surprisingly, the "usual care" group had also improved, with 40% fewer deaths than expected statistically: Their serum cholesterol had declined by nearly 5%, despite minimal dietary changes; 20% had quit smoking on their own initiative, and typical BP was only 4% higher. There was no significant difference in deaths between the "usual care" and "special intervention" groups (Shekelle et al., 1985).

The MRFIT intervention was an ambitious attempt to identify effective means of heart disease prevention, but unfortunately it did not resolve many questions. Why were the "usual care" group so much healthier than expected? Were they "regressing to the mean" in risk terms? Were the risk factors identified for special intervention the wrong ones? Or were the effects of minimal treatment and the cessation of smoking by 3 out of 10 enough? Many problems remain unresolved, but the weight of evidence in this chapter allows conclusions to be drawn about eating habits, arousal, and activity.

CONCLUSION

The maintenance of circulatory health is likely to involve the following life-style skills. Eating habits over the majority of the life-span will need to emphasise a high proportion of vegetables, and fats should form a small proportion (perhaps 20%–30%) of total calories. The ability to achieve emotional intimacy with a partner and to obtain social support in general are important during grief and other protracted emotional demands. Pacing of work, both paid and domestic, needs to ensure that leisure and relaxation can be experienced and arousal kept at moderate levels. Such abilities will avoid the need to use tobacco to achieve well-being and reduce the risk of reaching a state of exhaustion. The use of tobacco is greatly detrimental to cardiovascular health, while alcohol is harmful in excess, but mildly beneficial in moderation. An exercise habit will contribute to pacing and moderation of arousal. Exercise tolerance also improves cardiovascular response to peak arousal and helps with weight control.

REFERENCES

Appels, A. (1989). Loss of control, vital exhaustion, and coronary heart disease. In A. Steptoe & A. Appels (Eds.), *Stress, personal control, and health*. Chichester: John Wiley.

Appels, A., Falger, P., & Schouten, E. (1993). Vital exhaustion as a risk indicator for myocardial infarction in women. *Journal of Psychosomatic Research, 37* (8), 881–890.

Barefoot, J.C, Dahlstrom, G., & Williams, R.B. (1983). Hostility, CHD incidence, and total mortality: A 25-year follow-up of 255 physicians. *Psychosomatic Medicine, 45,* 59–63.

Bennet, G. (1970). Bristol floods 1968: Controlled survey of effects on health of local community disaster. *British Medical Journal, 3,* 454–458.

Berkman, L.F. (1984). Assessing the physical health effects of social networks and social support. *Annual Review of Public Health, 5,* 413–32.

Byrne, D.G. (1987). *The behavioral management of the cardiac patient*. Hove: Lawrence Erlbaum Associates Ltd.

Carruthers, M.E. (1969). Aggression and atheroma. *The Lancet, 2,* 1170–1171.

Chesney, A., & Rosenman, R.H. (1985). *Anger and hostility in cardiovascular and behavioral disorders*. New York: Hemisphere.

Conduit, E. (1992). If A–B does not predict heart disease, why bother with it? *British Journal of Medical Psychology, 65,* 289–296.

Doyle, J.T., & Kannel, W.B. (1970). Results of the National Pooling Project. *Circulation, 42.* Cited in D.G. Byrne, *The behavioral management of the cardiac patient*. Hove: Lawrence Erlbaum Associates Ltd, 1987.

Dumitrascu, D., Hopulele, S., & Baban, A. (1993). *Medicine and War, 9* (1), 45–51.

Dunbar, F. (1947). *Mind and body: Psychosomatic medicine*. New York: Random House.

Eysenck, H., & Grossarth-Maticek, R. (1990). Personality, stress, and disease: Description and validation of a new inventory. *Psychological Reports, 66,* 355–373.

Findlay, I., Cunningham, D., & Dargie, H. (1994). Coronary heart disease, the menopause, and hormone replacement therapy (Editorial). *British Heart Journal, 71,* 213–214.

Friedman, M., & Powell, L.H. (1994). The diagnosis and quantitative assessment of type A behaviour: Introduction and description of the videotaped structured interview. *Integrative Psychiatry, 2,* 123–136.

Friedman, M., Powell, L, Price, V., & Dixon, T. (1984). Alteration of type A behaviour and reduction in cardiac recurrence in post myocardial infarction patients. *American Heart Journal, 108* (2), 237–248.

Friedman, M., & Rosenman, R. (1974). *Type A behaviour and your heart.* New York: Knopf.

Gentry, W.D., Chesney, M.A., Gary, H., Hall, R., & Harburg, E. (1982). Habitual anger-coping styles: I. Effect on mean blood pressure and risk for essential hypertension. *Psychosomatic Medicine, 44,* 195–202.

Haines, A.P., Imeson, J.D., & Meade, T.W. (1987). Phobic anxiety and ischaemic heart disease. *British Medical Journal, 295* (1), 297–299.

Hart, J.T. (1980). *Hypertension.* London: Churchill Livingstone.

Haynes, S.G., Feinlieb, & Kannel, W.B. (1980). The relationship of psychosocial factors to coronary heart disease of the Framingham study: III. Eight-year incidence of coronary heart disease. *American Journal of Epidemiology, 111,* 37–58.

HPAW (1990). *Health for all in Wales.* Cardiff: Health Promotion Authority for Wales.

Hayano, J., Takeuchi, S., Yoshida, S., Jozuka, H., Mishima, N., & Fujinami, T. (1989). Type A behaviour pattern in Japanese employees: Cross-cultural comparison of major factors in Jenkins Activity Survey (JAS) responses. *Journal of Behavioral Medicine, 12* (3), 219–231.

Hearn, M.D., Murray, D.M., & Luepker, R.V. (1989). Hostility, coronary heart disease, and total mortality: A 33-year follow-up study of university students. *Journal of Behavioral Medicine, 12* (2), 105–121.

Hecker, M., Chesney, M., Black, G., & Frautschi, N. (1988). Coronary-prone behaviours in the Western collaborative group study. *Psychosomatic Medicine, 50,* 153–164.

Helgeson, V. (1991). The effects of masculinity and social support on recovery from myocardial infarction. *Psychosomatic Medicine, 53,* 621–633.

Helsing, K.J., Szklo, M., & Comstock, G. (1981). Factors associated with mortality after widowhood. *American Journal of Public health, 71,* 802–809.

Julius, M., Harburg, E., Cottington, E., & Johnson, E., (1986). Anger-coping types. Blood pressure and all-cause mortality: A follow-up in Tecumseh, Michigan. *American Journal of Epidemiology, 124 ,* 220–233.

Katsouyanni, K., Kogevinas, K., & Trichopoulos, D. (1986). Earthquake-related stress and cardiac mortality. *International Journal of Epidemiology, 15,* 326–330.

Keys, A., Taylor, H.L., et al. (1971). Mortality and coronary heart disease among men studied for 23 years. *Archives Internal Medicine, 128,* 201–214. Cited in K.

Matthews, S. Weiss, T. Detre, T. Dembrowski, B. Falkner, S. Manuck, & R. Williams, *Handbook of stress, reactivity, and cardiovascular disease*. London: Wiley, 1986.

Kornitzer, M., Kittel, F., De Backer, G., & Dramaix, M. (1981). The Belgian heart disease prevention project: Type A behavior pattern and the prevalence of coronary heart disease. *Psychosomatic Medicine, 43*, 133–145.

Krantz, D.S., Davia, J.E., Dembroski, T.M., MacDougall, J.M, Schaffer, R.T., Schaeffer, M.A. (1981). Extent of coronary atherosclerosis: Type A behaviour and cardiovascular response to social interaction. *Psychophysiology, 18*, 654–64.

Kraus, A.S., & Lilienfield, A.M. (1959). Some epidemiological aspects of high mortality rate in the young widowed group. *Journal of Chronic Disease, 10*, 207–217.

Kumar, P.J., & Clark, M.L. (1990). *Clinical medicine* (2nd ed.). London: Bailliere Tindall.

Kristensen, T. (1989). Cardiovascular diseases and the work environment. *Scandinavian Journal of Work and Environmental Health, 15*, 166–179, and 245–264.

Lawn, R.M. (1992). Lipoprotein(a) in heart disease. *Scientific American, 266* (6), 26–33.

Leeder, S.R., Dobson, A.J., Gibberd, R.W., & Flynn, S.J. (1983). Attack and case fatality rates for acute myocardial infarction in the Hunter region of New South Wales, Australia in 1979. *American Journal of Epidemiology, 118*, 42–51.

Manuck, S.B., Kaplan, J.R., & Clarkson, T.B. (1983). Behaviorally-induced heart-rate reactivity and atherosclerosis in cynomolgus monkeys. *Psychosomatic Medicine, 45*, 95–108.

Marmot, M.G., Syme, S.L, Kagan, A., Kato, H., Cohen, J., & Belsky, J. (1975). Epidemiologic studies of coronary heart disease and stroke in Japanese men living in Japan, Hawaii and California. *American Journal of Epidemiology, 102* (6), 514–525.

Marmot, M.G., & McDowell, M.E. (1986). Mortality decline and widening social inequalities. *The Lancet, 2*, 274–276.

Marmot, M.G. (1987). Look after your heart: Stress and cardiovascular disease—a studiable case? *Health Trends, 19* (August).

Marmot, M.G. (1989). General approaches to migrant studies: The relation between disease, social class, and ethnic origin. In Cruickshank, J.K, & Beevers, D.G. (Eds.), *Ethnic factors in health and disease*. London: Butterworth.

Matthews, K.A., Glass, D.C., Rosenman, R.H., & Bortner, R.W. (1977). Competitive drive, pattern A, and coronary heart disease: A further analysis of some data from the Western Collaborative Group Study. *Journal of Chronic Diseases, 30*, 489–498.

Matthews, K.A., Weiss, S., Detre, T., Dembrowski, T., Falkner, B. Manuck, S., & Williams, R. (1986). *Handbook of stress, reactivity, and cardiovascular disease*. London: Wiley.

Medalie, J.H., & Goldbourt, U. (1976). Angina pectoris among 10,000 men. *American Journal of Medicine, 60*, 910–921.

Meehl, P. (1954). *Clinical versus statistical prediction*. Minneapolis, MN: University of Minnesota Press.

Mendes de Leon, C.F. (1992). Anger and impatience/irritability in patients of low socioeconomic status with acute heart disease. *Journal of Behavioral Medicine, 15* (3), 273–284.

Minuchin, S. (1977). *Families and family therapy*. London: Tavistock.

Muldoon M.F., Manuck S.B., & Matthews K.A. (1990). Lowering cholesterol concentrations and mortality: A quantitative review of primary prevention trials. *British Medical Journal, 301* (6747), 309–314.

Osler, W. (1896). Lectures on angina pectoris and allied states. *New York Journal of Medicine, 4*, 224.

Paffenberger, R.S., Jr, Hyde, R.T., Wing, A.L., & Misch, C. (1986). Physical activity, all-cause mortality, and longevity of college alumni. *New England Journal of Medicine, 314* (10), 605–613.

Paffenberger, R.S., Jr, Hyde, R.T., Wing, A.L., Lee, I-M., Dexter, L.J., & Kaampert, J.B. (1993). The association of changes in physical-activity level and other lifestyle characteristics with mortality among men. *New England Journal of Medicine, 328* (8), 538–540.

Parkes, C.M., Benjamin, B., & Fitzgerald, R.G. (1969). Broken heart: A statistical study of increased mortality among widowers. *British Medical Journal, i*, 740–743.

Patterson, S.M., Zakowksi, S.G., Hall, M.H., Cohen, L., Wollman, K., & Baum, A. (1994). Psychological stress and platelet activation: Differences in platelet reactivity in healthy men during active and passive stressors. *Health Psychology, 13* (1), 34–38.

Powell, L., Shaker, L., Jones, B., Vaccarino, L., Thoresen, C., & Pattillo, J. (1993). Psychosocial predictors of mortality in 83 women with premature acute myocardial infarction. *Psychosomatic Medicine, 55*, 426–433.

Price, V.A. (1982). *Type A behaviour pattern*. New York: Academic Press.

Ragland, D.R., & Brand, R.J. (1988). Type A behaviour and mortality from coronary heart disease. *New England Journal of Medicine, 318*, 65–69.

Rees, W.D., & Lutkins, S.G. (1967). Mortality of bereavement. *British Medical Journal, 4*, 13–16.

Rofé, Y., & Goldberg, J. (1983). Prolonged exposure to a war environment and its effects on the blood pressure of pregnant women. *British Journal of Medical Psychology, 56* (4), 305–312.

Rosenman, R.H., Brand, R., Jenkins, C., Friedman, M., Strauss, R., & Wurm, M. (1975). Coronary heart disease in the Western Collaborative Group study: Final follow-up experience of eight and a half years. *Journal of the American Medical Association, 233*, 872–877.

Rosenman, R.H., Friedman, M., Straus, R., Wurm, M., Kositchek, R., Hahn, W., & Werthessen, N. (1964). A predictive study of coronary heart disease. The Western Collaborative Group Study. *Journal of the American Medical Association, 189* (1), 103–110.

Roskies, E. (1987). *Stress management for the healthy Type A: Theory and practice*. New York: Guilford.

Roskies, E., Kearney, H., Spevack, M., Surkis, A., Cohen, C., & Gilman, S. (1979). Generalizability and duration of treatment effects in an intervention program for coronary prone (type A) managers. *Journal of Behavioral Medicine, 2,* 195–207.

Ruberman, W., Weinblatt, E., Goldberg, J., & Chaudhary, B. (1984). Psychosocial influences on mortality after myocardial infarction. *New England Journal of Medicine, 311,* 552–559.

Russek, H.I. (1973). Emotional stress as a cause of cardiovascular heart disease. *Journal of the American College Health Association, 22* (2), 120–123.

Russek, H.I., & Russek, M.A. (1976). Is emotional stress an etiologic factor in coronary heart disease? *Psychosomatics, 17* (2).

Sandvik, l., Erikssen, J., Thaulow, E., Erikssen, G., Mundal, R., & Rodahl, K., (1993). Physical fitness as a predictor of mortality among healthy, middle-aged Norwegian men. *New England Journal of Medicine, 328* (8), 533–537.

Schwartz, P.J., Zaza, A., Locati, E., & Moss, A.J. (1991). Stress and sudden death. The case of the long QT syndrome. *Circulation, 83* (4. Suppl.), 1171–1180.

Seraganian, P., Roskies, E., Hanley, J., Oseasohn, R., & Collu, R. (1987). Failure to alter psychophysiological reactivity in Type A men with physical exercise or stress management programs. *Psychology and Health, 1* (3), 195–213.

Shekelle, R.B., Gayle, M., Ostfeld, A.M., & Paul, O. (1983). Hostility, risk of coronary heart disease, and mortality. *Psychosomatic Medicine, 45,* 109–114.

Shekelle, R.B., Hulley, S.B., Neaton, J., Billings, J., Borhani, N., Gerace, T., Jacobs, D., Lasser, N., Mittlemark, M., & Stamler, J. (1985). The MRFIT behaviour pattern study, II: Type A behaviour and incidence of coronary heart disease. *American Journal of Epidemiology, 122* (4), 559–570.

Siegman, A.W., & Dembroski, T.M. (1988). *In search of coronary-prone behaviour: Beyond Type A.* Hove: Lawrence Erlbaum Associates Ltd.

Spielberger, C.D., Johnson, E.H., Russell, S.F., Crane, R.J., Jacobs, G.A., & Worden, T.J. (1985). The experience and expression of anger: Construction and validation of an anger expression scale. In A. Chesney, & R.H. Rosenman (Eds.), *Anger and hostility in cardiovascular and behavioral disorders.* New York: Hemisphere, 1985.

Steptoe, A. (1990). The value of mental stress testing in cardiovascular disorders. In L.R. Schmidt, P. Schwenkmezger, J. Weinman, & S. Maes, *Theoretical and applied aspects of health psychology.* London: Harwood.

Taggart, P., & Carruthers, M. (1971). Endogenous hyperlipidaemia induced by emotional stress of racing driving. *Lancet, i,* 363.

Thoresen, C.A., & Ohman, A.(1987). The Type A Behaviour Pattern: A person-environment interaction perspective. In D. Magnusson & A. Ohman (Eds.), *Psychopathology: An interaction perspective.* New York: Academic Press.

Truswell, A. Stewart (1986). *ABC of nutrition.* London: British Medical Association.

Welin, L., Tibblin, G., Svardsudd, K., Tibblin, B., Ander-Perciva, S., & Larsson, B. (1985). Prospective study of social influences on mortality. The study of men born in 1913 and 1923. *The Lancet, 8434,* 915–918.

Williams, R.B., Barefoot, J.C., Haney, T., Harrell, F. Jr., Blumenthal, J., Pryor, D., & Peterson, B. (1988). Type A behaviour and angiographically-documented coronary atherosclerosis in 2289 patients. *Psychosomatic Medicine, 50* (2), 139–142.

9

Circulation: After Illness

In chapter 8 we saw that circulation is maintained by lifestyle factors. Some degree of arterial reduction is inevitable with ageing, and heart disease becomes increasingly common in the second half of life. In this chapter we examine the extent to which the progression of ischaemia can be slowed down and the risk of recurrence of major cardiac events reduced. The issues of diet, arousal, and so forth remain the same after a heart attack or a stroke, but the relative importance of preventive strategies may change, in at least two ways. Risk of a major cardiac event is not strongly correlated with the degree of ischaemia, so prevention of overarousal may become more important than reduction of atherogenic processes. As arterial obstruction progresses, lifestyle changes may not be sufficient to achieve a return to full health, so adherence to medical strategies becomes an issue.

HYPERTENSION REDUCTION

High blood pressure is an asymptomatic physiological state warranting treatment to prevent a variety of hazards, including stroke and infarct. Comprehensive reviews from a medical standpoint are provided by Hart (1980), and from a psychological standpoint by Blanchard, Martin, and Dubbert (1988). Some conventions are used in the following section, which will be described briefly. Blood pressure is usually measured by the force the artery in one arm can exert against a pressure cuff, although a cannula inserted into the artery may give a more accurate measure. The peak pressure is at systole and is referred to as systolic; the diastolic pressure occurs between heartbeats. Only diastolic figures are quoted in the following research to simplify data, and because this figure appears more frequently as a prognostic sign. Pressures are given as the height in millimetres of a mercury column (mm Hg). Many factors elevate blood pressure, including previous activity, full bladder, the "white coat" effect, startle as the cuff tightens, choice of arm, and others. Reactivity to demand may be a more useful measure, but BP at rest is taken as the standard.

Physiology

Elevated blood pressure increases the risk not only of heart attack, but also of stroke, kidney damage, retinal bleeding, and several other serious illnesses. It is also highly prevalent: Using the cut-off of 140/90, about 50% of people over the age of 55 years have hypertension. Dietary restriction, stress management, and increased exercise tolerance can all contribute to hypertension reduction, although the effect of each of these alone is generally smaller than that achieved by pharmacological means. Blood pressure is a function of cardiac output and peripheral vascular resistance, and lifestyle changes affect one or both of these elements. Stress management can lower vascular resistance by reducing sympathetic input, restriction of fat intake can lower resistance by reducing atheroma, and exercise can both increase cardiac output and reduce resistance of blood vessels in muscle. However, the most powerful influence on blood pressure is the fluid electrolyte balance achieved by the kidneys (Blanchard et al., 1988). Normally the kidneys can reduce BP by excreting water from the circulatory system, and this is the principal mechanism for maintaining BP homeostasis. Although this homeostatic mechanism is extremely efficient, the level of stasis can be reset at a higher level by excessive sodium ions or by insulin distortions associated with being overweight, and does not spontaneously reset to a lower level.

Relaxation

The research on controlled anger might suggest that instrumental strategies such as assertion training would reduce hypertension, but there is virtually no literature on this. Research on behavioural management of hypertension in the United Kingdom has been pioneered by Chandra Patel and colleagues at University College London, using simple relaxation. An early report (Patel, Marmot, & Terry, 1981) described the effects of relaxation in 204 employees of a large factory. Subjects were randomly assigned to relaxation assisted by biofeedback or to a control group, and both received a 10-minute talk and health-education literature on smoking and diet. Eight weeks later, the relaxation group had achieved a 7.2-mm reduction in diastolic BP, compared with 1.4 mm in the controls; at eight months, the reductions were 6.8 and 0.63 mm. In this study the plasma levels of renin and aldosterone, which are partly controlled by the ANS, were measured as well: These had fallen significantly more in the relaxation group at eight weeks, but the difference was non-significant at eight months.

A 4-year follow-up (Patel, Marmot, & Terry, 1985; Patel & Marmot, 1987) showed that relaxation and stress-management training was associated with a sustained reduction in blood pressure. Quality of life had improved in that significantly more subjects in the relaxation group reported improved relationships at work, general health, enjoyment of life, and personal and family relationships than those in the control group. There was no consistent relationship between the degree of reduction in BP and improvement in quality of life, but those who practised relaxation regularly, who integrated relaxation in everyday activities, and who used cognitive reappraisal as part of their stress-management strategies showed greater reduction in BP than did those who did not. Patel and Marmot (1988) report evidence that general practitioners can use training in relaxation and management of stress to reduce mild hypertension.

Van Montfrans et al. (1990) give a more sceptical account of a similar method with patients at Amsterdam University medical centre, where 35 subjects with initial diastolic BP between 95 and 110 were given muscle relaxation, yoga, and stress management, or attended with the instruction to "sit and relax twice a day". The novel feature of this study was the use of intra-arterial ambulatory measurement of BP via a cannula. No overall reduction had taken place in either group during the daytime and evening at one year follow-up. However, a night-time reduction of about 5 mm in the diastolic was evident in both groups. These medical practitioners conclude that "relaxation therapy was an ineffective method of lowering 24-hour blood pressure, being no more beneficial than non-specific advice, support, and reassurance—themselves ineffective as a treatment for hypertension".

Johnston (1989) reviewed 25 randomised controlled studies of stress management and hypertension and concluded that in the clinic the average reduction in systolic BP is about 9 mm, and in diastolic BP 6 mm. Generalisation to the outside was measured in fewer studies, and the reductions in these were estimated as 6 mm and 4.5 mm, respectively. Controls who did not receive stress management experienced an average reduction of about 2 mm, which is probably the effect of habituation of the startle response when the sphygmomanometer cuff is inflated. There are substantial individual differences in uptake of stress management, so appropriate selection is important. Steptoe (1990) reports on mental stress testing in the investigation of cardiovascular disorders, and reactivity to noise or other stresses is one indicator. Vinck (1990) attempted to select "good" candidates for relaxation training. Regression equations for increase or decrease in BP were made using sex, extroversion, and neuroticism, reactivity on a Stroop task, and reactivity within sessions as variables. Belief about causes of hypertension (stress or disease) and the ability to perceive one's BP were predictors of the response to training, in mildly hypertensive subjects.

Dietary control

The most important dietary remedies for hypertension are weight loss, sodium restriction, and reduction of excess alcohol. Moderate intake of alcohol has little effect on blood pressure, but intakes above 20 units a week are associated with a progressive rise in BP.

The association between being overweight and having raised blood pressure is well documented, though imperfectly understood. On average, a reduction of 1 mm Hg in diastolic BP is achieved for each kilogram of weight loss. Behavioural programmes for calorie restriction are the preferred method, as described in greater detail in chapter 11. Appetite suppressants such as fenfluramine are also sometimes prescribed, but they are only effective while the drug is being taken. Stunkard, Wilcoxon-Craighead, and O'Brien (1980) compared the two methods in a population of 57 hypertensives. After six months, patients receiving only behaviour therapy had lost 10.9 kg, those having appetite suppression had lost 14.5 kg, and those receiving both had lost 15.3 kg. However, the patients who had received pharmacotherapy or the combined approach regained most of their weight (8.2 and 10.7 kg) over the follow-up year, while those who had had behaviour therapy gained only 1.9 kg.

The evidence that sodium intake contributes to hypertension is mainly from cross-national comparisons. Sodium is found in salt used in bread and cooking, as well as in baking soda and monosodium glutamate. In Western Europe the daily intake is equivalent to about 10 grams of salt, which is ten times the dietary requirement; low-salt societies, on the other hand, have low levels of hypertension. There are few good studies in which sodium is the only restricted food, but available data suggest that a minority of hypertensives (30%–50%) will benefit from sodium restriction but the others will be unaffected. Reisin et al. (1978) in Israel were able to compare the relative influence of weight loss and salt intake with 81 obese hypertensives. Patients were told to restrict their diets to an average of 1000 calories, but they were encouraged to eat pickled vegetables and other low-calorie salty foods and to drink at least 2½ litres of water a day. Over two months, the diastolic BP dropped on average 20 mm despite the salt, contingent on an average weight loss of 9 kg. Heavy alcohol use is an important contributor to hypertension, especially where used to reduce arousal after work in occupations such as air traffic control.

Exercise

The difficulty of separating aerobic exercise from obesity, salt intake, etc. for research on hypertension is considerable. Blanchard et al. (1988) found only six studies that achieved waiting-list control, and none of these included comparisons with alternative treatments of attention placebo. The mean decrement in diastolic BP for the 65 hypertensives was 6 mm. Another study of 56 males at the Cooper Institute for aerobics research allowed separate evaluation of the effects of catecholamines on hypertension. Those with elevated plasma catecholamines achieved a mean reduction of 8.1 mm by exercise, compared with 6.4 mm for the normoadrenergic, and an increase of 2.9 mm for the controls receiving BP checks only. The effect of exercise was estimated as between 5 and 15 mm on diastolic BP, with lesser and variable effects on systolic BP.

Drug adherence

Apart from prevalence and seriousness, the other salient fact about hypertension is the extremely low level of adherence to effective antihypertensive strategies as mentioned in chapter 1. It is fairly easy to see why this would be so by considering the four elements of the Health Belief Model. Hypertension is usually symptom-free, with only the remote threat of disease, and as a result perceived susceptibility is often low. No immediate benefits are apparent, but immediate barriers are. Drug treatment may involve increased urination, sexual impotence, and various other unpleasant effects. Yet the benefits of antihypertensive therapy are well established. The Veterans Administration Cooperative Study Group (1967) gave the first strong evidence that antihypertensive agents prevent premature death. In the study, 143 males with severe hypertension were randomised to placebo or a combination of hydrochlothiazide, reserpine, and hydralazine. The treated group experienced a drop in diastolic pressure of 43 mm, while the placebo group remained unchanged. In the placebo group four had died, ten were removed following serious illness, and seven were removed because of continuing increase of BP, while only one treated patient was removed. The trial was discontinued after 2 years on ethical grounds, as the morbidity was significantly worse in the untreated group. Good communication with physicians is essential for hypertension control. Inui, Yourtee, and Williamson (1976) assigned two groups of physicians to tutorials and strategies based on HBM. After only one session, these doctors increased their amount of teaching time, and patients were observed to increase their knowledge about hypertension, which later turned into better adherence.

The great difficulty in persuading hypertensives to take their condition seriously was described in chapter 1 and has been addressed as a "marketing" issue by Ward (1984). The National High Blood Pressure Education Program in the United States was analysed using the four Ps of marketing: Product, Price, Promotion, and Place. A process of "market segmentation" was used to identify key change agents for future blood pressure education, and demonstration projects were set up in schools and workplaces. The following changes in public awareness between 1973 and 1979 were reported:

- 16% more people knew that hypertension is a very serious disease

- 33% more people knew that high blood pressure and hypertension mean the same thing

- 19% more people knew that hypertension can cause strokes

- 66% more people knew that normal BP is less than 140/90

- 27% fewer hypertensives had trouble getting life insurance

- 43% fewer hypertensives missed work due to high blood pressure

- 83% of the public had had BP checked within a year, compared with 78% in 1973

- 82% of hypertensives still took the prescribed medication, compared with 77% in 1973

High blood pressure continues to be major source of morbidity in Britain and other European countries, and preventive approaches need continuous improvement.

CHOLESTEROL REDUCTION

Cholesterol—or, more generally, the level of circulating lipids—has a strong loading on CHD risk in most epidemiological research. Reduction of the proportion of fat in diet might in principle slow or reverse the progression of atherosclerosis. The effect of a diet in which total fats constituted 27% of energy was compared with the cholesterol-reducing agent cholestyramine by Watts et al. (1992). Patients referred to St. Thomas' Hospital for coronary angiography were randomised to either "usual care", "diet", or "diet plus drug". Cine-frames of coronary artery segments were rated for mean absolute width of each segment. After 39 months, the mean artery width in the "usual care" group had decreased by 0.2 mm, was virtually unchanged in the "diet" group, and had increased by 0.1 mm in the "diet-plus-drug" patients. This suggests that a diet with 27% of energy as fats can arrest the progression of atherosclerosis, though the Ornish diet (described later) advocates 10% fat.

Despite the statistical risk associated with cholesterol, it does not appear to follow that medical strategies to reduce cholesterol as an isolated risk factor actually reduce premature deaths. At the University of Pittsburgh, Muldoon, Manuck, and Matthews (1990) undertook a meta-analysis of trials based on lowering cholesterol concentrations and their effect on mortality. A meta-analysis was undertaken of total mortality from coronary heart disease, cancer, and causes not related to illness in six primary prevention trials of cholesterol reduction (mean duration of treatment = 4.8 years); 24,847 male participants with a mean age of 47.5 years were followed for mortalities. Follow-up periods totalled 119,000 person years, during which 1147 deaths occurred. Mortality from coronary heart disease tended to be lower in men receiving interventions to reduce cholesterol concentrations compared with mortality in control subjects ($p = 0.06$), although total mortality was not affected by treatment. No consistent relation was found between reduction of cholesterol concentrations and mortality from cancer. There was a significant increase in deaths not related to illness (deaths from accidents, suicide, or violence) in groups receiving treatment to lower cholesterol concentrations relative to controls ($p = 0.004$). When drug trials were analysed separately, the treatment was found to reduce mortality from coronary heart disease sig-nificantly ($p = 0.04$). The treatment implications of this are confusing: Cholesterol-reducing drugs may be appropriate for those with hereditary lipid accumulation problems, but not for general use (Davey-Smith & Pekkanen, 1992). The case for viewing lipid circulation in the context of the circulatory subsystem and the arousal of the human organism as a whole is clearly strengthened.

Remarkably little is known about the relation between behaviour and lipid levels in the blood, apart from isolated reports such as that of Carruthers on racing drivers. Cholesterol is involved in synthesis of the hormones testosterone and oestradiol, but the significance of the connection between lipids and sex hormones is unclear. As cholesterol is such an important marker for CHD risk, it is surprising that so little research has been has been undertaken to see whether behavioural methods can reduce lipids. Cooper and Aygen (1979) have reported one study connecting SAM activity and lipid level. This study is fairly small, and experimental control imperfect, but it would certainly be worth replication. These authors used transcendental meditation, a form of meditation taught at that time by the Maharishi Mahesh Yogi, involving the use of a mantra sound during two 20-minute sessions per day. Subjects were Israelis who volunteered after lectures on meditation and had only slightly elevated cholesterol levels; subjects with diagnosed CHD, taking medication, or who had changed diet considerably were excluded. Twelve subjects were included in the relaxation group, and the 11 controls included 4 who had not persisted with medication, and 7 attending as outpatients for minor complaints. The fasting cholesterol of the meditation subjects was 6.5 mg per 100 ml at the start, compared with 6.64 for the controls. At follow-up about a year later, the subjects had a mean of 5.77, significantly lower than the controls' mean of 6.51.

REVERSING ISCHAEMIC HEART DISEASE

Plaque deposition on arterial walls continues throughout life, resulting in some reduction of the diameter of each artery, and hence increased resistance to the flow of blood. Atherogenesis in the body as a whole leads to an increase in peripheral vascular resistance, which, in turn, leads to an increase in the blood pressure. Some reductions of flow are possible without much loss of exercise tolerance or increased risk of disease, but the process becomes hazardous when the blood supply to particular organs is much reduced. This is particularly true of the arteries that supply the heart muscle itself, since the myocardium has to have a continuous supply of energy in proportion to its pumping rate. A shortage of oxygenated blood will lead to angina from the heart muscle under conditions of high exertion or high emotion. The same constriction is also a possible location for a clot to form. The possibility of slowing or reversing these processes is therefore of considerable importance for preventing these three hazards—angina, myocardial infarction, and hypertension.

Ornish (1991; Ornish et al., 1990) reports on "The Lifestyle Heart Trial", which assessed the effects of a non-medical approach to reduction of ischaemia. Participants were required to adhere to lifestyles that reduced the main risk factors, as follows:

- *low-fat vegetarian diet:* 10% of calories as fat; no animal products except 1 cup/day each of fat-free milk, and egg white
- *stopping smoking* (plasma cotinine monitoring was used to check)
- *stress management training:* stretching exercises, breathing techniques, meditation, progressive relaxation, imagery
- *moderate exercise:* 3 hours/week, 30 mins per session at target of 50– 80% of max. heart rate
- *other inputs:* no caffeine; alcohol 2 units/day; extra vitamin B_{12}; cholesterol less than 5 mg/day; salt unrestricted unless hypertensive; group support, twice-weekly, psychologist-led

The experimental group consisited of 28 subjects (mean age = 56.1), 27 of whom were male; the "usual care" control group consisted of 20 subjects (mean age = 59.8), 16 of whom were male. Entry criteria were: coronary artery disease in at least 1 vessel (any measurable atherosclerosis in a non-dilated, non-bypassed artery); age 35–75; male or female; San Francisco resident; no other life-threatening illnesses; no MI in previous 6 weeks; no history of Streptokinase or Alteplase; no current lipid-lowering drugs; left ventricular ejection fraction over 25%; not scheduled for bypass grafting; permission given by patient's cardiologist and physician; angiograms being used for other purposes.

Angiographic assessment (in which a probe reaches the heart via the femoral artery) for follow-up comparison was made 15 months later. Data were incomplete for 7 patients, but complete for 22 experimental subjects and 19 controls. The main finding was that compliance with the targets was significantly related to arterial diameter. Among subjects with "most adherence" (judged to have complied 125% to 161% with targets), arterial diameter actually widened by an average of 4%; those whose compliance was near the target had essentially stationary artery diameter; while those whose compliance was between 14% and 74% of target had an average of 8% decrease in arterial diameter (see Figure 9.1). This finding is encouraging, in the sense that healthy living can in principle slow and even reverse the process of atherogenesis. However, the scale of lifestyle change is hardly compatible with employment: The healthiest subjects were exercising for an hour and meditating for an hour a day, and the fat target was a quarter of that found in the traditional British diet. Many patients choose to take early retirement after MI, and perhaps only those with a highly internal locus-of-control could achieve the targets of the lifestyle heart trial.

HEART ATTACK

The concept of risk factors for MI was described at length in the chapter 8, but less is known of the immediate precursors for infarction. Fracturing of plaque in a coronary artery seems to be the commonest pathological mechanism, rather than a circulating clot being trapped. Atheromatous plaque is more brittle than the artery on which it is deposited, and the brittle surface layer may crack as the artery flexes; exposure of the underlying material to the blood may lead to a sequence of clotting events, which can completely obstruct the artery. Shearing forces on plaque are higher during vigorous heart activity, so we might expect MIs to be more common during high exertion or emotional arousal. Exhaustion seems to be a common precursor of MI, and overexertion is occasionally a trigger. Heavy physical exertion in the hour before MI was reported by 4.4% of 1228 MI survivors interviewed by

Change in percentage
diameter stenosis
(after–before intervention)

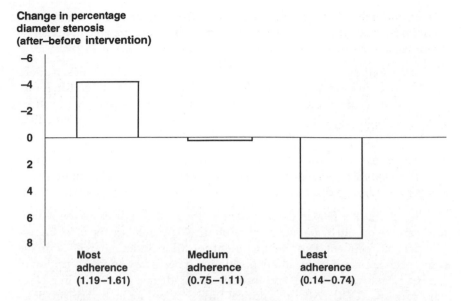

Figure 9.1 Compliance and arterial diameter in the lifestyle heart trial

Mittleman et al. (1993). Sexual intercourse was at one time thought to be a trigger for MI, but Ueno (1963) found only 18 related to coitus in a survey of 5559 sudden deaths, and 14 of these were associated with heavy alcohol use and a much younger extra-marital partner. Vital exhaustion was reported to increase risk of MI by a factor of 10 (see study by Appels discussed in chapter 8). Nixon (1989) hypothesises that CO_2 reduction caused by hyperventilation can trigger MI, e.g. after an industrial accident. Diurnal variation in incidence of MIs seems to show a morning peak about two hours into the working day, with a second afternoon peak in countries which have a siesta. A heavy bout of drinking or insults from the failure of other organ systems can also trigger a clotting event. In many cases, no immediate trigger can be identified, and the formation of a clot that is the thickness of a human hair appears to be a random biological event.

Myocardial infarction should be distinguished from the following related conditions:

- *Angina pectoris* involves a restriction of the blood supply; this condition is not itself fatal, but it recurs during episodes of high exertion or emotion. Lactic acid and other toxins build up and pain ensues, analogous to cramp in skeletal muscles.

- *Cardiac arrest* involves the inability of the heart to maintain good output and may arise through mechanical or electrical causes. It is usually fatal unless resuscitation occurs within minutes. Heart attacks are not necessarily accompanied by cardiac arrest.

- *Sudden death syndrome* occurs in about 1% of the population and is responsible for between 50,000 and 100,000 deaths a year in the United Kingdom. Myocardial infarction is usually absent, and no clear pathology can be demonstrated. It is likely that ventricular fibrillation (VF) is the immediate cause of most such deaths.

- *Cerebrovascular accident* (stroke) is a neurological deficit arising from either a thrombosis of a cerebral vessel, a haemorrhage into the brain, or an embolism from a distant site.

A heart attack is fatal in the first hour in about 40% of cases, so immediate intervention on site by paramedical or medical specialists is the most important part of treatment. Hospital treatment for MI includes emergency procedures such as resuscitation and defibrillation if necessary and prescription of anticoagulant, vasodilating, and thrombolysing drugs, preferably in a coronary care unit (CCU). After this critical time, risk reduction by aspirin, beta-blockade, etc. are used, as for patients who have not had MIs. The risk of fatality declines considerably over the three days after MI, but it is still appreciable. Some patients go home to bed, and the MI is only recognised some time later from changes in ECG. Others who are known to have had an MI receive treatment at home from their GP. Home treatment will not normally include these more intensive procedures, so it might be expected that patients in coronary care would have a better prognosis than those having care at home.

The findings of Mather et al. (1971) are, therefore, somewhat surprising. They observed 1203 MI episodes in four centres in the south west of England. In their study, 343 cases were randomly assigned either to home care under the family doctor or to an intensive care unit. The groups did not differ in age, CHD history, or hypertension, but there were slightly more poor-risk hypotensives (i.e. with low blood pressure) in the hospital group. The mortality rate was 15% (12 in each randomised group) at 28 days, but there was no difference between home and hospital groups. A further 754 patients elected to be treated in hospital, and 106 elected to be treated at home, and results for them were analysed separately from those randomly allocated. Of the "elective hospital" group, 16.8% died within the next 28 days, compared with 11.3% of the "elective home" group. Similar findings on the lack of prognostic advantage from coronary care have been reported in other surveys in the 1970s.

Removal by ambulance for hospital care may cause migration of clots or induce arrhythmias. An alarming experience in coronary care is the sight of attempts to resuscitate another patient after a cardiac arrest. Resuscitation is a rare event in every area of healthcare, except for the CCU, where cardiac arrests can occur every day. It is therefore quite likely that the CCU patient will witness an attempted resuscitation and possibly a death. Schwartz's research on fear and ventricular fibrillation in pigs may be relevant in the human context. In the coronary care unit at Dudley, considerable efforts are made to retain a calm and dignified atmosphere during resuscitation or defibrillation.

Anxiety may be regarded as a normal response to a heart attack. The narrow escape from death and the implications for the remainder of life weigh heavily on most patients. Lack of overt anxiety may be more problematic than anxiety, in that it may indicate denial. Croog, Shapiro, and Levine (1971) reported that 20% of men who had suffered a heart attack denied the medical significance of this 18 days and one year later. This has disadvantages in the sense of underestimating the risk of smoking, but may also be protective against overwhelming anxiety. Further discussion of the value of denial is given by Bennett and Hobbs (1991). Management of the psychophysiology of the person with an MI or arrhythmia is largely intuitive, and good research on this might make a substantial improvement to prognosis of cardiac problems.

Anxiety after MI is associated with arrhythmias and with difficulty in resuming tasks such as paid work or disciplining children. The prognostic significance of anxiety and TABP after hospitalisation with MI (Julkunen et al., 1990) is one of a small number of reports by psychologists working with heart patients. A questionnaire measure was given 8 to 10 days after MI and consisted of 14 TABP items and a Present Affect Reactions Questionnaire (PARQ) with 10 cognitive-worry items and 10 autonomic-emotional items. The 92 subjects were followed up over one year, during which there were 5 reinfarctions and 3 cardiac deaths. The authors did not show any prognostic significance of TABP, but reactive anxiety during the acute phase was predictive of poorer outcome: The mean PARQ for the 8 patients with recurrences was 46, compared with a mean of 32 for the 55 who survived without complications. Anxiety increased during the period up to 3 months after MI.

Depression is frequent after a heart attack, and its presence affects the risk of reinfarction. This finding is reported by Kavanagh (1984), Langosch (1988), Frasure-Smith, Lesperance, and Talajic (1993), and the present author. Complete MMPI data was available for 24 Dudley patients who attended stress-management courses led by the author in 1990–91. Their mean depression score was 1.8 standard deviations (SD) above the mean of the American mental health norms. Hs (bodily concern) and Hy (somatisation of emotional need) were about 1.5 SD above the mean. Anxiety and Cook-Medley hostility were at the population mean, and time-urgency and job involvement were much below the mean. TABP and hostility-inwards were criteria for referral, and all subjects accepted for stress management viewed their heart attacks as disposed by stress, so the low scores on TABP components and hostility were surprising.

STABLE ANGINA

Pain in the chest and arm associated with increased cardiac demand is known as angina. Most commonly, angina is stable and can be managed independently by the sufferer. Angina that becomes more severe over several days, on the other hand, may be associated with an impending major cardiac event. Psychosocial influences are strong: The effects of attention and arousal on pain (see chapter 13) also apply to pain from the myocardium, and arousal may also lead to vasoconstriction. In the research of Williams, Haney, and McKinnis (1986), "hypochondriasis" emerged as the main predictor of episodes of angina pain. This appears to mean that anxiety about bodily function, as well as anger and overarousal, are stronger influences on subjective pain than are physical measures such as artery diameter. Emotional intimacy, which probably affects the frequency and duration of anger, reduces angina. Medalie and Goldbourt (1976) report that "love and support by wives" emerged as a preventive factor against the emergence of new angina pectoris.

Medical treatment of angina involves the use of vasodilating drugs such as nitrates. These may be absorbed through the mouth for immediate relief of symptoms, or taken as tablets for a sustained level of artery widening. Severe headache is a common side-effect, as a result of the diverted blood supply. The following self-talk approaches are recommended by the author, in conjunction with restrained use of nitrates:

Catastrophic thought	Coping thought
"My doctor called it a mini heart attack!"	"It's like a cramp or stitch."
"It's a warning that I should be resting!"	"Rest for a few minutes, then carry on."
"There's no-one to help if I have an attack!"	"I can manage this by breathing slowly."

SUDDEN CARDIAC DEATH

Sudden cardiac death may be responsible for up to 100,000 deaths a year in the United Kingdom, but remarkably little is known about it. Our knowledge of events preceding sudden death comes mainly from coronary care units and more recently from some animal studies, but the same process may occur quite commonly in sudden deaths outside hospital. Kamarck and Jennings (1991) review a large number of reports on the physiology of sudden death.

Under conditions of very high arousal, the level of catecholamines at the beta-receptors in the myocardium may be high enough to initiate local foci for depolarisation, so that an ectopic or premature contraction occurs. Ectopic beats are fairly common in healthy hearts, but if several occur in sequence, the ventricles will contract in an uncoordinated fashion, independently of the atria, and the output of blood becomes insufficient for the body's needs. These brief partial contractions are referred to as fibrillations, and the most serious form is when the larger chambers or ventricles are contracting irregularly. Such ventricular fibrillation (VF) is the commonest reason for cardiac arrest. In hospital, prompt defibrillation can often restore sinus rhythm during an arrest, but otherwise it is invariably fatal.

In patients with recent infarctions of myocardial tissue, muscle cells near the scar site are thought to be particularly irritable and may start to fire in synchrony, starting a wave of depolarisation independent of that initiated by the SA node. The coincidence of episodes of VF in coronary care units with high stress events has been noted by several authors (Jarvinen, 1955; Cay et al., 1972). The first reported that significantly more patients died in conjunction with ward rounds conducted by the chief surgeon than at other times. However, sudden death can also occur in healthy young adults with no myocardial damage. Myocardial infarction is usually absent, and no clear pathology can be demonstrated at post mortem. Several syndromes associated with long recovery times of heart muscle increase the risk of VF (Schwartz et al., 1991). One is called long-QT syndrome, and sufferers are very vulnerable to VF after relatively small emotional shocks; fortunately they can be protected by drugs or surgical procedures that block sympathetic activity.

Sudden cardiac death is, by definition, difficult to study, but occasional anecdotal evidence arises when patients are being monitored medically at the onset of VF. Olsson and Rehnqvist (1982) report the case of a 70-year-old MI survivor who died while wearing a portable ECG monitor on discharge from hospital. He became agitated on noticing his wallet missing, and he telephoned the hospital to try to locate it; he was heard to be excited on the telephone, and after 15 minutes he sighed, and nothing more was heard. When the ECG was recovered after his death, it was seen that his heart rhythm had changed from normal sinus rhythm to a rapid rhythm (sinus tachycardia), with some ventricular ectopics; 15 minutes later a single premature ventricular contraction occurred, which rapidly degenerated into VF and death. Brackett and Powell (1988) found that predictors of sudden cardiac death after healing of acute myocardial infarction in the RCPP (see below) were mainly psychosocial rather than physiological. Kallio et al.

(1979) reported that cardiac rehabilitation mainly affected sudden death rates rather than MI recurrences.

Lown et al. (1980) attempted to identify psychological triggers for arrhythmias in 19 patients who had experienced ventricular arrhythmias previously. Carotid sinus stimulation, posture changes on a tilt table, Valsalva's manoeuvre, hyperventilation, breath-holding, and dive-reflex activation all failed to provoke ventricular ectopic activity. Premature beats were reported to fall dramatically while patients were asleep at home, but to increase again during REM sleep. A structured psychological test was found to increase the frequency of ventricular premature beats in 11 of the 19 patients. The test consisted of mental arithmetic for 5 minutes, reading Stroop colour cards for 5 minutes, and 10 to 15 minutes' discussion of financial and work-related problems, the significance of illness, and the possibility of death. The psychological interview was considered to be only mildly stressful, but the frequency of ventricular ectopic activity was significantly ($p < 0.05$) greater than in random control hours in an extended series of 31 patients.

Sudden and unexplained death in sleep (SUDS) is a significant cause of death of young adults in several Asian populations, especially in northeastern Thailand. Tatsanavivat et al. (1992) conducted a survey by mail of SUDS (known as "laitai" in the local dialect) that occurred in adults during 1988–89 in 3867 villages in northeastern Thailand, and 68% of village headmen replied. The verified SUDS victims were all men, with a mean age of 35.9 years ($SD = 7.8$). A family history of SUDS was reported in 40.3% of index cases, and 18.3% had brothers who had died similarly; no such deaths were reported among sisters. The estimated annual rate of death from SUDS among men aged 20–49 years was 25.9 per 100,000 person years. The sudden deaths were seasonal, with 38% occurring during March–May and 10% during September–October. Sudden death among Thai migrant workers in Singapore has been the focus of speculation about the role of cultural and linguistic isolation and the associated level of fear. Thiamine deficiency may be a cause of prolonged QT interval, which increases risk of sudden death. Munger et al. (1991) found that the mean heart-rate–corrected QT interval was significantly greater among 123 Laotian refugees in Thailand at high risk than in 77 Laotian refugees in the United States at lower risk and 199 non-Asian US residents at negligible risk. Among refugees in Thailand, prolonged QT interval was associated with poor thiamine status and a history of seizure-like episodes in sleep.

Sudden cardiac death has been observed in animals that normally run from threat—the example of a zoo giraffe that became stuck in a straddled position was widely reported. Pigs often "die of fright" en route to market. Pigs are believed to have similar circulation and nervous control to humans, though dogs have different ANS control. Lown et al. (1980) describes a technique for assessing threshold for VF by applying gradually increasing current during the heart's recovery phase, until two or more extra systoles are observed. This technique was applied to dogs restrained in Pavlovian harnesses, where fear had been previously induced by mild electrical shocks. Dogs with intact hearts had a VF threshold 40% to 50% lower than their threshold before fear was induced. Dogs that had experienced a coronary artery occlusion in the stressful harness had a three-times-higher incidence of VF than those who recovered from the same occlusion in a non-stressful environment.

Parker et al. (1990) simulated heart attacks in pigs by tying off a coronary artery, and the ischaemia thus produced resulted in VF and death in most cases. Injection of a beta-adrenergic blocking agent into the brain was found to reduce the probability of VF. It was observed that pigs unfamiliar with the laboratory would withdraw from the scientists, and all would go into ventricular fibrillation and die. If, on the other hand, the pigs had been previously introduced to the lab and had been fed, petted, and handled there, none of them died during the simulated heart attack. Schwartz et al. (1991) have shown that stimulation of the vagus nerve in dogs, which increases the parasympathetic influences on heart rate, can antagonise VF.

MEDICAL TREATMENT OF CHD RISK FACTORS

Medical strategies may be contrasted with lifestyle approaches, but the risks of CHD require appropriately serious comparisons. Half of all hospital deaths are related to cardiovascular disease (Kumar & Clark, 1990), and this risk of mortality makes the selection of treatment a sharp concern. Such powerful interventions in one part of the cardiovascular system often have undesirable effects elsewhere in the system. Some of these unwanted as well as protective effects are shown in Table 9.1.

Behavioural and lifestyle interventions entail few such side-effects, but their efficacy needs to be demonstrated because of the high risks associated with CHD. The assessment of the value of behavioural and lifestyle interventions after a cardiac event will often be by comparison with pharmacological or surgical treatments.

STRESS REDUCTION AS SECONDARY PREVENTION

The medical consensus at the present time places "stress" as an additional factor, but it is considered much less important than the classical risk factors in terms of risk of recurrence. Various services to survivors of MI are pro-

Table 9.1 Medical treatments for CHD risk

Treatment and intended effect	Unwanted effect
anti-clotting agents (e.g. Aspirin)	slow wound healing, ulceration
beta-adrenergic blockade (e.g. Inderal, Trasicor): reduces BP, pulse, some arrhythmias	sexual impotence; lower exercise tolerance
diuretics (e.g. Frusemide, Lasex, Moduretic): reduce fluid in circulation, hence BP	frequent urination
vasodilators (e.g. Hypovase)	cold extremities
sodium ion blockers (e.g. Lignocaine): anti-arrhythmic	cause arrhythmia in overdose
calcium blockers (e.g. Verapamil): anti-arrhythmic	cause arrhythmia in overdose
lipid-lowering drugs (e.g. Nicotinic acid): convert cholesterol to bile acids	increased violence (Muldoon)
atheroplasty (compression of the atheroma on coronary arteries by inflatable balloon)	surgical risk
coronary artery bypass graft (surgical insertion of arterial graft to bypass 1–3 blocked coronary arteries)	neuropsychological deficits; atheroma recurs
heart/lung transplant (graft of organs from donor)	immune rejection; mortality risk

vided, usually under the heading of "cardiac rehabilitation". These tend to focus on medical treatments and exercise (Horgan et al., 1992). The question of preventability is central: An MI is likely to occur during strain or arousal, such as pushing a stalled car in snow, protracted sleep disturbance, or being in a rage. Such demand situations are difficult to avoid completely, and if the effects of overarousal are mediated this way, psychological change will have minimal effect on CHD rates. The most substantial evidence of the role of stress management in the prevention of MI recurrence is found in the major Type-A reduction study described later. It would hardly be practical for people who have had not had a heart attack to devote much effort to the avoidance of exhaustion (Conduit, 1988). Yet in those who have survived an MI, the evidence is that this is one of the more effective ways of preventing a recurrence. Ruberman et al. (1984) showed that the combination of social isolation and stress greatly increased the risk of reinfarction.

Some cardiologists take a psychological view of rehabilitation. For example, Dr Peter Nixon, formerly of Charing Cross Hospital in London, says in his foreword to *The heart attack recovery book* (Wilde McCormick, 1984):

A large number [of people] are driven by panic and rage to struggle mindlessly against the heart's limitations and warnings . . . the heart attack usually makes its appearance when the individual is drained of strength and resilience by effort which has carried him beyond the limits of his endurance for a year or more.

The rehabilitation strategy implied by this view concentrates on adequate sleep and rest and avoidance of hyperventilation, and gives less emphasis to smoking abstinence and physiological factors. The main features of the psychosocial model of rehabilitation (Nixon, 1989; King & Nixon, 1988) are summarised in the acronym SABRES:

- Sleep: awareness of the quantity and quality required and how to get it

- Arousal: learning to relax and modulate the effects of rage and struggle, despair and defeat well enough to keep out of catabolic disarray (i.e. predominance of metabolic breakdown, without compensating anabolic repair processes)

- Breathing: awareness and control to prevent hyperventilation

- Rest: achieving the ability to be still and calm when the heart needs to be rested

- Effort: recognising and respecting the limits of beneficial physical and mental effort and the onset of healthy tiredness

- Self-esteem and confidence, restored by close support of the occupational therapist trainer and the successful employment of SABRE

THE RECURRENT CORONARY PREVENTION PROJECT

The Recurrent Coronary Prevention Project (RCPP) attempted to prevent reinfarctions by alteration of Type A behaviour pattern. This is a large study and provides by far the best research to date on prevention of recurrence in which the role of behaviour can be separated (Friedman et al., 1984; Powell & Friedman, 1986; Suinn, 1975). The subjects were 862 post-MI patients who volunteered to be randomly allocated into either: (1) a control cardiologic counselling group (n = 270), or (2) an experimental group receiving TABP counselling and cardiologic counselling (n = 592). Group training included relaxation, but considerable emphasis was given to the avoidance of "hooks". This metaphor was used to capture the idea of cues for episodes of overaroused behaviour without adequate consideration, such as a fish experiences if it is unfortunate enough to swallow a fishing hook. The two groups were initially very similar in age, height and weight, cholesterol, and several cardiac measures including angina and infarction history; the largest discrepancy was in hypertension (42.5% and 35.8%). Every subject had a Videotaped Structured Interview, and questionnaires about Type A habits were completed by self, spouse, and a work colleague. Counselling was intensive, with 24 sessions for the control group and 44 group sessions for the TABP counselling group over 3 years. The dropout rate was 97 voluntary withdrawals from cardiologic counselling, and 200 withdrawals from the TABP intervention group, which included 36 who had not complied with the exercises; none of these 36 had had MI recurrence prior to exclusion.

Type A behaviour reduced significantly in the TABP counselling group, with VSI scores falling from a mean of 28.0 to a mean of 17.0. The control group also became less Type A, reducing from 29.2 to 23.1 over 3 years. Cardiac recurrence rates were examined among those 181 subjects of either group whose self-rated Type A behaviours declined by more than one standard deviation in the first year. The MI recurrence rate in the second and third years was 1.7% among those who moved significantly towards Type B, compared with an 8.6% recurrence (28 MIs) in the less changed subjects. The cumulative cardiac recurrence rate was 7.2% in the group who initially enrolled to receive Type A counselling, significantly less (p < 0.005) than the 13% in those who initially enrolled for cardiologic counselling. The RCPP study appears to have achieved reasonable control of most influences on MI recurrence other than behaviour, and their claim to have reduced recurrences by half is the best evidence available to date of prevention of MI by psychological means (see Figure 9.2).

A stress management programme for post-MI patients in Dudley was conducted in 1986–87 by Williams and colleagues. This utilised stress-inoculation methods (Meichenbaum, 1985), but not the drills and Type A self-monitoring of the RCPP. Patients were taught the role of the sympathetic nervous system; a further 11 patients received information to form a control condition. The present author followed up these patients three years later, and all 23 were traced. The most significant change during the programme had been a reduction in anxiety, and this effect was increased at follow-up. There was little change in TABP, depression, and most health beliefs. This disclosed a tendency in referrers and patients to equate stress with anxiety, although driven behaviour, exhaustion, and controlled hostility are regarded as more pathological. Three patients had died in the three-year interval to

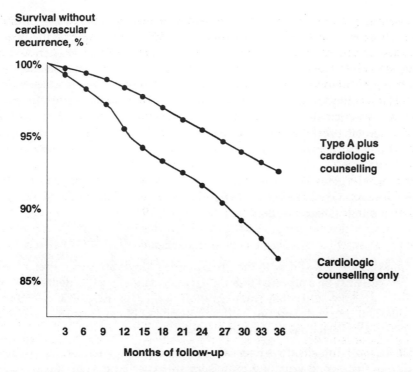

Figure 9.2 The Recurrent Coronary Prevention Programme: MI recurrences over three years

follow-up, giving a survival rate of 87%. This rate is somewhat better than that estimated from baseline morbidity measures. On the basis of Peel indices (Peel, 1960) the survival rate was predicted as 60%. However, medical treatment for MI has improved the prognosis since Peel's observations in the 1950s, so the survival rate reported by Greenland et al. (1991) on 5000 Israelis is probably a better reflection of the risk of reinfarction for patients in the mid 1980s. The 87% survival rate is slightly but not significantly better than these baselines.

AEROBIC EXERCISE AS SECONDARY PREVENTION

Fitness emerges in epidemiological studies as a moderate protective factor, reducing MI risk by 30% in older adults and more in younger adults. Although this is a relatively small protective factor, exercise programmes are the most common rehabilitation strategy after MI. Exercise training provides a well-defined structure, and the American Association of Cardiovascular and Pulmonary Rehabilitation (1991) has produced guidelines for cardiac rehabilitation programmes. The general rationale is to exercise the large muscles of the body sufficiently to force the heart to circulate energy and oxygen to replace energy at peripheral muscles. Achievement of an exercise effect usually involves running, brisk walking, or other large-muscle activity for over 20 minutes. Shorter durations, even of strenuous activity, do not achieve this circulatory effect. More strenuous exercise forces the muscles into anaerobic breakdown of glucose into lactic acid, and the incidence of undesirable cardiac events increases steeply at above 85% of maximal exercise.

Kavanagh (1984) has developed one such programme in Canada, and the same principles are used in the "Action Heart" programme in Dudley in the West Midlands (Dugmore, Bone, & Kubik, 1986).

The Action Heart programme

- *Fitness to exercise.* Entry to the programme follows an exercise tolerance test with ECG on a powered treadmill; abnormalities such as depression of S–T segment would entail a more cautious level of exercise. ECG telemetry is used during early sessions, and monitoring of blood pressure and chest pain before each exercise session is used.

- *Attendance.* Initially three times a week, the number of sessions is reduced during the second year, and exercisers are expected to continue on their own; agreement specifying a minimum level of attendance is in the form of a written contract.

- *Warm-up.* Sessions start and finish with stretching and suppleness exercises to prevent muscle strains or tears; the vigorous phase of exercise is followed by 10 minutes of stretching to cool down and prevent sudden venous return pressure on cessation.

- *Graded exercise.* Brisk walking, sit-ups, bench-steps, and some other tasks that mainly utilise the quadriceps are carried out in rotation to achieve 60–80% of calculated physical capacity for each person; sessions last about 70 minutes.

- *Stress reduction.* The psychosocial aspects of the programme are enhanced by scheduling the session between 5.00 and 6.30 p.m., i.e. after work for many, and by "club" activities that increase the opportunities for sharing feelings.

The mechanisms by which "fitness" achieves its effects are by no means simple. In principle, the myocardial muscle fibres can increase in number and length as a result of demand, and this would be expected to increase the stroke volume of the heart. However, this central cardiovascular effect has not been clearly demonstrated in post-MI exercise programmes, and peripheral changes in oxygen uptake at the muscles may be more important. Various psychosocial influences also occur, including the group support that develops among exercisers, the cathartic effects of fatigue on accumulated tension, and lowered reactivity of blood pressure. Sinyor, Schwartz, and Peronnet (1983) reported that reactivity to psychosocial stress is lower in those with higher aerobic fitness. Exercise programmes are popular with heart-attack survivors, who usually achieve a considerable improvement in well-being (Prosser et al., 1981). However, this may be through a placebo effect (see chapter 6). Research on mood among participants in post-MI exercise programmes has been reviewed by Langosch (1988). He reports that participants placed great value on their programmes, but negative effects were a tendency to avoid rather than confront their problems and increased anxiety when discharged from the structured programme.

Meta-analysis has been used to pool the results of exercise programmes. Where research reports include the mean and standard deviation of treated and control groups, it is possible to combine trials statistically in a procedure called meta-analysis. Oldridge et al. (1988) analysed 10 randomised trials involving 2145 controls and 2202 exercisers. These trials included a WHO multi-centre trial and a report by Carson in Stoke-on-Trent. The trials included variable amounts of risk factor management. O'Connor et al. (1989) undertook a similar meta-analysis involving about the same number of patients, including the WHO multi-centre trial and the reports by Carson and Bethell in Britain. These analyses will be compared with the results for the RCPP and IHD monitoring programmes.

The effects of exercise rehabilitation programmes on depression and anxiety were calculated in a meta-analysis of 15 trials by Kugler, Seelbach, and Kruskemper (1994). The mean depression score for exercisers was 0.46 standard deviations lower than the mean for controls in the case of depression, and the corresponding effect size was 0.31 for anxiety. The authors comment that these effects are modest by comparison with psychotherapeutic interventions.

COMPARISON OF REHABILITATION PROGRAMMES USING DIFFERENT PRINCIPLES

Although it is clear that lifestyle factors substantially affect the risk of cardiac recurrence, it is much less clear what kind of programme will minimise this risk. Smoking abstinence is the most important factor, but there is little evidence on how best to achieve this. An audit of in-patient post-MI education in Dudley found that 70% of smokers reported that they had been totally abstinent in the seven months following discharge, and 22% reported that they had smoked "at least once". Patients are now reluctant to admit smoking to hospital staff, so such a high figure must be treated cautiously. In face-to-face interviews, two factors were most frequently mentioned by ex-smokers. All had seen the film "Suckers" while they were in-patients, and most recalled the scene in which a pathologist demonstrates in a matter-of-fact way the "gruel" texture of a smoker's lung. The second factor was the perception of communication with coronary-care nurses, which was rated as "very good" by nearly all patients in the audit. This combination of an aversive health message, loyalty to the coronary-care staff, and the normal anxiety of surviving a heart attack seems to be highly effective.

Cardiac rehabilitation programmes usually have exercise as a major focus, but a few North American programmes have evaluated stress reduction. A comparison of programmes using two different stress-reduction rationales with the meta-analysis of exercise was made by the present author (Conduit, 1993). One programme was the Recurrent Coronary Prevention Programme, described above; the other was the IHD Life Stress Monitoring Program (Frasure-Smith & Prince, 1989), which involved monthly telephone monitoring of 20 cognitive and behavioural stress symptoms. Where 5 or more symptoms were reported or re-admission occurred, a home nursing intervention followed. Nurses were trained in coronary care but not in counselling, and they had the support of peers, a psychiatrist, and a psychologist. Patients were 461 males admitted between 1977 and 1981 to McGill Hospital, Montreal. Table 9.2 shows the odds-ratio: that is, the number of treated patients who experienced that event as a proportion of all treated patients, compared with the same proportion for control patients. Two major cardiac events—reinfarction and sudden cardiac death—are reported. Results have been calculated for two years after intake. The RCPP presented results for the most adherent patients under the heading "active in group treatment", as well as for all patients enrolled.

The patients are probably comparable in medical care terms, as they were seen in the 1980s in North America, but there are several difficulties in this comparison: The two-year figure was extracted from the results curve for the RCPP; "cardiac deaths" may not have exactly the same meaning in different studies; and age and morbidity may not be strictly comparable. The figures can only be treated as indicators, but the trend is interesting. The baseline mortality rate at that time was about 5% a year, and mortality was reduced considerably in RCPP participants. Exercise programmes seem to have little effect on risk of reinfarction but do give protection against lethal arrhythmias. The IHD programme seemed to have given some protection against both major cardiac events, though in this study other factors, such as better adherence to drugs, may have given the benefit. The strongest

Table 9.2 Comparison of cardiac rehabilitation programmes

	Non-fatal recurrence		Cardiac deaths	
	Odds ratio	% in treated group	Odds ratio	% in treated group
IHD Life Stress Monitoring Program	0.59	8.6%	0.61	7.8%
Exercise programmes (Oldridge)	1.15	10.1%	0.75	9.9%
RCPP ("intention to treat" principle)	0.61	4.1%	1.2	3.1%
RCPP ("active in group treatment")	0.31	5.0%	1.3	4.0%

effect is clearly among patients who worked hard in the RCPP groups to be less driven. Patients tended to recall this programme in terms of the need to avoid "hooks"—a metaphor for cues that elicited sequences of driven behaviour. Although there are considerable difficulties with the Type A concept, the evidence that reducing driven behaviour reduced mortality is strong.

CONCLUSION

Recurrence prevention involves smoking abstinence, a low-fat diet, exercise, and the achievement of intimacy and moderate arousal, as does circulation maintenance. In MI survivors some atheroma is already established, so the relative importance of these factors changes. Adherence to the four principal lifestyle factors can in principle reverse atheroma, but the dietary restriction and the necessity for calm and fitness are very strict. Blood pressure may be reliably reduced by weight loss, aerobic exercise, and relaxation, but adherence to antihypertensive drugs is very necessary if these lifestyle changes are not being achieved, and for more severe hypertension. Lipid reduction can in principle also reverse atheroma, though it is not clear that medical strategies for cholesterol-lowering actually increase life expectancy. The probability of recurrence of heart attack and sudden cardiac death can be substantially reduced by lifestyle influences. Motivation for stress reduction, smoking abstinence, etc. usually results in much higher adherence than it does in asymptomatic people. Exercise programmes have a positive effect on morale, and structured stress management can reduce the risk of MI recurrence.

REFERENCES

American Association of Cardiovascular and Pulmonary Rehabilitation (1991). *Guidelines for cardiac rehabilitation programs*. Leeds: Human Kinetics Publishers.

Bennett, P., & Hobbs, T. (1991). Counselling in heart disease. In H. Davis & L. Fallowfield (Eds.), *Counselling and communication in health care*. Chichester: Wiley.

Blanchard, E.B., Martin, J.E., & Dubbert, P.M. (1988). *Non-drug treatments for essential hypertension*. Oxford: Pergamon.

Brackett, C.D., & Powell, L.H. (1988). Psychosocial and physiological predictors of sudden cardiac death after healing of acute myocardial infarction. *American Journal of Cardiology, 61*, 979–983.

Cay, E.L., Vetter, N., Philip, A., & Dugard, P. (1972). Psychological status during recovery from an acute heart attack. *Journal of Psychosomatic Research, 16*, 425–435.

Conduit, E. (1988). Modifiability of hostility and heart disease. In R. Shute & G. Penny (Eds.), *Proceedings of BPS Welsh Branch Conference*. Cardiff: British Psychological Society Welsh Branch.

Conduit, E. (1993). Psychological principles in cardiac rehabilitation. *British Association for Cardiac Rehabilitation Conference*, Oxford.

Cooper, J., & Aygen, M. (1979). A relaxation technique in the management of hypercholesterolaemia. *Journal of Human Stress* (December), 24–27.

Croog, S.H., Shapiro, D.S., & Levine, S. (1971). Denial among male heart patients. *Psychosomatic Medicine, 33*, 385–397.

Davey-Smith, G., & Pekkanen, J. (1992). Should there be a moratorium on the use of cholesterol-lowering drugs? *British Medical Journal, 304*, 431–434.

Dugmore, D., Bone, M.F., & Kubik, M. (1986). The organisation and implementation of a cardiac rehabilitation programme in the District General Hospital. In R.H. Fagard & I.E. Bekaert (Eds.), *Exercise in health and cardiovascular disease*. Berlin & Dordrecht: Martinus Nijhoff.

Frasure-Smith, N, Lesperance, F., & Talajic, M. (1993). Depression following myocardial infarction. *Journal of American Medical Association, 20* (15).

Frasure-Smith, N., & Prince, R. (1989). Long-term follow-up of the Ischemic Heart Disease Life Stress Monitoring Program. *Psychosomatic Medicine, 51*, 485–513.

Friedman, M., Thoresen, C., Gill, M., Powell, L., Ulmer, D., Thompson, L., Price, V., Rabin, D., Breall, W., Dixon, T., Levy, R., & Bourg, E. (1984). Alteration of Type A behaviour and reduction in cardiac recurrences in post-myocardial infarction patients. *American Heart Journal, 108*, 237–248.

Greenland, P., Reicher-Reiss, H., Goldbourt, U., & Behar, S. (1991). In-hospital and 1-year mortality in 1,524 women after myocardial infarction. Comparison with 4,315 men. *Circulation, 83* (2), 484–491.

Hart, J. Tudor (1980). *Hypertension*. London: Churchill Livingstone.

Horgan, J., Bethell, H., Carson, P., Davidson, C. Julian, D., Mayou, R., & Nagle, R. (1992). Working party report on cardiac rehabilitation. *British Heart Journal, 67*, 412.

Inui, T., Yourtee, E., & Williamson, J. (1976). Improved outcomes in hypertension after physician tutorials: A controlled trial. *Annals of Internal Medicine, 84*, 646–651.

Jarvinen, K.A.J. (1955). Can ward rounds be a danger to patients with myocardial infarction? *British Medical Journal, 1*, 318–320.

Johnston, D. (1989). Can stress management affect heart disease? *The Psychologist, 2* (7), 275–278.

Julkunen, J., Idönpäön-Heikkilä, & Saarinen, T. (1990). Type A Behaviour, Anxiety, and the first-year prognosis of a myocardial infarction. In L.R. Schmidt, P. Schwenkmezger, J. Weinman, & S. Maes, *Theoretical and applied aspects of health psychology*. London: Harwood.

Kallio, V., Hamalainen, H., Hakkila, J., & Luurila, O.J. (1979). Reduction in sudden deaths by a multifactorial intervention programme after acute myocardial infarction. *The Lancet, 2*, 1091–1094.

Kamarck, T., & Jennings, J.R. (1991). Biobehavioral factors in sudden cardiac death. *Psychological Bulletin, 109* (1), 42–75.

Kavanagh, T. (1984). Distance running and cardiac rehabilitation. Physiologic and psychosocial considerations. *Clinics in Sports Medicine, 3* (2), 513–525.

King, J., & Nixon, P. (1988). A system of cardiac rehabilitation: Psychophysiological basis and practice. *British Journal of Occupational Therapy, 51* (11), 378–384.

Kugler, J., Seelbach, H., & Kruskemper, G. (1994). Effects of rehabilitation exercise programmes on anxiety and depression in coronary patients: A meta-analysis. *British Journal of Clinical Psychology, 33* (3), 401–410.

Kumar, P.J., & Clark, M.L. (1990). *Clinical medicine* (2nd ed.). London: Baillière Tindall.

Langosch, W. (1988). Psychological effects of training in coronary patients: A critical review of the literature. *European Heart Journal, 9* (Suppl. M), 37–42.

Lown, B., de Silva R., Reich, P., & Murauski, B. (1980). Psychophysiologic factors in sudden cardiac death. *American Journal of Psychiatry, 237*, 1325–1355.

Mather, H.G., Pearson, N., Read, K., Shaw, D., Steed, G., Thorne, M., Jones, S., Guerrier, Grant C., McHugh, P., Chowdhury, N., Jafary, M., & Wallace, T. (1971). Acute myocardial infarction: Home and hospital treatment. *British Medical Journal, 3* (7), 334–338.

Medalie, J.H., & Goldbourt, U. (1976). Angina pectoris among 10,000 men. *American Journal of Medicine, 60*, 910–921.

Meichenbaum, D. (1985). *Stress inoculation training*. New York: Pergamon.

Mittleman, M., Maclure, M., Tofler, G., Sherwood, J., Goldberg, R., & Muller, J. (1993). Triggering of acute myocardial infarction by heavy physical exertion. *The New England Journal of Medicine, 329* (23).

Muldoon M.F., Manuck S.B., & Matthews, K.A. (1990). Lowering cholesterol concentrations and mortality: A quantitative review of primary prevention trials. *British Medical Journal, 301* (6747), 309–314.

Munger R., Prineas R., Crow R., Changbumrung S., Keane V., Wangsuphachart, V., & Jones M. (1991). Prolonged QT interval and risk of sudden death in South-East Asian men. *The Lancet, 338* (8762), 280–281.

Nixon, P.G.F. (1989). Human functions and the heart. In D. Seedhouse & A. Cribb, *Changing ideas in health care*. Chichester: John Wiley.

O'Connor, G.T., Buring, J.E., Yusuf, S., Goldharber, S., Olmstead, B., Paffenberger, R. Jr., & Hennekens, C. (1989). An overview of randomized trials of rehabilitation with exercise after myocardial infarction. *Circulation, 82*, 234–244.

Oldridge, N.B., Guyatt, G.H., Fischer, M.D., & Rimm, A.A. (1988). Cardiac rehabilitation after myocardial infarction: Combined experience of randomized clinical trials. *Journal of the American Medical Association, 260*, 945–950.

Olsson G., & Rehnqvist, N. (1982). Sudden death precipitated by psychological stress. *Acta Med. Scand., 212*, 437–441.

Ornish, D. (1991). *Dr. Dean Ornish's programme for reversing heart disease.* London: Random Century.

Ornish, D., Brown, S.E, Schwerwitz, L.W., Billings, J., Armstrong, W., Ports, T., McLanahan, S., Kirkeeide, R., Brand, R., & Gould, K. (1990). Can lifestyle changes reverse coronary heart disease? The Lifestyle Heart Trial. *The Lancet, 336*, 129–133.

Parker, G.W., Michael, L.H., Hartley, C.J., Skinner, J.E., & Entman, M.L. (1990). Central beta-adrenergic mechanisms may modulate ischemic ventricular fibrillation in pigs. *Circulation Research, 66* (2), 259–270.

Patel C., & Marmot M.G. (1987). Stress management, blood pressure and quality of life. *Journal of Hypertension, 5* (1, Supplement), S21–S28.

Patel C., & Marmot, M. (1988). Can general practitioners use training in relaxation and management of stress to reduce mild hypertension? *British Medical Journal, 296* (6614), 21–24.

Patel, C., Marmot M., & Terry, D.J. (1981). Controlled trial of biofeedback-aided behavioural methods in reducing mild hypertension. *British Medical Journal, 282*, 2005–2008.

Patel C, Marmot M., & Terry, D.J. (1985). Trial of relaxation in reducing coronary risk: Four-year follow-up. *British Medical Journal, 290*, 1103–1106.

Peel, A. (1960). A coronary prognostic index for grading the severity of infarction. *British Heart Journal, 24*, 743–760.

Powell, L.H., & Friedman, M. (1986). Alteration of type A behaviour in coronary patients. In M.J. Christie & P.G. Mellett, *The psychosomatic approach: Contemporary practice in whole-person care.* London: John Wiley.

Prosser, G., Carson, P., Phillips, R., Gelson, A., Buch, N., Tucker, H., Neophytou, M., Lloyd, M., & Simpson, T. (1981). Morale in coronary patients following an exercise programme. *Journal of Psychosomatic Research, 25* (6), 587–593.

Reisin, E., Abel, R., Modan, M., Silverberg, D.S., Eliahou, H., & Modan, B. (1978). Effect of weight loss without salt restriction in overweight hypertensive patients. *New England Journal of Medicine, 298*, 1–5.

Ruberman, W., Weinblatt, E., Goldberg, J., & Chaudhary, B. (1984). Psychosocial influences on mortality after myocardial infarction. *New England Journal of Medicine, 311*, 552–559.

Schwartz, P.J., Zaza, A., Locati, E., & Moss, A.J. (1991). Stress and sudden death. The case of the long QT syndrome. *Circulation, 83* (4, Supplement), 1171–1180.

Sinyor, D., Schwartz, S.G., & Peronnet, F. (1983). Aerobic fitness level and reactivity to psychosocial stress: Physiological, biochemical, and subjective measures. *Psychosomatic Medicine, 45*, 205–217.

Steptoe, A (1990). The value of mental stress testing in the investigation of cardiovascular disorders. In L.R. Schmidt, P. Schwenkmezger, J. Weinman, & S. Maes, *Theoretical and applied aspects of health psychology.* London: Harwood.

Stunkard, A.J., Wilcoxon-Craighead, L., & O'Brien, R. (1980). Controlled trial of behaviour therapy, pharmacotherapy, and their combination in the treatment of obesity. *The Lancet, 1,* 1045–1047.

Suinn, R.M. (1975). The cardiac stress management program for Type A. *Cardiac Rehabilitation, 5,* 13–15.

Tatsanavivat, P., Chiravatkul, A., Klungboonkrong, V., Chaisiri, S., Jarerntanyaruk, L., Munger, R.G., & Saowakontha, S. (1992). Sudden and unexplained deaths in sleep (Laitai) of young men in rural northeastern Thailand. *International Journal of Epidemiology, 21* (5), 904–910.

Ueno, M. (1963). The so-called coital death. *Japan Journal of Legal Medicine, 17,* 535.

Van Montfrans, G.A., Karemaker, J.M, Wieling, W, & Dunning, A.J. (1990). Relaxation therapy and continuous ambulatory blood pressure in mild hypertension: A controlled study. *British Medical Journal, 300,* 1368–1372.

Veterans Administration Cooperative Study Group on Antihypertensive Agents (1967). Effects of treatment morbidity in hypertension: Results in patients with diastolic pressures averaging 115 through 129 mm Hg. *Journal of the American Medical Association, 202,* 1028–1034.

Vinck, J. (1990). Borderline hypertension and relaxation training. In L.R. Schmidt, P. Schwenkmezger, J. Weinman, & S. Maes, *Theoretical and applied aspects of health psychology* (pp. 339–350). London: Harwood.

Ward, G. (1984). The National High Blood Pressure Education Program: An example of social marketing in action. In L. Frederiksen, L. Solomon, & K. Brehony (Eds.), *Marketing health behavior: Principles, techniques, and applications.* London: Plenum Press.

Watts, G., Lewis, B., Brunt, J., Lewis, E., Coltart, D., Smith, L. Mann, J., & Swan, A. (1992). Effects on coronary artery disease of lipid-lowering diet, or diet plus cholestyramine, in the St. Thomas' Atherosclerosis Regression Study (STARS). *The Lancet* (7 March), 563–569.

Wilde McCormick, E. (1984). *The heart attack recovery book.* London: Coventure.

Williams, R.B., Haney, T.H., & McKinnis, R.A. (1986). Psychosocial and physical predictors of anginal pain relief with medical management. *Psychosomatic Medicine, 48* (3/4), 200–210.

10

Breathing

This chapter describes the normal processes of respiration and talking. Deviations from normality occur when the airways are partly obstructed, as in obstructive airways disease or asthma, but also through misuse; hyperventilation and vocal abuse are common patterns of misuse that can be remedied by appropriate education. Asthma is a common condition, which can be largely prevented by adherence to appropriate drugs; breathing training and emotion expression may also help.

NORMAL BREATHING

Respiration serves the biological purpose of taking in oxygen and expelling carbon dioxide. Normal respiration involves the vertical movement of the diaphragm and upward and outward movement of the ribs by the intercostal muscles. (The airways and muscles used for breathing are shown in Figure 10.1.) During quiet inspiration the diaphragm is pulled down and tidal air is pulled in by the lowered pressure inside the body. In deep respiration the diaphragm is pulled down further, and intercostal muscles contract as well. Expiration is by passive relaxation, and this is why breathing out is one of the most effective parts of relaxation and meditation methods. Normal respiration at rest occurs about 14–16 times per minute (Fried, 1990). In forced expiration, such as blowing against a resistance, muscles of the abdominal

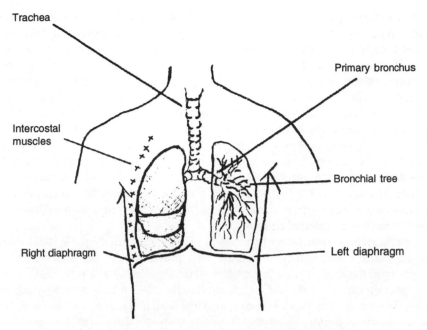

Figure 10.1 The airways and muscles of breathing

wall contract for expiration; positive pressure can be 30 mm Hg above atmospheric. Coughing and sneezing are sudden forced expirations, which expel non-self substances from the airways. Demand for oxygen is strongly related to the workload of the body as a whole, and as a result exertion and emotion have a considerable effect on breathing. Voluntary muscles of the diaphragm and chest are involved, and smooth muscles of the airways are under adrenergic control, so breathing is susceptible to the influence of emotion.

Emotion has considerable effects on breathing, though scientific knowledge of the relationship is unsystematic at present. Yoga teaches that of all the physical effects accompanying emotion, breathing changes the most rapidly. Morse et al. (1984) found that respiratory changes preceded GSR and heart-rate changes in 48 subjects as they came out of deep yoga meditation, and also during mental arithmetic. Inhibition of the rate of breathing seems to occur during anticipation of aversive events in dogs, and perhaps in anticipation of high demands in humans. Haythornthwaite, Anderson, and Moore (1992) used transducers in elastic bands around the chest, and found that episodes of breathing at less than 12 breaths per minute occurred in contexts where other people were present, and also during desk work and reading. Rapid shallow breathing occurs during exertion and with high emotional arousal.

Maladaptive patterns of breathing include sleep apnoea, hyperventilation, and forced expiration. There is an adaptive increase in oxygen uptake by rapid breathing, but this may progress to hyperventilation if forced expiration continues for a few minutes; this has profound physiological consequences, which are discussed later. Sleep apnoea is a recently identified pattern in which airway obstruction leads to very frequent waking from sleep. Low muscle tone in the soft palate or base of the tongue leads to constriction and turbulent airflow, which is heard as snoring. Oxygen deficiency is only remedied by waking for 1–5 seconds—too short to be remembered, but occurring up to 100 times an hour. Apnoea leads to an increased rate of daytime accidents, but also to hypertension and other coronary syndromes (Douglas, 1993). Forced expiration occurs as a long-term compensation for airway obstruction, and chronic asthmatics and emphysema sufferers tend to have over-inflated chests.

Impairment in respiratory function is usually measured by the reduction in the volume and velocity of in-and-out movement of air. Forced Vital Capacity is the total volume of air that can be expelled after a full breath and forced expiration. Height and weight obviously affect this: In a healthy adult male the peak flow is about 4.5 litres, and in a female it is about 3.2 litres. Rate of expiration is a more important measure in respiratory disorders that involve airway narrowing, such as asthma. Peak Expiratory Flow Rate is one such measure, and Forced Expiratory Volume in the first second (FEV1) is the most commonly used measure of asthmatic severity. FEV1 in a healthy male is about 75% of the vital capacity. The difficulty in expiration characteristic of asthma may result in an FEV1 of 2 litres or less.

Several diseases can reduce the air-exchange capability of the lungs. Tar in cigarette smoke damages the upward movement of airborne debris by the hairs of the large airways ("mucociliary escalator") and clogs the alveoli. This leads to a reduction in efficiency and to the development of "smoker's cough" as a compensatory process for mucus escalation. Prolonged occupational exposure to dust in mines, brick-works, etc. can also lead to a permanent reduction in the efficiency of gaseous exchange. Chronic Obstructive Airways Disease (COAD) is the name given to the relatively permanent reduction in gaseous exchange and includes chronic bronchitis and emphysema. Quite often the inflammation caused by one infection can allow a second infection to become established: Antibiotic "cover" is often given during influenza infections to prevent bacterial infections starting in the lungs.

VOCAL HYGIENE

The vocal folds are muscles that resonate to produce the basic speech waveform, which is then modified by the positions of tongue and lips to produce speech sounds. Increasing speech volume is most appropriately achieved by increasing the volume of the resonant cavity. This involves initiating speaking with the diaphragm pulled down, the lungs full, and the voluntary muscles of breathing in a non-tense state. However, many people produce speech with tense muscles and a small resonant cavity, and they increase volume by shouting—that is, by increasing the range of movement of the vocal folds. Singing, teaching, and other "professional voice uses" make particular demands on the muscles involved in voice production, and inflammation of the vocal folds is a frequent problem in such occupational groups.

The following principles of vocal hygiene are adapted from Colton and Casper (1990):

- *Smoking abstinence:* cigarette smoke irritates the vocal folds, dries mucus, and leads to inflammation. Chalk and other airborne dusts should also be avoided.

- *Avoidance of vocal abuse:* untrained singers, teachers in a noisy environment, or families who communicate between rooms, all tend to increase volume by shouting. This has the effect of banging the folds together hard, possible resulting in inflammation or ulceration.

- *Relaxation:* regular deep breathing and unforced vocal fold movement are essential to voice production, and these muscles are particularly prone to tension. Some techniques for relaxation can restore voice in a person who is becoming hoarse or showing pitch changes.

- *Breathy voice:* most people can achieve a "confidential" tone of voice, which actually involves the vocal folds remaining slightly open. This deliberate use of a breathy voice is incompatible with shouting and reduces inflammation in a person suffering from vocal abuse. Alternative techniques include whispering, saying "um–hum", and starting to voice while pushing energetically against a wall.

- *Breath support:* singers or lecturers may need to practise starting to speak on a full inspiration and maintaining the flow of words evenly with expiratory flow.

- *Optimum pitch:* sometimes the carrying power of a flat voice can be increased by raising the pitch; the voice adjusts to the perceived distance of the listener, so singing towards a wall some distance away has been used as a practice technique.

- *Swallowing* rather than coughing: coughing is another form of vocal abuse, and it is often initiated through nervous tension; swallowing is the normal method of mucus disposal and can be used when dryness or a lump is felt.

Treatment of voice problems is usually carried out by speech therapists; proper feedback on the use of these techniques requires the therapist's trained ear and perhaps electronic measurement of vocal-fold activity. Singing teachers use similar techniques. Voice techniques are mainly a matter of experience, and there is little formal evaluation of their efficacy.

HYPERVENTILATION

Hyperventilation is the term for exaggerated depth and rate of respiration of such magnitude that it produces an abnormal drop in the carbon dioxide tension and a corresponding increase in the alkalinity of the arterial blood (Groen, 1982; Fried, 1987, 1990). In mountain climbing, hyperventilation is an adaptive response to the lower air pressure, which requires a much increased breathing rate; failure to hyperventilate can lead to fluid collecting in the lungs. However, Hyperventilation Syndrome (HVS) is usually maladaptive and is the mechanism for symptoms in many phobias, pseudo cases of myocardial infarct, and even fits in temporal-lobe epileptics (Fried & Fox, 1990).

We think of carbon dioxide as a waste substance, so it is rather surprising that the body needs a constant minimum level of it. Deep and rapid breathing for several minutes will expel too much carbon dioxide from the blood, and fainting will follow. Once unconscious, the person's breathing will become slower and shallower, the carbon dioxide level will be restored, and the person will recover with no ill effects. Other symptoms of excessive alkalinity include tingling around the mouth, tremors, and muscle cramps in the hands.

Quite different patterns (Hough, 1991) can lead to alkalosis, including:

- *excessive expiration:* such as screaming in pop concerts

- *panting:* shallow, fast, apical breathing

- *sighs and yawns*

- *excessive control:* heard as "statue" or "cogwheel" breathing

Hyperventilation is fairly easy to counteract, but it is difficult to diagnose. The rate of breathing may be 20 times per minute in a chronic hyperventilator, but expiratory force must also be present. Authors such as Tavel (1990) estimate that as many as 10% of referrals to physicians present with

HVS, but most of them are given diagnoses such as peripheral neuropathy, heart attack, or multiple sclerosis. There is no foolproof diagnostic test, but HVS sufferers are not able to hold their breath for more than a few seconds, and an "emphasis on exhaling" and "time pressure" have some validity as questionnaire items for diagnosing HVS. A hyperventilation provocation test has been widely used for reproducing symptoms of panics, so Lindsay, Saqi, and Bass (1991) asked subjects to breathe at 30 breaths per minute on two occasions. Dizziness, tingling, dry mouth, and fainting were reported by at least 20 of the 28 subjects on both occasions. However, symptoms such as cold hands, head warmth, and feelings of unreality had much lower test–retest reliability, so provoking hyperventilation does not reliably reproduce HVS sensations.

Hyperventilation and emotional arousal may be major exacerbating factors in asthma. Fried (1990) focuses on hyperventilation as the central mechanism in asthma maintenance; this view was put forward as long ago as 1946 by Herxheimer, and restated by Clarke in 1982. According to this theory, emotion, including the suggestion or even the memory of asthma, can trigger hyperventilation, which brings on asthma, which leads to further hyperventilation. Hibbert and Pilsbury (1988) report on the case of a 20-year-old male whose asthma followed a period of stress-induced hyperventilation; anxiety about his health led to breathlessness. A technique of controlled breathing was taught to prevent hyperventilation. However, several other aggravating mechanisms may operate in asthma, as discussed below.

ASTHMA: PHYSICAL MECHANISMS

Asthma is a respiratory disease that is differentiated from chronic obstructive disease (e.g. emphysema) and acute infections by the reversibility of the airway obstruction: Inhalation of a bronchodilating drug will cause dilatation of the airways. The term is derived from the Greek for "hard breath". The American Thoracic Society offers a comprehensive definition:

> Asthma is a disease characterised by an increased responsiveness of the trachea and bronchi to various stimuli, and manifested by a widespread narrowing of the airways that changes in severity, either spontaneously or as a result of therapy.

This bronchospasm is reversible by beta-agonist drugs—that is, substances that mimic adrenalin. The ability of beta-agonists to increase forced expiratory volume in 1 second (FEV1) can be used as the diagnostic test of asthma. Since the 1980s, the medical consensus has shifted towards viewing the inflammatory process as primary and the bronchoconstriction as a consequence. Antibodies of the immunoglobulin E class (see chapter 14) are important in the inflammatory process.

The prevalence of asthma is high: About 10% of adults would show the characteristic reversibility with bronchodilating drugs if tested, though most do not recognise a slight breathing problem as asthma. The prevalence has been generally agreed to be about 5% in industrialised countries, but it may be higher. Incidence in children is about twice as high, but about half these remit with age; incidence rises again in the second half of life. About one person in 80 needs daily drug therapy for asthma. Most asthmatics experience the condition as a minor nuisance, but the condition can be fatal. The UK mortality rate has been in the region of 1500 per annum since the 1950s but appears to be rising. Intensive study in New Zealand found that over-reliance on beta-agonist drugs, failure to treat inflammation, and panic without seeking hospital care were important contributors to premature asthma deaths. Similar findings for England and Wales are reported by Burney (1986). The premature death rate also rose, especially in males aged 15–34, in the decade up to 1986. The natural history of asthma is usually more benign, resulting in inconvenience rather than threat to life. Public and commercial costs are also high. In 1987, asthma cost the National Health Service an estimated 100 million and accounted for 5.7 million days' certified absence from work (1.6% of all lost working days), resulting in an estimated £223 million lost-production earnings (Teeling-Smith, 1990).

The best-known triggers for asthma are allergic, but such sensitivity is absent in many cases. In an influential study. Rees (1964) assessed the etiological role of allergic, infective, and psychological factors with regard to 388 asthmatic children. Psychological factors included emotions such as anxiety, anger, tension, depression, and anticipated pleasurable excitement. The relative importance of allergic, infective, and psychological factors in the etiology of asthma shown in Table 10.1.

Since that time, several additional allergic sources have been identified, including the spores of aspergillus, fumes of rape-seed, and isocyanates in car paints. The proportion of allergen-triggered episodes may be somewhat higher. Triggering by cold air and by stopping exercise were not reliably differentiated among the psychological triggers and might not involve higher mental processes.

Table 10.1

	Dominant	Subsidiary	Unimportant
allergic (e.g. house dust mite, pollen)	23%	13%	64%
infective ('flu, colds, etc.)	38%	30%	32%
psychological (anxiety, excitement)	37%	33%	30%

ADHERENCE TO ASTHMA MEDICATION

Asthma is a condition in which most treatment is undertaken by the sufferer without the presence of healthcare professionals. There is thus considerable scope for divergence between the sufferer's view of appropriate treatment and the medical view. Although the rate of prescription of anti-asthma drugs increased steadily in the 1980s, the premature death rate also rose. This is one indication of a considerable non-adherence problem in asthma medication. Adherence behaviours will be given in some detail for asthma, to indicate the level of biological knowledge required by the client to achieve control. This, though not as high as the level of knowledge required for diabetes, is still equivalent to a substantial part of a secondary-school examination syllabus—which most asthma sufferers have not gained.

Partnership. Since most of the responsibility for administration falls to the patient, the prescriber needs to have a detailed awareness of the asthmatic's health beliefs and lifestyle. Rejection of the recommended treatment may arise through dislike of anti-inflammatory agents, and misunderstandings about dosage and inhaler technique are common. Conservatism and reluctance to take risks were found to accompany high adherence in a study by Pritchard and the author. Cattell's 16PF questionnaire was administered to 21 asthmatics, and these personality traits were found to be correlated with accuracy of peak-flow estimates and knowledge of symptom-guided remedies. The introverted person with strong bodily concern seems more likely to achieve good control than is the sociable person who likes excitement and change, as also found in diabetes (see chapter 11).

Correct inhaler use. To receive an adequate body dose of the drug, the sufferer needs to keep most of the dose in the lungs, rather than breathing it out into the atmosphere. This can be achieved by:

- shaking inhaler vigorously
- exhaling first
- breathing in deeply while depressing the inhaler button
- holding the breath for 10 seconds, exhaling slowly

Positive attitude to prevention by steroids. The use of anti-inflammatory drugs for prophylaxis in the absence of asthma symptoms is relatively recent, so many sufferers who learned about their asthma some decades ago do not distinguish these drugs from beta-agonist relievers. Side-effects such as thrush in the throat or developing a round face also deter people from using them. Timing differs between the two main drug classes:

- *Brown container:* inhaled steroids; use by the clock
- *Blue containers:* beta-agonists; use when wheezing

Respiratory fitness. During healthy periods, those with a tendency to asthma can increase their respiratory efficiency through exercise such as running or other aerobic activity. This will increase the use of lower areas of the lungs. Some sufferers start to wheeze with exertion, although this may happen when stopping rather than at maximum exertion.

Awareness of allergic triggers. A minority of people with asthma have an allergic sensitivity. This can sometimes be determined by skin tests, but many people can make their own diagnosis by systematically varying their domestic arrangements for a few weeks to see whether the symptoms diminish. Airborne allergens include:

- house dust mite faeces (found in blankets, etc.)
- dog or cat hair
- cigarette smoke
- flour, coal dust, etc.
- spores of the fungus aspergillus fumigatus
- aromatic oils, e.g. rape-seed
- paint chemicals—isocyanates
- platinum salts

Food allergies are unusual as asthma triggers.

Peak flow monitoring. The rate of expiration is the most useful measure of severity of bronchoconstriction, and this can be monitored by the sufferer using a commercially available hand-held tube. The amount of treatment needed can be directly related to the peak flow, using a scheme such as the following (Beasley, Cushley, & Holgate, 1989). The ideal peak flow for a woman would be between 300 and 400 litres/min, and for a man it would be between 500 and 600 litres/min. This increases with height and decreases with age. The following guidelines for self-administration require different action, depending on the percentage of ideal peak flow the asthmatic is achieving:

- 70%–100%: inhaled corticosteroid twice daily + bronchodilator as required

- 50%–70%: double dose of corticosteroid; bronchodilator every 2–3 hours

- 30%–50%: start oral steroids—prednisolone 40 mg

- Below 30% or 120 litres/min: go to hospital or GP for nebuliser, etc.

A comparison of peak-flow–guided and symptom-guided treatment was undertaken in a Norfolk general practice by Charlton et al. (1990). The 46 children and 69 adults achieved reductions in the number of GP consultations, courses of oral steroids, and short-term nebulised Salbutamol over the next year. Use of a peak-flow meter was not crucial, and teaching of appropriate action in relation to symptoms was the essential variable.

Managing panic. Inability to breathe is very frightening, and panic has been implicated as a factor in status asthmaticus deaths. Most sufferers report that the presence of someone who can continue to give calming instructions will reduce the panic, and hence the oxygen demand. Fear of suffocation is a very strong motive, and prolonged practice of the arousal control methods described in chapter 2 is necessary for many asthmatics to achieve calm without direct medical help.

LIFE-EVENTS AND SUGGESTIBILITY

A frequent observation about the triggers for asthma is that the thought is often as potent as an allergenic substance. For example, the patient allergic to pollen may wheeze at the picture of a flower. Dekker and Groen (1956) attempted to reproduce the "special emotional meaning" of asthma-inducing situations in the laboratory. The patients who wheezed and showed reduced FVC when seeing a goldfish in a bowl also wheezed at the sight of a toy goldfish or even of the empty bowl. The process looked very similar to that of stimulus generalisation, which occurs in classical conditioning. Even more interesting is the observation that wheezing can be reversed by the belief in the bronchodilating properties of the aerosol. Luparello et al. (1968) gave inhalers containing saline to asthmatic children: The children's breathing and FEV1 measures improved just as well as with the pharmacologically active substance. In another condition saline was given with the suggestion of bronchoconstriction, and with this suggestion wheezing ensued. However, saline may, in fact, be mildly bronchoconstrictive. Isenberg, Lehrer, and Hochron in 1992 found a much weaker effect of suggestion on airways of asthmatic subjects, with only two of 19 subjects showing more than 20% changes in mid-expiratory flow. Suggestibility was found to be related to cognitive but not to hypnotic susceptibility, and to feelings of physical vulnerability and anxiety.

Onset of asthma in adulthood may be related to major life-changes. Teiramaa (1977) examined psychosocial factors in the onset and course of asthma. In this study, 100 patients and 100 controls were given a psychiatric interview, MMPI, Beck Depression Inventory, Wartegg test, etc. Subjects were found to have been introverted and to have had respiratory symptoms before the onset of asthma, and they had "less favourable childhood milieux". Of females, 19% had developed asthma during pregnancy or soon after delivery; and 19% of males had developed asthma around the same period of their partner's pregnancy. Teiramaa (1986) went on to study gender differences in life-stress factors and onset of asthma. Results of questionnaires and a psychiatric interview suggest that the challenges of different ages represent an important factor in onset of asthma. Jacobs et al. (1970) provided some evidence that life situations characterised by failure, unresolved role crisis, and social isolation are associated with respiratory illness. They assessed 106 male college subjects with various degrees of dysfunction and 73 normal subjects on questionnaire measures of life change, manifest affect, and personality. Ago et al. (1982) reported on asthma onset in 209 Japanese adults, who were interviewed about life-events at the time of onset of their asthma. Among those with early-onset asthma, there was a raised proportion of first-borns. Among women whose asthma started in their twenties or thirties, many women suffered problems with their mother-in-law after marriage or found that their husbands were interested only in work.

The psychosomatic view of asthma some decades ago resulted in exaggerated emphasis on the causal role of parental behaviour in maintaining the symptom, often resulting in unhelpful "blaming". Some evidence for a causal relationship between early parental behaviour and the later onset of asthma was reported by Mrazek et al. (1991). Judgements of both parenting problems and maternal coping in a cohort of 150 children who were genetically at risk for developing asthma were made during a home visit when the infant was 3 weeks old. The sample was divided into two groups based on the presence or absence of concerns about coping and parenting. During the following two years, the respiratory status of the children was monitored. Early problems in coping and parenting were associated with the later onset of asthma. Viewing asthma as a frightening physical reaction that requires a calm response is more likely to be constructive than an approach that assigns blame.

Optimum parental strategies for children with asthma have not been well defined, but reducing any sense of "pressure" (see further on) seems valuable. Separation from parents, sometimes called "parentectomy", either in institutions or in their own homes, often has a striking effect of symptom reduction. However, many environmental changes—such as in amount of dust and exertion—also accompany such separations from family. Similar effects can sometimes be achieved in the family home by slight relaxation of some aspect of discipline that is seen as oppressive, such as bedtimes, smoking, or work. Purcell et al. (1969), report the beneficial effects of such treatment for children in whom psychological factors were deemed the principal precipitants of asthma. The successful combination of parentectomy and individual and family therapy at the Roth Pediatric Psychosomatic Unit in California (Steiner et al., 1982, 1987) was held to support the view that general dysfunctional family and coping strategies may maintain asthma in at least some children. However, no one type of maternal personality was implicated, but, rather, generally inappropriate attention and reinforcement transactions.

PSYCHOPHYSIOLOGY OF ASTHMA

Asthma is now thought of as a mainly inflammatory rather than a psychosomatic disease, but emotion still has strong effects. As with any physical illness, anxiety and distress may be higher than for healthy people, but there is little evidence that anxiety is a principal cause of asthma. Goreszny et al. (1988) asked 12 asthmatic and 12 obstructive airways patients to monitor anxiety level on the STAI, perceived severity of stressors, and severity of airways symptoms. There were no differences between groups on symptom severity or between high- and low-anxiety days. Symptoms were different between high and low stress for both groups, which suggests that factors other than anxiety mediate between stress and airways symptoms. Jones et al. (1976) also found neurotic characteristics to be related to age, sex, and duration of illness, rather than to asthma per se. Attempts to characterise personality traits of asthmatics have shown little consistency (Steptoe & Holmes, 1985).

Several possible pathways exist between mental events and the inflammation and broncho-constriction of asthma. Drug treatments mimic ordinary bodily processes in a fascinating way. They are usually administered by inhalation, so they can act quickly and need only small doses. Steroids—i.e. substances that mimic the natural hormones produce by the adrenal cortex—stabilise mast cell secretions. These slow-acting drugs in inhaled forms, including Pulmicort and Becotide, are currently regarded as a long-term preventive treatment, in contrast to the previous recommendation of the symptom-determined use of beta-agonists. Relieving agents, e.g. Ventolin/Salbutamol, are analogous to adrenalin and promote beta-adrenergic effects, notably bronchodilation. Parasympathetic antagonists, e.g. Ipratroprium, which are the mirror image of beta-agonists, work best in older people. The interesting question here is whether the asthma pathology is a specific parasympathetic anomaly, whether it is an aspect of more general autonomic changes, or whether bronchospasm is a consequence of inflammatory processes not much affected by the ANS. Several possible psychophysiological pathways will be examined: paradoxical breathing, adrenergic deficiency, inhibition of sobbing, airway cooling, and oppressed posture.

No simple model of anxiety or emotion in asthma is well supported. Interpretative psychotherapy does not bring about desired results according to most reports (e.g. Forth & Jackson, 1976). Therapists such as de Boucaud and Groen who have worked this way report on the extreme reluctance of the asthmatic to talk about feelings and on the desire to appear normal and to be treated for an isolated lung problem. These therapists speak of "disguising" therapy as a chat. Devoted medical care, as and when the patient wants it, are reported to have the best psychotherapeutic effect. The effects of a permanent sense of oppression associated with fear of suffocation are discussed further on. Group discussion therapy was reported to be of benefit by Groen and Pesler (1960); this may be because the group consensus limits the depth of disclosure of feelings while reinforcing the sense of permanent availability of medical help. Relaxation usually helps a little in improving flow (Alexander, 1972). Counter-suggestion under hypnosis has frequently been reported as an effective remedy for wheezing. Brown and Fromm (1988) report on the hypnotic treatment of asthma; anger or fear were viewed as triggers, and counter-suggestion was sometimes effective.

Paradoxical breathing

People with long-term airway obstruction tend to develop a pattern of breathing with the upper thorax only. The shoulders are held in an elevated position, and the arms are kept rigid to act as a point of leverage for the ribcage. The ribcage is elevated during inspiration, and little use is made of the diaphragm. Expiration is achieved with positive pressure rather than relaxation. Eventually overinflation of the chest becomes permanent, and the sufferer's chest develops a barrel-like appearance. The term "paradoxical breathing" is used to describe the deviant pattern where the abdomen is seen to be drawn in during inspiration, rather than being pushed out by the descending diaphragm. Physical therapy designed to restore relaxed breathing is used, and physiotherapists are involved in this re-educative process. Hough (1991) suggests the following strategies:

- *Achieving abdominal breathing* (previously called diaphragmatic breathing): While sitting or half-lying, rest the dominant hand on the abdomen; keep shoulders relaxed; allow the hand to rise gently; visualise air filling abdomen like a balloon; sigh out. Gradually increase depth while remaining relaxed.

- *Decreasing the work of breathing:* While sitting or standing, lean forward with arms loosely folded on a support, such as a chair back; do not lock the hands on the support, which creates a rigid shoulder fulcrum for chest movement.

- *Singing or sport:* Participation with enjoyment may be beneficial, perhaps because the patient then "forgets" his oppressed state and pressed breathing.

Adrenergic deficiency

The efficacy of adrenergic drugs in relieving asthma might suggest that response to adrenalin is deficient in some way. Some sufferers from asthma who also have medical training have reported that expressing anger actually reduces wheezing. The vagus nerve of the parasympathetic ANS innervates the bronchial tree, but the smooth muscles of these airways are not actually supplied by adrenergic (sympathetic) nerves. However, they have beta adrenergic receptors, regulated by circulating catecholamines, adrenalin being primary for bronchodilation. Effective interaction of adrenalin and beta receptors promotes bronchodilation. Weiner (1987) compares specific and general adrenergic hypotheses about nervous control in asthma. The cholinergic bronchoconstrictor reflex hypothesis is that stimulation of rapidly adapting receptors initiates a parasympathetic vagal reflex, which in turn causes acetylcholine release and subsequent bronchospasm. The beta-adrenergic blockade hypothesis (Szentivanti, 1968) suggests that BA responses and receptors are deficient, perhaps associated with low adrenalin and catecholamines.

Evidence that the asthmatic has an insufficient adrenal response to stress has been found in a few studies. Mathe and Knapp (1971) examined physiological measures of arousal including cortisol, vanylmandelic acid (an adrenalin derivative), and cardiovascular indices. Subjects were 6 male students with asthma and 6 controls, free of drugs at the time of the study. Stress was induced by mental arithmetic and a film. Asthmatics had significantly lower adrenalin (but not noradrenalin or cortisol) during stress and control periods. Cardiac acceleration training with biofeedback was shown to reduce airway resistance of asthmatic volunteers by Harding and Maher (1982). Increasing heart rate must entail adrenergic effects and antagonise parasympathetic inputs, so voluntary increase of heart rate or other SAM effects may have therapeutic potential for asthmatics.

Attempts to study possible parasympathetic excess have included measures of salivary volume, although this correlates only weakly with autonomic activity. Grilliat et al. (1983) used a more direct method, involving the raising of tone in the vagal nerve by carotid massage, which raises the pressure at the baroreceptors in the main arteries from the heart. An atropine challenge was given to the 69 subjects half an hour after return to baseline of pulse and BP. On the basis of responses, subjects were divided according to whether their vagal tone was above (hypervagotonic) or below (hypovagotonic) the global mean, and whether bronchial sensitivity to atropine was above the mean (hyperreactive) or below it (hyporeactive). When the allergic factor was compared across these groups, it was found that 62% of the non-allergic subjects had vagal tone above the global mean, while 85% of those with allergic factor had a vagal tone above the global mean. In other words, higher vagal tone was associated with allergic asthma.

Inhibition of sobbing

Asthma was thought by the Chicago school to be a classic psychosomatic illness. The psychoanalyst Alexander noted a low frequency of crying in asthmatic children and proposed the view that the asthmatic attack develops as a substitute for crying. Sobbing is a particularly powerful action of the chest muscles, which greatly alters respiration. The fundamental emotional conflict underlying asthma was held to concern a cry for the mother figure, suppressed through fear of rejection, aroused by her ambivalent attitude, "simultaneously seductive and rejecting" (Alexander, French, & Pollack, 1968). The asthmatic attack was regarded as an attempt to "discharge the tension along an abnormal pathway" (Groen, 1982), and thus as an abnormal respiratory expression of the suppressed sob. Regarding crying as "the first communication of the child with the mother", Alexander suggests that the inhibition of sobbing subsequently extends to an inhibition of the verbal communication of emotions (Alexander et al., 1968). However, it seems doubtful that children with asthma cry less than do others. Weinstein (1984) reports on 104 cases with crying-induced bronchospasm out of a sample of 268 children aged between 6 months and 19 years. The most frequent questionnaire finding was that parental discipline precipitated crying.

Donald Winnicott (1957), a paediatrician and psychoanalyst, drew attention to the way respiratory changes associated with anger or independence may be perceived by the mother in terms of illness rather than independence strivings. He used a "spatula game" as a paediatric assessment tool, and he gives this vignette of his view of the psychological triggers for asthma in a 7-month-old girl referred for asthma:

The baby sat on her mother's lap with the table between them and me. It was therefore very easy to see when at a certain point the child developed bronchial spasm. The mother's hands indicated the exaggerated movement of the chest, both the deep inspiration and the prolonged obstructed expiration were shown up, and the noisy expiration could be heard. . . . The asthma occurred on both occasions over the period in which the child hesitated about taking the spatula. She put her hands to the spatula and then, as she controlled her body, her hand and her environment, she developed asthma, which involves an involuntary control of expiration. At the moment when she came to feel confident about the spatula which was at her mouth, when saliva flowed, when stillness changed to the enjoyment of activity and when watching changed into self-confidence, at this moment the asthma ceased.

Although the psychosomatic view of asthma is not widely held in Britain, in France psychoanalytic treatment for asthma is quite common. The French asthma research group GREPA (1977) regularly brings together psychiatrists and physicians who treat from this standpoint. At the second GREPA conference, Alby pointed out that the physician may play an iatrogenic role, in that the symptom may express the wish to seek refuge from internal conflict. Grilliat at the same seminar discussed the asthmatic's need for refuge, while Gachie discussed the dependence of patient on doctor that becomes essential in asthma.

Expression of emotion in asthma was studied by Steele in collaboration with the present author, comparing 17 patients with asthma with 13 patients with COAD or other respiratory problems. Crying was described in terms of sobbing, tears flowing, eyes pricking, and lump in throat. Crying was slightly lower in asthmatics, but not significantly lower on any of the four types of crying. However, overall expression of emotion (sum of 10 scales, each of 5 points) was significantly lower in the asthma group, and asthmatics were significantly more likely to report coping inwardly. Of the 10 emotions, "worry", and the related qualities of "inscrutability" and "toleration of unhappiness caused by another" each produced significantly lower figures in the asthma group.

Airway cooling

There is considerable evidence that asthmatics express emotion less than do others. This could be a causal psychophysiological process, but control of stronger emotions might be a learned mechanism for avoiding wheezing. Cold air can trigger bronchospasm for many asthmatics, so learning to inhibit emotion might have an adaptive value.

Kagan and Weiss (1976) found an inverse relationship between allergic precipitants and emotionally toned respiratory precipitants (laughing and crying). This relationship was not supported in the 47 6–16-year-olds studied when the index of emotional precipitants included only worry, anger, upset, and excitement. Florin et al. (1985) studied facial expression of emotion and physiological reactions in children with asthma. In their study, 18 asthmatics and 18 normal controls were shown a comic film, and given a stress-inducing achievement task. The asthmatics showed significantly fewer expressions of facial emotion than did controls in the stress-inducing, but not in the joy-inducing, condition. Forced expiratory volumes of asthmatics decreased significantly, and heart rate increased significantly, under both conditions. Hollaender and Florin (1983) examined the relation between expressed emotion and airway conductance. Fourteen asthmatics aged 9–11 were matched with controls, and each was subjected to a stress-inducing competitive achievement situation. Video recordings showed significantly fewer and shorter expressions of facial emotion in the asthmatics. Anger/rage, enjoyment/joy, and surprise/startle, in particular, were lower. Duration of overall expressed emotion showed a significant negative correlation with peak expiratory flow reduction in the asthmatic group.

Oppressed posture

Having a tendency to asthma entails having had episodes of struggling for breath, resulting in a fear of suffocation. This fear may recur in response to suggestion, and postural changes associated with fear of suffocation may be adopted. Groen (1982), a doctor working in Holland and Israel, advanced a voluntary breathing theory of asthma. He saw the obstruction to expiration as occurring in the large airways, which are distorted by positive pressure within the thorax brought on by forced expiration. Groen reported that many asthmatics can reproduce the wheeze if asked to do so by voluntary means. In an experiment by Dekker, Defares, and Heemstra (1957), measurements were taken of pressure in the oesophagus and a middle-sized bronchus, and of air-flow at the mouth. During normal "sighing" (expiration without effort), pressure and flow varied together, but during voluntary wheezing the pressure in the large airways rose, and the air-flow did not rise. Groen concluded that the airway obstruction lies higher up and consists of a long stretched narrowing of the larger bronchi and trachea. Re-education of breathing to prevent "pressed" breathing during feelings of "oppression" can remove the pattern in the presence of the physiotherapist, but generalisation to everyday cues is difficult. The habitual forced expiration may resume as soon as the patient is alone again. Reduction of facial tension by feedback of frontalis EMG activity was found helpful in the treatment of asthma in children by Kotses et al. (1991). Facial muscle tension seems to influence lung airway resistance, but limb muscle tension does not (Glaus & Kotses, 1983).

There are very few controlled comparative studies of non-drug treatments for asthma. One exception is the Ph.D. dissertation of Frank (1986). She compared three conditions for self-regulation of asthma: breathing training, autogenic training, and assessment only. Dependent measures were respiratory rate, FVC and FEV (1), state anxiety, intensity of asthma response, and skill utilisation. Six asthmatic subjects were assigned to each of the three conditions, along with 18 non-asthmatic volunteers. As predicted, subjects in the Breathing Training group were more effective in achieving decreased respiratory rates, fewer asthma episodes, and increased skills. Expiratory effort was equally improved in autogenic and breathing training groups, and anxiety reduced in all three groups.

In a study involving the author (Conduit et al., 1993), asthmatics were either given breathing training or participated in an emotion-expression group. Subjects who were able to attend regularly and keep diaries were randomly assigned to one of these treatments and instructed to continue their drug treatments as before. The emotion-expression group had weekly meetings with a focus on one emotion, such as anger, grief, or worry. The breathing group had individual sessions with a physiotherapist, where they learned to use breathing with the abdomen and to reduce the work of breathing during exacerbations of asthma. Detailed monitoring included videotapes of chest movement, diaries of symptoms, and questionnaires about coping skills and emotion expression. Most variables, including anxiety, quality of life, drug use, and peak flow did not change significantly. Voluntary control of breathing was better in the breathing group, and emotion expression was better in the expression group, as expected. There was considerable reduction in wheezing and coughing and a statistically significant reduction in night waking in both groups. The most interesting finding was that the use of the chest muscles changed significantly towards the pattern associated with lower abdominal breathing in both groups. The elevation of the shoulders was seen to drop on videotapes, without an accompanying reduction in general relaxation, or any hints having being given that this was a desirable change. Some evidence was provided for the hypothesis of a habitual "oppressed stance" in the person with asthma.

Pragmatic approaches to asthma

It is difficult to disentangle the different influences on asthma, and the above theories are weakly supported. Creer and Wigal (1985) list various pragmatic strategies that may be helpful. The evidence for most of these strategies is anecdotal, and postural and psychological management of asthma remains an art rather than a science. Strategies that normalise breathing are useful, and a self-talk strategy such as the following is used by the author:

"Let shoulders droop and your head rest back. When breathing in, feel the navel coming out. Open the mouth and sigh out. Do not push. Count the breath out, 1 . . . 2 . . . 3 . . . If the count reaches 4, even better. Keep breathing in slowly, with the tummy, and sighing out."

This strategy is appropriate to low-demand situations, and the counts would be shorter during physical or emotional demands. The instruction to "breathe deeply" sometimes brings about overinflation and expiratory force, but it may be used once the normal pattern is established. Such deliberate strategies are difficult to maintain when there are external demands on attention, but they can be used to restore the normal pattern at pauses during public speaking, rock-climbing, or other high-demand situations. Discussion of feelings of pressure, such as duty to care for an elderly person or being the only trained person present during an emergency, has resulted in easier breathing for several asthmatic patients seen by the author.

CONCLUSION

Breathing responds rapidly to emotional changes, and deviant breathing can have powerful physical effects. Hyperventilation and sleep apnoea cause marked changes in blood chemistry and may be implicated in accidents and cardiovascular problems. Misuse of the speaking voice can cause vocal-fold inflammation. Asthma is a common condition involving inflammation and a reversible obstruction of airways. It is not a "stress-related" disease in the simple sense but may involve adrenergic deficiency, hyperventilation, or oppressed posture. Strategies to restore adaptive breathing are helpful in preventing a variety of recurrent illnesses.

REFERENCES

Ago, Y., Sugita, M., Teshima, H., & Nakagawa, T. (1982). Specificity concepts in Japan. *Psychotherapy and Psychosomatics, 38* (1–4), 64–73.

Alexander, A.B. (1972). Systematic relaxation and flow rates in asthmatic children. *Journal of Psychosomatic Research, 16,* 405–410.

Alexander, F., French, T.M., & Pollack, G.H. (Eds.) (1968). *Psychosomatic specificity, Vol. 1.* Chicago, IL: University of Chicago Press.

Beasley, R., Cushley, M., & Holgate, S. (1989). A self-management plan in the treatment of adult asthma. *Thorax, 44,* 200–204.

Brown & Fromm (1988). Hypnotic treatment of asthma. *Advances, 5* (2), 15–27.

Burney, P.J. (1986). Asthma mortality in England and Wales: Evidence for a further increase. *The Lancet, 2,* 323–326.

Charlton, I., Charlton, G., Broomfield, J., & Mullee, M. (1990). Evaluation of peak-flow and symptoms only self-management plans for control of asthma in general practice. *British Medical Journal, 301,* 1355–1359.

Clarke, P.S. (1982). Emotional exacerbations in asthma caused by overbreathing. *Journal of Asthma, 19,* 249–251.

Colton, R.H., & Casper, J.K. (1990). *Understanding voice problems: A physiological perspective for diagnosis and treatment.* London: Williams & Wilkins.

Conduit, E., Atherden, M., Conduit, J., & Bone, M. (1993). Behavioural management of asthma. *Proceedings of the European Respiratory Society Conference,* Florence, Italy.

Creer, T.L., & Wigal, J.K. (1985). Respiratory disorders. In S. Pearce & J. Wardle (Eds.), *The practice of behavioural medicine.* Leicester: The British Psychological Society.

Dekker, E. & Groen, J. (1956). Reproducible psychogenic attacks of asthma. *Journal of Psychosomatic Research, 1,* 58–67

Dekker, E., Defares, & Heemstra (1957). Cited by J.J. Groen, *Clinical research in psychosomatic medicine.* Assen, The Netherlands: Van Gorcum, 1982.

Douglas, N.J. (1993). The sleep apnoea/hypopnoea syndrome. *Proceedings of the Royal College of Physicians of Edinburgh, 23,* 132–139.

Florin, I., Freudenberg, G., & Hollaender, J. (1985). Facial expressions of emotion and physiologic reactions in children with bronchial asthma. *Psychosomatic Medicine, 47* (4), 382–393.

Forth, M. & Jackson, M. (1976). Group psychotherapy in the management of bronchial asthma. *British Journal of Medical Psychology, 49,* 257–260.

Frank, E. (1986). *Breathing training as a self-regulatory stress reduction method for asthma prone individuals.* Ph.D. thesis, University of Southern Mississippi.

Fried, R. (1987). *The hyperventilation syndrome—research and clinical treatment.* Baltimore, MD: Johns Hopkins University Press.

Fried, R. (1990). *The breath connection.* New York: Plenum Press.

Fried, R., & Fox, M. (1990). Effect of diaphragmatic respiration with end-tidal CO_2 biofeedback on respiration, eeg, and seizure frequency in idiopathic epilepsy. *Annals of the New York Academy of Sciences, 602.*

Glaus, K., & Kotses, H. (1983). Facial muscle tension influences lung airway resistance; limb muscle tension does not. *Biological Psychology, 17,* 105–120.

Goreczny, A.J., Branthey, P., Buss, R., & Waters, W. (1988). Daily stress and anxiety and their relation to daily fluctuations of symptoms. *Journal of Psychopathology & Behavioral Assessment, 10* (3), 259–267.

GREPA (1977). L'asthmatique et ses médecins. Conference proceedings. Reproduced in *Psychologie Médicale, 10* (1978, No. 6).

Grilliat, J.P, LeVan, D., Mayeux, D., & Kohler, C. (1983). Tonus vagal et reactivité bronchique [Vagal tone and bronchial reactivity]. *Psychologie Médicale, 15* (7), 1071–1076.

Groen, J.J. (1982). *Clinical research in psychosomatic medicine.* Assen, The Netherlands: Van Gorcum.

Groen & Pesler (1960). Cited by J.J. Groen, *Clinical research in psychosomatic medicine.* Assen, The Netherlands: Van Gorcum, 1982.

Harding, A.V., & Maher, K.R. (1982). Biofeedback training of cardiac acceleration; effects on airway resistance in bronchial asthma. *Journal of Psychosomatic Research, 26* (4), 447–454.

Haythornthwaite, J., Anderson, D., & Moore, L. (1992). Social and behavioral factors associated with episodes of inhibitory breathing. *Journal of Behavioral Medicine, 15* (6).

Hibbert, G., & Pilsbury, D. (1988). Demonstration and treatment of hyperventilation causing asthma. *British Journal of Psychiatry, 153,* 687–689.

Hollaender, J., & Florin, I. (1983). Expressed emotions airway conductance in children with bronchial asthma. *Journal of Psychosomatic Research, 27,* 307–311.

Hough, A. (1991). *Physiotherapy in respiratory care.* London: Chapman & Hall.

Isenberg, S.A., Lehrer, P.M., & Hochron, S. (1992). The effects of suggestion on airways of asthmatic subjects breathing room air as a suggested bronchoconstrictor and bronchodilator. *Journal of Psychosomatic Research, 36* (8), 769–776.

Jacobs, M., et al. (1970). Life stress and respiratory illness. *Psychosomatic Medicine, 32,* 233–242.

Jones, N., et al. (1976). Personality profile in asthma. *Journal of Clinical Psychology, 32,* 285–291.

Kagan, S., & Weiss, J. (1976). Allergic potential and emotional precipitants of asthma in children. *Journal of Psychosomatic Research, 20* (2), 135–139.

Kotses, H., Harver, A., Segrets, J., Glaus, K., Creer, T., & Young, G. (1991). Long term effects of biofeedback-induced facial relaxation on measures of asthma severity in children. *Biofeedback Self Regard, 16* (1), 1–21.

Lindsay, S., Saqi, S., & Bass, C. (1991). The test–retest reliability of the hyperventilation provocation test. *Journal of Psychosomatic Research, 35* (2/3), 155–162.

Luparello, T.H., Lyons, H.A., Bleeker, B.A., & McFadder, E.R. (1968). Influences of suggestion on airway reactivity in asthmatic subjects. *Psychosomatic Medicine, 30,* 819–825.

Mathe, A., & Knapp, P. (1971). Emotional and adrenal reactions to stress in bronchial asthma. *Psychosomatic Medicine, 33,* 323–340.

Morse, D.R., Cohen, L., Furst, M.L., & Martin, J.S. (1984). A physiological evaluation of the yoga concept of respiratory control of autonomic nervous system activity. *International Journal of Psychosomatics, 31* (1), 3–19.

Mrazek, D., Klinnert, M., Mrazek, P., & Macey, T. (1991). Early asthma onset: Consideration of parenting issues. *Journal of the American Academy of Child and Adolescent Psychiatry, 30* (2), 277–282.

Purcell, K., Brady, K., Chai, H., Muser, J., Molk, L., Gordon, N., & Means, J. (1969). The effects of asthma in children of experimental separation from family. *Psychosomatic Medicine, 31,* 144–164.

Rees, L. (1964). The importance of psychological, allergic and infective factors in childhood asthma. *Journal of Psychosomatic Research, 7,* 253–262.

Steiner, H., Fritz, G., Hilliard, J., & Lewiston, N. (1982). A psychosomatic approach to childhood asthma. *Journal of Asthma, 19* (2), 111–121.

Steiner, H., et al. (1987). Defense style and the perception of asthma. *Psychosomatic Medicine, 49,* 35–44.

Steptoe, A., & Holmes, R. (1985). Mood and pulmonary function in adult asthmatics. *British Journal of Medical Psychology, 58,* 87–94.

Szentivanti (1968). Cited by J.J. Groen, *Clinical research in psychosomatic medicine.* Assen, The Netherlands: Van Gorcum, 1982.

Tavel, M.E. (1990). Hyperventilation syndrome—hiding behind pseudonyms? *Chest, 97,* 1285–1288.

Teiramaa, E. (1977). Psychological and psychic factors and age at onset of asthma. *Journal of Psychosomatic Research, 23,* 27–37.

Teiramaa, E. (1986). Psychosocial factors, personality and acute-insidious asthma. *Journal of Psychosomatic Research, 25,* 43–49.

Teeling-Smith, G. (1990). *Asthma.* London: Office of Health Economics.

Weiner, H. (1987). Stress, relaxation and asthma. *International Journal of Psychosomatics, 34,* 21–24.

Weinstein, A.G. (1984). Crying-induced bronchospasm in childhood asthma. *Journal of Asthma, 21,* 161–165.

Winnicott, D. (1957). The spatula game. In *Collected papers.* London: Hogarth.

11

Digestion

Problems of digestion, weight control, and glucose metabolism are almost as common as are those of the heart and arteries. They may cause more pain and distress, but they are generally less life-threatening. Like the cardiovascular system, the gut is made up of smooth muscle, in the form of a tube from mouth to anus, and autonomic innervation is extensive. Digestion involves activation of the parasympathetic system, whereas SAM activity inhibits digestion. Whitehead and Schuster (1985) have presented a behavioural approach to gastrointestinal diseases that can hardly be bettered, and further details of treatments described in this chapter can be found there. Digestive problems have received little attention from clinical psychologists to date, while dietitians take a major role in preventive strategies. This chapter starts with the behavioural act of eating and moves on to describe normal and deviant processes in the mouth and oesophagus, the stomach, the pancreas, and the small and large intestines. A diagram showing the organs involved in the digestive process is presented in Figure 11.1.

WEIGHT AND SIZE

Body weight is a major determinant of health and is influenced by food intake, exercise, and heredity. Obesity is a significant risk factor for heart disease and diabetes, and complicates surgical treatment.

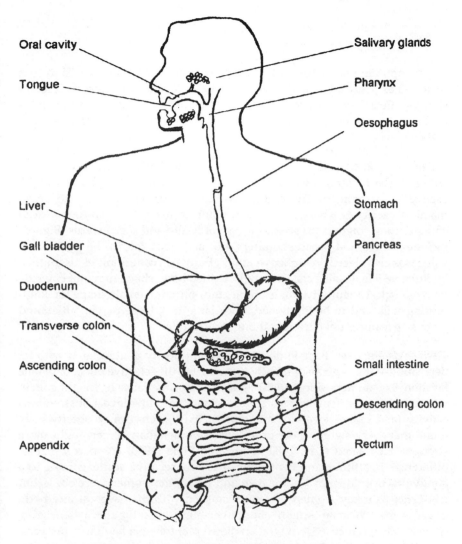

Figure 11.1 Organs involved in the digestive process

Definition by life expectancy. Medical definitions of optimum weight are mainly informed by data on life expectancy in relation to weight. The actuarial tables of the Metropolitan Life Company are widely used. Using life expectancy criteria, ideal weight may be defined for a given height, with smaller corrections for bone length and density. A widely used formula is the Body Mass Index (BMI), defined as follows:

$$BMI = \frac{\text{Weight (kilograms)}}{\text{Height}^2 \text{ (metres)}}$$

The optimum range for BMI is regarded as between 20 and 25; 25 to 30 is regarded as overweight, and over 30 as obese. Additional measures such as skin-fold thickness or the relative distribution of fat cells in different regions of the body may be used as predictors of specific risk for heart disease or diabetes.

Cultural differences. Concepts of ideal weight and appearance are strongly cultural. The cultural ideal in Western Europe is for a low body weight, especially for women. The cultural value on leanness appears to apply mainly to societies where food is abundant. In many modern-day African communities, "bigness" is seen as a sign of health and social status. Bigness includes height and broad shoulders, but also body fat. In the past, social value was also placed on higher weight in European communities, as implied by Rubens' female subjects. Culturally valued body shape may not coincide with biological adaptivity. For example, the optimum female shape for child-bearing will tend to be big-boned, with large feet, large pelvic outlet, and other size features not currently thought attractive.

Gender differences. Female development at puberty is associated with fat deposition at the expense of muscle growth, and the selective effect of female hormones on fat deposition might be seen as a prime cause of weight gain in women. However, female roles are associated with low levels of strenuous activity (and higher levels of moderate activity). Surveys of obesity have found that overweight is more prevalent in women than in men and is more strongly age-related (Ley, 1980). Seim and Fiola (1990) compared gender differences in attitude and behaviour of 198 consecutive adults coming to a family practice clinic; 25% of the men and 10% of the women were obese, but five times as many women were not satisfied with their weight and body image as men. Women thought about overeating and felt guilty when eating twice as often as men; 68% of women dieted monthly to a few times per year, but 75% of men dieted once yearly or never dieted. Trait anxiety or depression were not significantly different between obese and non-obese among 393 adolescent girls from lower-middle to middle-class families (Wadden et al., 1989). Obese girls reported significantly greater dissatisfaction with their weight and figure than did non-obese girls, but many of the latter also expressed dissatisfaction with their weight, supporting the view that women's dissatisfaction with weight is a "normative discontent". Nearly 70% of the total sample had attempted to lose weight in the past year.

Class differences. There is a strong connection between obesity and lower social class among women in developed societies, according to a review by

Sobal and Stunkard (1989) of 144 published studies. The relationship is inconsistent for men and children in developed societies. In developing societies, however, a strong direct relationship exists between social and economic status (SES) and obesity among men, women, and children. Reasons for the lower levels of obesity with higher social class may include dietary restraint, physical activity, social mobility, and inheritance. Jeffery et al. (1991) tried to establish how class relates to BMI, but SES remained a significant predictor of BMI after controlling for all measured health behaviours. Obesity and health behaviours that influence energy balance (diet, exercise, and dieting to lose weight) were examined in a population of several thousand working men and women in relation to SES. Body mass index, as expected, was found to be inversely related to SES. Higher SES was also associated with several behaviours that contribute importantly to energy balance, including a lower fat diet, more exercise, and a higher prevalence of dieting to control weight. However, lower smoking rates were observed in upper SES men and women, and higher alcohol consumption was reported in upper SES women. Both alcohol and tobacco associations appear to be inconsistent with the inverse association between SES and obesity.

Age differences. Across the life-span there is a tendency to increase fat stores in middle life and for this subcutaneous fat to be withdrawn in later life: This is seen as the characteristic "middle-age spread" and the loose skin folds of old age. Maintaining a moderate level of subcutaneous fat in later life may be protective against brittle bones.

Metabolic differences. Hereditary influences are relatively strong and appear to be partly related to levels of brown adipose tissue. This tissue has the effect of metabolising fat rapidly and releasing heat. The habitually thin person is likely to feel a rise in temperature after a large meal around the major sites of adipose tissue, notably on either side of the thoracic spine. A high thermic response to protein meals, though not necessarily to fat or carbohydrate meals, has been reported for lean subjects. This research cannot be interpreted to mean that obese people can maintain weight on a lower energy intake, according to the review by Garrow (1986). Metabolic disorders associated with lethargy and low activity level, such as hypothyroidism, tend to entail weight gain.

OVEREATING

Inactivity and overeating are the two main behavioural influences on weight, though heredity also has a strong influence. Eating disorders have been grouped into overeating, bulimia, and anorexia, though overeating and bulimia are now seen often to be linked. Anorexia nervosa involves fasting or food avoidance and requires interpersonal avoidance and needs for control that are rather beyond the scope of this book. A recent review can be found in Brownell and Foreyt (1986). Bulimia nervosa is a pattern of excessive eating alternating with purging; it may also be described as "compulsive eating", "dietary chaos syndrome", "bulimarexia", etc. (Wardle & Beinart, 1981). It was previously seen as an aspect of anorexia nervosa, but it is now seen as an eating pattern that is present in people of normal and obese weight, as well as underweight. Loro and Orleans (1981) made a special study of binge eating in 280 overweight adults attending a dietary rehabilitation clinic in the United States. Just over half the sample reported consuming "large or enormous quantities of food in short periods of time" at least once a week, and only 20% of respondents said that this never happened.

It has proved difficult to identify any consistent psychological patterns associated with overeating, so any of the following topics may be relevant in weight control programmes. Many factors hypothesised as causal in obesity, such as field dependence, lack of impulse control, inability to delay gratification, or a maladaptive eating style have not been supported by experimental evidence. Lack of emotional expression (alexithymia) in obese people is one of the stronger effects to emerge from the following research.

Hunger and craving. Lappalainen et al. (1990) suggest that the frequency of hunger and craving and reactivity to food stimuli decrease during fasting, but no changes occur during dieting. One group of fasting obese patients and one group of dieting obese patients were instructed to report their feelings of hunger and craving on a continuous basis before and during a three-week treatment period. Once a week they were also exposed to food slides to measure their reactivity to food stimuli. The frequency of hunger/craving responses and reactivity to food stimuli showed radically different changes over time in the fasting and dieting groups. During the last week of fasting, reactivity to food slides was completely abolished, and the frequency of hunger/craving responses was close to zero. Only slight changes of frequency of hunger/craving responses and reactivity to food stimuli were observed in the dieting group.

Portion cues. Most researchers have concluded that inaccurate estimation of portion size is a major problem in calorie restriction, but not noticeably worse in obese people. Portion estimation was studied by Blake, Guthrie, and Smiciklas-Wright (1989), who found no definitive differences in the ability of overweight and normal-weight subjects to estimate food portions accurately—serious errors were made by all subjects. The overweight sample was homogeneous as to education, income, and ethnicity.

Body image. Overweight subjects may be less accurate than normal-weight subjects in their perception of their own size. A video TV monitor was used with 42 obese and normal-weight subjects by Gardner et al. (1988). Subjects manipulated the width of their body image on TV. Subjects rated their full body, body regions that included face, waist, and thighs, and two inanimate control objects. Results from the continuous task revealed that obese subjects overestimated body size, and also the four body regions, more than did normals. Obese subjects were poorer at detecting size distortions of the body regions. They found thin/normal discrimination more difficult than heavy/normal discrimination. Using a modification of the distorting camera technique (Craig & Caterson, 1990), 50 obese women (BMI 35.1), 40 obese men (BMI 38.2), and their respective normal-weight controls estimated their body size. The obese women, control women, and obese men overestimated their body size, whilst control weight men were accurate. The control men were satisfied with their body size, control women were less so, and the obese were unsatisfied.

Locus of control. External locus of control has been hypothesised as a factor in bingeing and purging, but results are inconsistent. In research by Shisslak, Pazda, and Crago (1990), bulimic women from underweight ($n = 20$), normal-weight ($n = 31$), and overweight ($n = 22$) categories were compared with restrictor anorexics ($n = 20$), normal controls ($n = 31$), and obese subjects ($n = 22$). Bulimic women in all three weight categories, but especially in the underweight group, exhibited greater psychopathology, more external locus of control, lower self-esteem, and a lower sense of personal effectiveness than did non-bulimic women at similar weight levels. A contrasting result was found by Mills (1991), who used Rotter's I–E Control Scale with 18 men in residential treatment for alcoholism and 13 men in intensive outpatient treatment for obesity. The obese sample scored significantly higher in internal locus of control, whereas the alcoholic sample was comparatively external in control orientation.

Alexithymia. Raynes, Auerbach, and Botyanski (1989) present evidence for "psychic structural deficit" and "external regulation" in food addiction. Families of 22 moderately obese and 24 normal-weight subjects were compared using the Blatt family interaction questionnaire. The mean level of object representation of both parents was lower for the obese subjects than for the normal-weight subjects. This was interpreted as support for the view that "addicts" do not have adequate psychic structure with which to regulate painful affects internally and use, instead, their drug of choice as an external regulator to self-medicate painful affects. Clerici et al. (1992) studied alexithymic characteristics in a group of 106 massive obese patients who requested a surgical intervention. Six alexithymia variables were measured by Rorschach ink-blot protocols of patients, and a reference group of 600 nonpatients was studied. Findings supported the presence of a striking alexithymic element among severely obese patients in comparison with their lean counterparts. Legorreta, Bull, and Kiely (1988) report a similar study of two overweight groups (moderately and morbidly obese) of 95 subjects divided into three groups. The results revealed that the two obese groups were generally more alexithymic and had a greater inhibition of symbolic function than did normal-weight controls. Nevertheless, the two alexithymia measures used in this study disclosed inconsistent results.

Coping with stress. Some people eat more when they are unhappy, others eat less. The evidence that overeating is related to short-term fluctuations in stress is not strong. Sympathetic arousal tends to reduce appetite, and, indeed, pharmacological anorexic agents have used this effect. Rothschild, Peterson, and Pfeifer (1989) report some increased depression in young obese men. There was a weak positive correlation (0.4) between Beck Depression Inventory score and BMI, though the those in the overweight group were not clinically depressed on average. Rosenfield and Stevenson (1988) looked at "oral behaviours" (e.g., eating, drinking, smoking) in three groups of women, aged 25 to 45. Subjects included 37 female normal alcohol users of normal weight, 23 recovering alcoholics of normal weight, and 37 normal alcohol users who were 25 to 100% overweight. The normals responded to daily stress levels by changing their oral behaviours in predictable and consistent ways: On unpleasant days, the normals and the recovering alcoholic women ate more sweet, starchy, and salty/spicy foods. By contrast, the overweight women ate more food, especially salty/spicy and sweet foods, regardless of the type of day. Both alcoholics and overweight women desired to or engaged in their habituated oral behaviours regardless of fluctuating daily stress levels.

Social reward. Overweight people are seen as unattractive, and hence have less rewards from others. This may increase reliance on food as a reward. Peternelj-Taylor (1989) studied the affective neutrality of 100 senior female students in their practice of nursing and examined the effect of patient weight and sex on evaluations, attributions, and care delivery decisions formed by nurses. Obese patients were rated as significantly less attractive, but not held more responsible for presumed transgressions, so "mutual withdrawal" reported in other studies of nursing was not strongly evident. Inability to find rewarding social exchanges is probably related to the alexithymic trait described above.

WEIGHT MAINTENANCE

Determinants of body weight include age and heredity, but those that can be brought under personal control are dietary restraint, exercise level, and the establishment of new food cues.

Dietary restraint. Strategies for this may involve a huge variety of patent dietary programmes. Of those programmes requiring attendance, most use the behavioural principle of social reinforcement for weight loss. Commercial weight-reduction organisations mainly use this principle for the reinforcement of weight targets. "Weight Watchers", "Take Off Pounds Sensibly" (TOPS), "Silhouette Slimming Clubs", and others run several thousand classes per week between them. Other behavioural techniques that have been used in professional healthcare contexts are reviewed by Foreyt (1977) and include aversive techniques as well as reinforcement: "aversion-relief therapy", "assisted covert sensitisation", and "contingency contracting". Aversive stimuli have included foul-smelling substances or pictures of the overweight subject in underwear.

Continued participation in a weight-reduction class tends to go with continuing restraint, while those not able to restrain themselves are likely to drop out. Nir and Neumann (1991) followed 116 women who participated in a 10-week weight reduction programme and lost, on average, 7 kg. Subjects with low self-esteem scores lost significantly less weight than did subjects with medium and high scores (4.3 kg vs. 8.7 and 6.4, respectively). No significant differences were recorded between Internals and Externals, and variables such as marriage and number of children did not directly affect weight loss.

Exercise. The effect of low activity level on weight gain has created most concern in relation to children, who in recent years have been much less likely to walk to school. For adults, keep-fit or aerobics will have an effect on weight maintenance, but adherence is particularly difficult for women in middle life, who usually have substantial commitments of time. Gillett (1988) investigated the factors which would maintain regular exercise in overweight middle-aged women. In the study, 38 moderately overweight women participated in a 16-week dance exercise programme. Participants were randomly assigned to an experimental group ($n = 20$) that received intensity-controlled, graded exercise and individual and group reinforcement, or to a control group ($n = 18$) that exercised at a moderate intensity typical of commercial fitness classes and received no special reinforcement. In both groups, 94% of the women adhered to the program—an exceptionally high adherence rate for this population. Eight participant-identified factors seemed to have influenced exercise adherence:

- group homogeneity
- car-pooling and social networks
- pleasurable feelings associated with increased energy and fitness
- leader with a health-related background
- time limitation of exercise programme
- commitment to an established goal
- desire to change body image
- desire to change health status and improve physical health

New food cues. the long-term strategy for the person with a tendency to become overweight must be dietary re-education, combined with increased activity. Establishment of eating habits based on effective control of internal and external cues is needed. Nutritional awareness will usually entail a shift in food preferences away from fats and starches towards foods with higher bulk in relation to calorific value, and most of these are green vegetables. A change towards a high-vegetable diet will involve exploration of the range of tastes and giving sufficient time for the old taste preferences for sugars and fats to become aversive. Emphasis on food preparation will be needed to overcome the use of ready-to-eat foods: This may entail keeping a supply of washed and sliced vegetables in the refrigerator and carrying fruit on journeys.

SWALLOWING AND NAUSEA

The mouth. We use our teeth to break the food down into pieces small enough to swallow safely, and in so doing, we mix the food with saliva, which serves several functions. It lubricates dry food and adds a digestive enzyme that begins the process of breaking down starches into sugars; it also dissolves molecules of the food, permitting the taste-buds and the olfactory receptors to be stimulated.

Swallowing. The action of swallowing involves a wave of muscle contraction passing down the tube. Breathing, feeding, and speaking all involve the use of a single passage through the mouth and throat. Normally the sphincters of the larynx close when the swallowing reflex is initiated, to seal the airway so that food enters only the oesophagus. The movements of speech and swallowing occur with no awareness of the intricate muscular adaptations that are required, but sometimes after a stroke or other neurological injury one or other of these muscle movements is impaired. Logemann (1983) describes some of the techniques needed to restore feeding movements when some component of the swallowing reflex is absent: positioning of material in the mouth; manipulating it with the tongue; chewing a bolus of varying consistencies; recollecting food into a ball before swallowing; and organising peristalsis of the tongue to propel the bolus backwards. Such muscle movements can be retrained separately, rather than asking the sufferer to masticate and swallow normally, with the risk of aspirating food into the lungs.

Globus. Globus pharyngeus is the persistent sensation of a lump in the throat. The former name, "globus hystericus", implies the complex psychodynamic mechanisms of hysteria (see chapter 4). Heightened awareness of the throat is often associated with depression, so antidepressants may be prescribed. Globus is usually associated with strong emotion, and many globus sufferers say it disappears with crying. Schatzki (1964) proposed a plausible hypothesis mechanism for this sensation, as follows: Under tension, the person becomes aware of swallowing saliva, focuses on it, and swallows several times in quick succession; his mouth is thus dry, he has difficulty swallowing further, and he experiences this as a lump in the throat, with the consequent urge to swallow more. Up to a third of patients presenting with lump in the throat would on closer examination turn out to have hiatus hernia.

Vomiting. Being sick starts with a forceful closure of the pylorus, causing stomach contents to be pooled near the opening to the oesophagus. The diaphragm then descends, and the abdominus rectus muscles are forcefully contracted. This sequence of reflexes is controlled from a reflex centre in the medulla, but some of the components are under voluntary control. Thus people with bulimia can vomit with minimal stimulation, while those who have to pass naso-gastric tubes can learn to inhibit gagging. Nausea and vomiting occur as an adaptive response to infections, in bulimia, psychogenic vomiting, and conditioned nausea associated with chemotherapy for cancer. In childhood an association between vomiting and foods eaten during the previous 12 hours is very easily acquired, in a process that can be described as classical conditioning.

Nausea and chemotherapy. Drugs used in chemotherapy for cancer are highly likely to induce nausea, retching, and vomiting, and this makes adherence to this treatment particularly difficult. This emesis can be controlled by drugs such as metoclopramide, and also by smoking high-purity cannabis. Conditioning of anticipatory nausea is strong, and many nurses working with cytotoxic drugs have an anecdote about encountering a former patient in the street, who was promptly sick. Scott et al. (1986) compared relaxation training and metoclopramide in the management of emesis in 17 women receiving chemotherapy. Both groups had preparatory education, and relaxation consisted of progressive relaxation, slow-stroke back massage, and guided imagery. Those receiving the drug had fewer emetic episodes, but duration of emesis was shorter in the relaxation group. In addition, there was more urine and diarrhoea in the drug-treated patients. Acupressure above the wrist has been shown to counteract nausea during pregnancy or after surgery (see chapter 13).

Psychogenic vomiting. This occurs at mealtimes, is not preceded by nausea, and causes the patient hardly any concern. Little research has been done on it, but Hill and Blendis (1967) observed the following in 20 patients: strong antagonism to spouse; loss of parent in childhood; family and childhood history of vomiting. Hill concludes that psychogenic vomiters are shy individuals who cannot tolerate confrontation.

Rumination syndrome. Frequent regurgitation of food into the mouth, where it is chewed and re-swallowed or spat out is called "rumination"; "pica", on the other hand, involves the eating of inappropriate objects. Pica is relatively common in infancy and persists in a proportion of institutionalised people with learning difficulties, but it is also found in adults of normal intelligence. Because it is rare and occurs predominantly in infants and in persons with learning difficulties, there are no published studies in which psychometric tests were administered. Kanner, known for his work on autism, observed that anxiety or lack of parental attention may increase the frequency of rumination. Both punishment of regurgitation and use of increased "mothering" (i.e. holding the ruminating infant) have been used successfully to treat rumination in children. Rumination in adults has been treated with biofeedback.

Diffuse oesophageal spasm. Many gastroenterologists believe this to be exclusively a manifestation of underlying physical disease, but there are several reports in the older literature that objectively document the elicitation of oesophageal spasm by stressful interviews in patients who presented with dysphagia and chest pain. There is an association between oesophageal contraction abnormalities and psychiatric diagnoses of depression, generalised anxiety disorder, and panic disorder. Treatment of oesophageal spasm by means of progressive muscle relaxation training has been reported.

THE STOMACH AND ULCERATION

Once food is swallowed and enters the stomach, this organ begins to secrete hydrochloric acid and the enzyme pepsin. Hydrochloric acid breaks the food into small particles, and pepsin breaks proteins in the food into their constituent amino acids. The muscles in the wall of the stomach become active, churning the food so that it becomes well mixed with the digestive juices. The wall of the stomach contains stretch receptors and chemoreceptors. These receptors respond to the bulk and chemical nature of the contents of the stomach, and their activity plays a role in the control of the digestive processes. The receptors in the wall of the stomach also provide feedback to the brain and control food uptake.

Peptic ulcer disease may occur either in the stomach (gastric ulcers) or the duodenum. They can be painful, but the process of re-growth of the mucous lining is sufficiently rapid that ulcers will often disappear with a week or two of rest and appropriate diet. However, there is a serious risk of perforation, which is still an important cause of death, so prompt pharmacological treatment is given if there is evidence of bleeding from an ulcer. Prophylaxis is now effective with H_2-receptor-antagonist drugs such as ranetidine, or omeprazole which blocks acid secretion. A strong placebo effect with ulcers is described in chapter 13. Infections with organisms such as helicobacter may prolong ulceration, and antibiotics are sometimes used to control this bacterium, which apparently can survive in the stomach.

In the case of peptic ulcers, occupational stressors are well documented. Cobb and Rose (1973) found that incidence was twice as high in air-traffic controllers as in second-class airmen controls, and incidence correlated with traffic density. The association between ulcer risk and demand was replicated in air-traffic controllers by Grayman (1972). Ulcers are also prevalent in policemen, and higher in wartime, according to Pflanz (1971). However, ulcers in air-traffic controllers may be associated with use of alcohol to reduce arousal, rather than through direct psycho-physiological effects (see chapter 6). Ulcer-preventive therapy is practised with patients in intensive care, as in this situation ulcers would otherwise often develop, apparently because of the stressfulness of the procedures.

The psychoanalytic view of peptic ulcers taken by Franz Alexander, popular in the 1940s and reprinted in 1987, is of a sufferer with "dependency, and a craving to be fed". Some support for this view was found by Weiner et al. (1957), who selected the 15% highest and 15% lowest pepsinogen subjects. They separately identified immature dependency (which included paranoia and pseudo-masculinity) by projective tests, and they predicted hypo- (51% correct) and hyper-secretors (71% correct) of gastric acid. They picked the 10 most dependent, and predicted future development of ulcers, which was borne out in 7 out of 10 cases.

Ulcers were later thought to be a typical feature of "executive stress". Brady et al.'s (1958) "executive monkeys" had to press a key every 20 seconds to avoid shock. They developed gastric ulcers, while yoked controls did not. Weiss (1972) found the opposite trend with rats and inferred that "controllability" predicted less ulceration. A discussion of control and ulceration is found in chapter 3. Animal models are interesting, but two discrepancies arise between humans and other species: Of human ulcers, 75% are in the duodenum, and human ulcers are associated with increased acidity.

Behavioural approaches have been neglected since drug treatments have improved, but a treatment that would nowadays be called cognitive–behavioural was developed more than half a century ago by Chappell and Stevenson (1936). Patients were taught that there was a link (which was, properly speaking, hypothetical) between emotion and gastric secretion, and they were given a distraction strategy during worry. Following training, 31 out of 32 were symptom-free, compared to 2 out of 20 controls. Preventive approaches at the present time concentrate on relaxed digestion: leisurely meals in moderate quantities during low arousal. Alcohol and tobacco both aggravate the tendency to ulceration, but it is not clear that any other ingested substances do so to any great extent.

THE PANCREAS AND DIABETES

The pancreas communicates with the duodenum by means of the pancreatic duct. Pancreatic enzymes, insulin and glucagon, break down proteins, lipids, starch, and nucleic acids, thus continuing the digestive process. The pancreas also secretes bicarbonate, which neutralises stomach acid. Utilisation of glucose by muscle cells requires the hormone insulin, which is produced by beta cells in the pancreas. Diabetes is a disorder of glucose metabolism that is potentially controllable at several levels: Affluent sedentary lifestyles may be a contributory cause; emotional stress may exaggerate glucose control problems; and insulin adherence may create more problems to extroverts.

Affluence and inactivity. When diabetes manifests in adult life, some beta cells in the pancreas continue to work, so the patient may not need insulin treatment, at least for several years. It is therefore known as Non-Insulin-Dependent or Type II diabetes. There is no evidence of immune or viral cause in this type, but hereditary factors are strong. The indication that affluence is a contributory factor comes mainly from epidemiology, as shown by the following prevalence rates for Type II diabetes:

United States–Mexican immigrants	17%
United States as a whole	6.9%
Malta	7.7%
Asian immigrants to United Kingdom	10%
United Kingdom as a whole	2%
New Guinea Highlands	0%

The effect of migration to a more affluent country greatly increases diabetes risk. Inactive but well-fed populations have been shown in various studies to be 2 to 20 times more likely to develop Type II diabetes than are those of similar ethnicity who remain in the food-deprived country. This strongly suggests that the homeostatic mechanisms that regulate insulin production in relation to energy demand are being disrupted. A diet that is high in refined carbohydrates creates rapid surges and declines in glucose. However, high consumption of fats is more likely to predispose to diabetes than is consumption of refined sugar. Complex carbohydrates from vegetables take longer to metabolise, thereby prolonging the rate of absorption into the blood stream. The influences of fat, starches, and refined sugars on diabetes are overviewed by Truswell (1986). Higher exercise levels may be valuable in prevention, by making sustained demands for glucose.

Personality and adherence. The requirement of matching dietary intake and insulin dose is quite demanding, and personality adjustments are to be expected. Bradley and Cox (1982) report that introverted persons are more likely to achieve balanced intake, and also to maintain sterile procedures. Bradley found a significant correlation of 0.51 between average blood glucose and the diabetic's extroversion score on the Maudsley Personality Inventory. The lifestyle of a highly social person is somewhat incompatible with the requirement to timetable food and insulin. It is likely that this higher blood glucose reflects the lower priority given to glucose regulation by the extrovert.

Stress and brittle control. It seems plausible that diabetics can utilise more of their blood glucose during stressful conditions. The possible role of emotional stress in precipitating episodes of keto-acidosis in insulin-dependent diabetes has attracted considerable research attention. Vandenbergh, Sussmann, and Vaughan (1967) induced emotion in diabetic subjects by hypnotic means, and by creating anticipation of electric shock. They reported finding decreases in blood glucose without increases in urinary glucose excretion, and some increase in free fatty acids. Vandenbergh and Sussmann went on to look at glucose levels in insulin-dependent diabetics during the naturally occurring stress of examinations. There were significant decreases in blood glucose during the pre-exam and exam weeks compared with a control week, and in five of the six students the decrease in blood glucose correlated positively with increased anxiety. Noise can be used to induce stress, and Bradley, Cox, and Mackay (1975) used this approach in studying the performance of insulin-dependent diabetic males. Diabetics who started with low blood glucose (below 180 mg%) showed a further fall in blood glucose. This was similar to Vandenbergh's finding, but diabetics whose glucose was initially above 180 mg% showed an *increase* in blood glucose, and performance dropped slightly during noise. Unger (1976) has argued that glucagon is the factor which mediates the unexplained fluctuations in blood glucose in early-onset diabetics. Levine (1976) cites studies showing that glucagon only leads to high blood glucose in diabetics deprived of insulin. In healthy subjects glucagon secretion in response to stress such as noise would, in turn, stimulate insulin secretion. In diabetics, however, the insulin response would be insufficient, so blood glucose would continue to rise through failure of the negative feedback loop.

THE INTESTINES

The meal passes through the small intestine, where most of the available nutrients are absorbed; the residue enters the large intestine. Hardly any nutrients are absorbed in the large intestine, but water and electrolytes are re-absorbed there. The stomach empties into the duodenum, the upper portion of the small intestine. The rate of gastric emptying is controlled by the composition of nutrients received by the duodenum. The walls of the duodenum contain chemoreceptors that regulate gastric activity by means of neural reflexes and by the release of various hormones. Proteins and carbohydrates are much more readily digested, so the duodenum permits the stomach to empty more quickly when it contains a meal that is low in fats. As the products of digestion begin to be absorbed into the bloodstream and as the acid is neutralised by the bicarbonate, the stomach empties more of its contents into the duodenum. In the digestive system, carbohydrates are broken down into simple sugars, and proteins are broken down into amino acids. These water-soluble nutrients enter the capillaries of the intestinal villi— finger-like structures that protrude into the interior of the intestine. These capillaries drain into the hepatic portal system and reach the liver before reaching any other portion of the body.

Fats are not soluble in water and must be emulsified before they can be absorbed. Emulsification refers to the breakdown of the globules into tiny particles. In the digestive system, emulsification is accomplished by bile—a substance produced by the liver and stored in the gallbladder. The duodenal receptors also stimulate secretion of the peptide hormone cholecystokinin (CCK), which causes the gallbladder to contract, releasing bile into the duodenum. When chemoreceptors in the duodenum detect the presence of fats, they initiate the secretion of CCK, which causes bile to be released into the intestine. Emulsified fats are absorbed into the intestinal capillaries that eventually empty the fats, via the lymph duct, into veins in the neck. There is a strong correlation between fat intake and national incidence rates for various cancers. The correlation is above 0.9 for cancers of the breast, prostate, and small intestine (Creasey, 1985).

The normal processes of peristalsis and absorption of food and water in the bowels can be interrupted by inflammatory bowel disease (IBD). Ulcerative colitis is the more common form of IBD, with a prevalence of 1.17%, while Crohn's disease, which involves thickening of the intestinal wall, has a prevalence of 0.34%. In considering the psychophysiology of colitis, the sequence of cause and effect is critical. The disorders discussed in this book always present a similar problem: Do pain, anxiety, and emotionality cause the disorder, or are these psychological states a result of a previously existing physical lesion? This question is particularly critical in relation to problems of digestion, and in colitis the direction of cause and effect is still a wide-open question. Patients with IBD show high levels of anxiety, depression, and hypochondriacal concern, but less than IBS patients, and similar to those with low back pain (Timmermans & Sternback, 1974). IBD patients do not see themselves as exposed to more stressors than do others (e.g. Fava & Pavan, 1976/77).

The psychoanalytic view of the Chicago school (e.g. Alexander, Engel) was that the IBD patient was emotionally dependent on the mother, so that symptoms arise at threatened separations. Engel (1955) claimed to have analysed a series of patients to the extent that colitis disappeared entirely. It could be argued that social conformity and inhibition works against reporting distress; IBD could be seen as at the repressed pole in Bahnson's repression-projection dimension in chapter 4 (see Figure 4.1). Two cases of inflammatory bowel disease treated by the author will illustrate this question:

Mr C was 22 when seen in hospital, where he had been admitted following increasingly painful diarrhoea and vomiting. The gastroenterologist gave a provisional diagnosis of Crohn's disease but included irritable bowel syndrome as an alternative. Mr C was treated with steroid drugs, and the more extreme symptoms remitted within two weeks. In hospital he had shown marked social avoidance, despite evidence that he was fairly intelligent, so psychological referral was initiated. His work was in the same unskilled post he had held for four years, and he had not progressed into skilled training in his work, suggesting some lack of assertion; he described digestive pain as arising during banter among his work-mates or when he had to see his supervisor. On psychometric testing his intelligence was found to be average, so he should easily have coped with the demands of a trade or more skilled occupation. Therapy consisted mainly of assertion training, involving the use of height, posture, and especially eye-contact. He became considerably more confident with male colleagues at his workplace and started study at an evening class, though he still had not progressed to a more satisfactory career by the end of treatment. Social avoidance was linked with retreats to the toilet in this case.

Mr D had chronic ulcerative colitis and worked hard to identify precipitants for relapses: He was knowledgeable about medication, was extremely careful about foods and alcohol, and had managed to give up smoking. Despite this, his unpredictable exacerbations caused him to spend several months each year in hospital for treatment. This made it impossible for him to keep a salaried job and severely restricted his social life. At the age of 42, he lived at his parents' home. He asked his GP for a psychological referral, and completed the Meichenbaum coping skills profile described in chapter 3, on life events. His answers here indicated much less depression and anger than in most men of his age, and only slight anxiety. He could be appropriately assertive and communicate in embarrassing situations, and he showed good instrumental skills. He could also relax and use other palliative strategies when needed, though some additional techniques were suggested for times of early colitis symptoms. It seemed unlikely that overt emotional stress was a significant contributor to his colitis, though it could be argued that there was covert avoidance of separation.

Both improved psychologically with training in coping skills, and this appeared to be accompanied by a reduction in digestive pain and diarrhoea. The real problem is to know whether the physical improvement was a consequence of psychological change or part of the random fluctuation of an organic disease of the colon. There is no easy way of answering that question. Whitehead and Schuster (1985) found themselves unable to decide on the psychophysiology of ulcerative colitis. The sensible approach seems to be to treat psychosocial problems and suspend judgement on their possible significance for the colon.

DEFAECATION

The final phase in the digestive process is elimination of residue via the anus. This is normally initiated by relaxation of the anal sphincter in response to sensed pressure in the rectum. Two problems may occur in this process, which are both amenable to behavioural management: irritable bowel and faecal incontinence.

Irritable bowel syndrome (IBS) is a diagnostic term used to describe pain and problems with defaecation. This term is mainly applied by gastroenterologists after exclusion of other diagnoses, so it has tended to be a rather vague descriptor of unwell feelings. The definition has been tightened recently (Whitehead, 1992) and now refers to pain that is relieved by defaecation or associated with variation in stools and lasting for more than three months. IBS must also include variation at least 25% of the time in at least two of the following: stool frequency, hardness or softness, straining or urgency, passage of mucus, or bloating. Prevalence is very high in the general population, since 12.8% of adults would agree to these symptoms.

There is no gross pathology in IBS. There may be changes in sensory receptors in particular portions of the bowel, so that pain is felt on slight pressure from food. Insertion into the rectum of an inflatable balloon to cause pressure elicits pain at some points and not at others, suggesting hypersensitivity of receptors in IBS (Dawson, 1985). Such sensitivity to pain is often associated with anxiety (see chapter 13), but IBS patients were not more sensitive to aversive stimuli applied to the skin. Of IBS patients, 50–75% score at caseness level on psychometric tests—usually anxiety and depression—but there are no particular distinctive patterns of moods. Half of patients report that stress exacerbates symptoms, and half report an acute stress episode prior to first onset. (Hislop, 1971). Remote trauma, including loss of a parent and sexual abuse in childhood, are reported more frequently by IBS patients than by other medical patients (Whitehead, 1992). However, the association between neurotic traits and IBS has been in people who consult. In two community samples reported by Whitehead, 70% or more of people who meet IBS criteria had not consulted. Anxiety is therefore more strongly linked with treatment-seeking than IBS.

Despite the prevalence of IBS, few controlled treatment trials had been carried out prior to 1980. Svedlund et al. (1983) randomly assigned 101 IBS patients either to medical therapy or to psychotherapy plus medical therapy. Medical therapy consisted of bulk laxatives, anticholinergics (to reduce spasm), and minor tranquillisers. Psychotherapy consisted of 10 one-hour sessions, aimed at monitoring of stress cues and developing alternative coping strategies. Eleven months after treatment, the psychotherapy group had significantly less abdominal pain. Systematic desensitisation, hypnosis, and dynamic psychotherapy have each been reported as effective, and more controlled studies are under way. Bennett (1987) and Thornton (1985) provide reviews of IBS treatments in a British context.

Faecal incontinence in adults has long been suspected to occur because of impairment of rectal sensation, and this has now been demonstrated by controlled studies. Other contributory causes are weak sphincter control, but leakage associated with faecal impaction can also occur. Biofeedback using transducers from balloons placed in the anal canal has proved to be a very effective behavioural treatment, according to Whitehead (1992), and it seems to be equally effective with elderly patients. Constipation is also subject to behavioural approaches, since it is commonly associated with inability to relax pelvic floor muscles.

CONCLUSION

Eating is influenced by needs for wholesomeness, control, comfort, relaxation, social contact, and body image, as well as nutrition. Problems of excess in eating are now more problematic than are those of deficiency. Behavioural influences on digestion are strong, both through parasympathetic effects and through eating habits. Excessive arousal can lead to inflammation or ulceration of smooth muscle, and to vomiting. Problems of excess apply to fats more than to starches and sugars, and a high proportion of fats in the diet can contribute to ulceration, cancer, and diabetes. Behavioural strategies can contribute to restoring normal function at every stage of food digestion.

REFERENCES

Alexander, F. (1987). *Psychosomatic medicine.* London: Norton.

Bennett, P. (1987). Psychological aspects of physical illness: Irritable bowel syndrome. *Nursing Times, 83* (46), 51–53.

Blake A.J., Guthrie, H.A., & Smiciklas-Wright, H. (1989). Accuracy of food portion estimation by overweight and normal-weight subjects. *Journal of the American Dietetic Association, 89* (7), 962–964.

Bradley, C., & Cox, T. (1982). Stress and health. In T. Cox, *Stress* (pp. 91–111). London: Macmillan.

Bradley, C., Cox, T., & Mackay, C.J. (1975). The effects of stress on the regulation of blood glucose levels. Cited in T. Cox, *Stress.* London: Macmillan, 1982.

Brady, J.V, Porter, R.W., Conrad, D.G., & Mason, J.W. (1958). Avoidance behaviour and the development of gastroduodenal ulcers. *Journal of the Experimental Analysis of Behaviour, 1,* 69–72.

Brownell, K.D., & Foreyt, J.P. (1986). *Handbook of eating disorders.* New York: Basic Books.

Chappell, M.N., & Stevenson, T.I. (1936). Group psychological training in some organic conditions. *Mental Hygiene, 20,* 588–597.

Clerici, M., Albonetti, S., Papa, R., Penati, G., & Invernizzi, G. (1992). Alexithymia and obesity. Study of the impaired symbolic function by the Rorschach test. *Psychotherapy and Psychosomatics, 57* (3), 88–93.

Cobb, S., & Rose, R.M. (1973). Hypertension, peptic ulcer, and diabetes in air traffic controllers. *Journal of the American Medical Association, 224,* 489–492.

Craig, P.L., & Caterson, I.D. (1990). Weight and perceptions of body image in women and men in a Sydney sample. *Community Health Studies, 14* (4), 373–383.

Creasey, W.A. (1985). *Diet and cancer.* Philadelphia, PA: Lea & Febiger.

Dawson, A.M. (1985). Origin of pain in the irritable bowel syndrome. In N. Read (Ed.), *The irritable bowel syndrome* (pp. 155–162). London: Grune & Stratton.

Engel, G.L. (1955). Studies of ulcerative colitis. III. The nature of the psychologic processes. *American Journal of Medicine, 17,* 231–256.

Fava, G.A., & Pavan, L. (1976/77). Large bowel disorders. I. Illness configuration and life events. *Psychotherapy and Psychosomatics, 27,* 93–99.

Foreyt, J. (Ed.) (1977). *Behavioural treatments of obesity*. Oxford: Pergamon.

Gardner, R.M., Martinez, R., Espinoza, T., & Gallegos, V. (1988). Distortion of body image in the obese: A sensory phenomenon. *Psychological Medicine, 18* (3), 633–641.

Garrow, J. (1986). Exercise, diet and thermogenesis. *Current Concepts in Nutrition, 15,* 51–65.

Gillett, P.A. (1988). Self-reported factors influencing exercise adherence in overweight women. *Nursing Research, 37* (1), 25–29.

Grayman, R.R. (1972). Air controllers syndrome: Peptic ulcer in air traffic controllers. *Illinois Medical Journal, 142,* 111–115.

Hill, O.W., & Blendis, L. (1967). Physical and psychological evaluation of "nonorganic" abdominal pain. *Gut, 8,* 221–229.

Hislop, I.G. (1971). Psychological significance of the irritable colon syndrome. *Gut, 12,* 452–457.

Jeffery, R.W., French, S.A., Forster, J.L., & Spry, V.M. (1991). Socioeconomic status differences in health behaviors related to obesity: The Healthy Worker Project. *International Journal of Obesity, 15* (10), 689–696.

Lappalainen, R., Sjoden, P.O., Hursti, T., & Vesa, V. (1990). Hunger/craving responses and reactivity to food stimuli during fasting and dieting. *International Journal of Obesity, 14* (8), 679–688.

Legorreta, G., Bull, R.H., & Kiely M.C. (1988). Alexithymia and symbolic function in the obese. *Psychotherapy and Psychosomatics, 50* (2), 88–94.

Levine, R. (1976). Glucagon and the regulation of blood sugar. *The Lancet, 294,* 494.

Ley, P. (1980). The psychology of obesity: Its causes, consequences and control. In S. Rachman (Ed.), *Contributions to medical psychology, Vol. 2.* Oxford: Pergamon.

Logemann, J.A. (1983). *Evaluation and treatment of swallowing disorders.* San Diego: College-Hill Press.

Loro, A.D., Jr, & Orleans, C.S. (1981). Binge eating in obesity: Preliminary findings and guidelines for behavioural analysis and treatment. *Addictive Behaviours, 6,* 155–166.

Mills, J. (1991). Control orientation as a personality dimension among alcoholic and obese adult men undergoing addictions treatment. *Journal of Psychology, 125* (5), 537–542.

Nir, Z., & Neumann, L. (1991). Self-esteem, internal-external locus of control, and their relationship to weight reduction. *Journal of Clinical Psychology, 47* (4), 568–575.

Peternelj-Taylor, C.A. (1989). The effects of patient weight and sex on nurses' perceptions: A proposed model of nurse withdrawal. *Journal of Advanced Nursing, 14* (9), 744–754.

Pflanz, M. (1971). Epidemiological and sociocultural factors in the aetiology of duodenal ulcer. *Advances in Psychosomatic Medicine, 6,* 121–151.

Raynes, E., Auerbach, C., Botyanski, N.C. (1989). Level of object representation and psychic structure deficit in obese persons. *Psychological Reports, 64* (1), 291–294.

Rosenfield, S.N., & Stevenson, J.S. (1988). Perception of daily stress and oral coping behaviors in normal, overweight, and recovering alcoholic women. *Research In Nursing and Health, 11* (3), 165–174.

Rothschild, M., Peterson H.R., & Pfeifer, M.A. (1989). Depression in obese men. *International Journal of Obesity, 13* (4), 479–485.

Schatzki, R. (1964). Globus hystericus (globus sensation). *New England Journal of Medicine, 270,* 676.

Scott, D.W., Donahue, D.C., Mastrovito, R.C., & Hakes, T.B. (1986). Comparative trial of clinical relaxation and an antiemetic drug regimen in reducing chemotherapy-related nausea and vomiting. *Cancer Nursing, 9* (4), 178–187.

Seim, H.C., & Fiola, J.A. (1990). A comparison of attitudes and behaviors of men and women toward food and dieting. *Family Practice Research Journal, 10* (1), 57–63.

Shisslak, C., Pazda, S., & Crago, M. (1990). Body weight and bulimia as discriminators of psychological characteristics among anorexic, bulimic, and obese women. *Journal of Abnormal Psychology, 99* (4), 380–384.

Sobal, J., & Stunkard, A. (1989). Socioeconomic status and obesity: A review of the literature. *Psychological Bulletin, 105* (2), 260–275.

Svedlund, J., Sjodin, I., Ottoson, J.O., & Dotevall, G. (1983). Controlled study of psychotherapy in irritable bowel syndrome. *Acta Psychiatrica Scandinavia* (suppl.), *306,* 1–86.

Thornton, S. (1985). Irritable bowel syndrome. In S. Pearce & J. Wardle, *The practice of behavioural medicine.* Leicester: British Psychological Society.

Timmermans, G., & Sternback, A. (1974). Factors of human chronic pain: An analysis of personality and pain reaction variables. *Science, 184,* 806–808.

Truswell, A.S. (1986). *ABC of nutrition.* (reprinted from the *British Medical Journal*). London: British Medical Association.

Unger, R.H. (1976). Diabetes and the alpha cell. *Diabetes, 25,* 136.

Vandenbergh, R.L., Sussmann, K.E., & Vaughan, G.D. (1967). Effects of combined physical-anticipatory stress on carbohydrate-lipid metabolism in patients with diabetes mellitus. *Psychosomatics, 8,* 16.

Wadden, T., Foster, G., Stunkard, A.J., & Linowitz, J. (1989). Dissatisfaction with weight and figure in obese girls: Discontent but not depression. *International Journal of Obesity, 13* (1), 89–97.

Wardle, J., & Beinart (1981). Binge eating: A theoretical review. *British Journal of Clinical Psychology, 20,* 97–109.

Weiner, H., Thaler, M., Reiser, M., & Mirsky, I. (1957). Etiology of duodenal ulcer. I. Relation of specific psychological characteristics to rate of gastric secretion (serum pepsinogen). *Psychosomatic Medicine, 19,* 1–10.

Weiss, J.M. (1972). Influence of psychological variables on stress-induced pathology. In R. Porter & J. Knight (Eds.), *Physiology, emotion, and psychosomatic illness* (CIBA Foundation Symposium 8). New York: Elsevier.

Whitehead, W.E. (1992). Behavioral medicine approaches to gastrointestinal disorders. *Journal of Consulting and Clinical Psychology, 60* (4), 605–612.

Whitehead, W.E., & Schuster, M.M. (1985). *Behavioral approach to gastrointestinal diseases.* London: Academic Press.

12

Movement

This chapter is concerned with maintaining suppleness of the musculo-skeletal system, particularly the spine. Movement is experienced in youth as effortless, free from pain, and requiring no forethought. With age and various sorts of degeneration, movement becomes increasingly difficult. Some of the disability that accompanies a "bad back" or stiff joints can be prevented if the mechanics of the body are understood and maintained. Overuse of particular musculoskeletal structures in the course of work is another cause of loss of movement, and much of this can be prevented by good ergonomic design of workplaces. This chapter concentrates on the following aspects of normal movement: providing knowledge on optimum biomechanics; ergonomic design; and maintaining suppleness in later life.

THE SPINE

The spine is a column of separate bones buffered by discs that cushion the rigid vertebrae and permit a small amount of movement. In the chest area the vertebrae form a relatively robust structure in conjunction with the ribs, but the lower back and neck have no collateral bony structures, so these areas are vulnerable to misuse. The lumbar spine is particularly at risk, and this may be partly understood by thinking of its evolutionary context. The human skeleton is essentially similar to that of other primates, which move on four limbs most of the time. In quadrupedal movement, the weight of the chest and head are taken on the front legs; in bipedal movement, the lumbar spine has to act as "scaffolding" for all the movements of the upper body. The evolutionary adaptations of the primate body for bipedal movement are mainly an increase in size of particular muscles, notably the gluteals or buttocks, without much change in the skeleton. Considerable flexing is needed between the lumbar vertebrae for bending, and most of the fixation against lateral movement has to be provided by relatively weak structures such as the erector spinae muscle.

The optimum configuration for the spine for sitting and bipedal walking is thought to be an S-shape when viewed from the side, with weight distributed symmetrically to left and right. One curve of the S is towards the front in the lower back, and the other curve is rearwards at the base of the neck. In this configuration the centre of the skull is directly above the centre of the pelvis, so that most of the weight of the upper body is supported by bones (see Figure 12.1). However, many positions that feel "comfortable" involve the use of relatively weak muscles to support weight, with a consequent risk of strain. The indent in the lower spine, or lumbar lordosis, is quite counter-intuitive to many people, and many settees, bucket chairs, and so forth tend to create an opposite, C-shaped curvature. The load-bearing structure of the neck is also a single column of bone and is vulnerable to excessive forward and rotatory forces and poor neck posture.

WORKPLACE ERGONOMICS

The design of workplaces suitable for the human body is given the name "biological ergonomics". General principles are reviewed by Wilson and Corlett (1990), and occupational therapists use such principles in recommending aids and appliances for various kinds of disability. The EEC rulings on health and safety at work, which have led to regulations in each member state, speak mainly of "workplace organisation", rather than giving very detailed rulings about ergonomics. Each workplace should have the organisation of its tasks assessed and approved by an appropriately trained person. Many people now work at desks or in seated positions, using a limited number of muscles. Only ergonomic features of sedentary work are described here. A support for sitting that minimises muscle work will have the following features:

- a convex seatback to prompt lordosis

- seat height that allows feet to be placed flat on the floor while supporting thighs

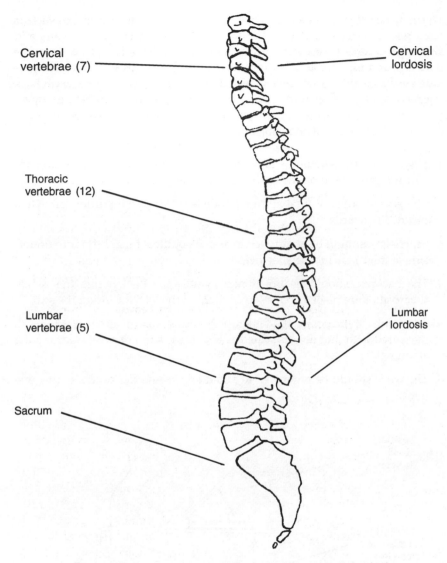

Cervical vertebrae (7)

Cervical lordosis

Thoracic vertebrae (12)

Lumbar vertebrae (5)

Lumbar lordosis

Sacrum

Figure 12.1 The spinal column, showing optimum lordosis

- seat depth that allows seat back to be reached with most of thigh supported
- seat back that allows arms to be rested, with elbows not restricted
- arm rests that allow elbows to rest at about a right angle

This may be regarded as a good chair for leisure use, though features such as head rest and arm rests are less suitable for work chairs. Balans chairs and similar structures take weight at the shin and lower thigh rather than the buttocks, and these tend to prompt lower lumbar lordosis. Such chairs provide an alternative for protracted seated work for those with long-term back injuries. Bendix (1986) recommends the following chair and table adjustments for a seated work station (see Figure 12.2); the principles involved combine biomechanical and subjective aspects:

1. Highest priority should be given to a mobile, slanting desk, inclining 35–45°, and positioned on the horizontal tabletop.

2. The seat should be tiltable and upholstered to avoid sliding off when inclined forwards.

3. Seat height should be about 3–5 cm above popliteal height (floor to underside of thigh), including shoe heels.

4. The backrest should be positioned against the back while the ischial tuberosities are placed about 4–6 cm behind the axis for tilting the seat.

5. The height of the horizontal tabletop should be 4–6 cm above elbow level, measured with the subjects seated as above, the shoulders relaxed, and the elbows at 90°.

6. The work should be organised to avoid any seated period exceeding one hour.

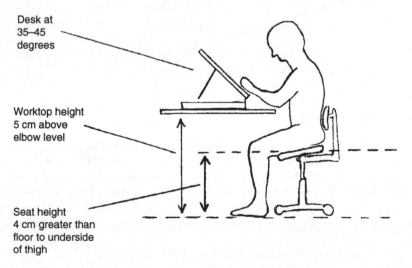

Desk at 35–45 degrees

Worktop height 5 cm above elbow level

Seat height 4 cm greater than floor to underside of thigh

Figure 12.2 Sitting at a workstation (redrawn from Bendix, 1986)

BACK INJURIES

Low back pain is the commonest source of disability and absence from work. Back injuries are estimated to cost the UK health service 764,000 working days a year, so safe lifting of patients should receive a high priority (Health Services Advisory Committee, 1992). A postal survey was undertaken by the author and Bereszczak of 1 in 300 people on the electoral register for wards within Dudley health authority, and some 250 usable responses were received. This found that 25% of respondents admitted to some degree of back pain, and this was four times the level of the next-most-frequent problem.

Injuries to the back at the level of the lumbar spine include:

- *support muscles tear*—the most frequent reason for back pain

- *facet joint injury* creating friction

- *slipped disc* prolapse of intervertebral disc—well known, but actually not a common cause

- *inflammation pressing on a sensory nerve root* may occur with prolapse or facet joint injury; this can cause referred pain, e.g. in the legs, known as "sciatica"

- *intervertebral disc* wear, causing bone-to-bone contact, as in arthritis

Each of these injuries tends to have ramifying effects. Each is likely to give rise to an involuntary protective spasm of surrounding muscles, experienced as "the back locking". Any pain is likely to give rise to a protective stance, which often means leaning to one side and forward. This will, in time, lead to further muscle pain, often well away from the original injury. For example, a person who has developed a lop-sided gait when using a walking-stick following a lower back injury may some years later experience pain in the neck.

BACK SCHOOLS

An increasingly popular early remedy for back problems is an educational approach, intended to allow the sufferer to optimise use of the body to reduce further problems. Although physiotherapy strategies had involved an educational approach for many years, the Swedish Back School (Forssell, 1980) is generally regarded as the first explicit use of this term. The system introduced at Danderyd Hospital near Stockholm in 1970 is now widely used. Some of the principles are:

- *Fitness to start.* Training is appropriate for back sufferers (called "students") with chronic or recurrent pain. Sudden pain or spasms will not be alleviated by this approach, and anti-inflammatory drugs and bed rest may be more appropriate.

- *Coping skills.* Students need to be committed to the development of knowledge and skills that will help them cope alone and avoid resorting to passive treatments by doctor or physiotherapist. Forssell's school requires patients to undergo a test at completion.

- *Teaching.* Four 45-minute sessions over two weeks are supervised by a physiotherapist. A videotape, plastic skeleton, and flip charts are used to teach anatomy and function of the back.

- *Psoas position.* This is regarded as the most restful and involves the sufferer lying on the back, with lower legs supported above floor level. Students adopt this, rather than sitting, during the first lesson. This can be used during exacerbations of pain.

- *Lordosis and symmetry.* The general aim is to use the S-shaped spine, without excessive effort on one side. Sitting should use a front or back rest, for short periods only. Standing with a forward lean is to be avoided unless the body can be supported.

- *Quadriceps use.* The thigh muscles are very strong by comparison with the weak spinal support muscles. A lifting action that involves bending at the knee, keeping a straight back, and standing close to the load is modelled and reinforced—for example, for lifting a child.

- *Abdominal strengthening.* The abdominal or tummy muscles are also fairly weak in most people, but they can be strengthened through isometric exercises such as pelvic tilting so that they form a brace for the lumbar spine. This takes about 40 seconds and is seen as homework for the rest of students' lives. Pool use is recommended for early phases of treatment.

A follow-up of 140 patients who had attended Danderyd Hospital at various times up to eight years previously was carried out; 75% of respondents to the questionnaire said that knowledge of anatomy had prompted them to change their working positions. A subsequent controlled prospective study of back schools for Volvo employees allowed comparison with manual physiotherapy and placebo treatment. The back school reduced absence from work, and the school and physiotherapy both had superior results to the placebo for low back pain. A back school was used by Von Hagen and Hierholzer (1991) in the treatment of 214 patients with vertebral fractures. Tests of knowledge and behaviour were held by the authors to be superior to physiotherapy alone. Klaber Moffett et al. (1986) examined the efficacy of a back school at the Nuffield Orthopaedic centre by comparison with an exercise-only control group. In this study, 78 patients were involved, with an average history of seven years' back pain. Levels of pain and functional disability were assessed, and both groups showed improvement after six weeks. At 16 weeks, patients who had attended the back school had significantly less pain and less disability.

Stankovic and Johnell (1990) compared a mini back school method with McKenzie exercises in the treatment of acute low back pain. (The exercises developed by the New Zealand physiotherapist Robin McKenzie, 1981, 1985, are intended to centralise posture and maintain lordosis.) This study involved 100 patients, all in work, mostly male, and with an average age of 34. The McKenzie methods were found to give better results on return to work, length of sick-leave during first occurrence, pain, pain recurrences during the next year, and movement. Patients' ability to self-help and sick leave during recurrences were found to be similar in the two groups.

Lindstrom et al. (1992) examined the effect of graded activity and an operant conditioning behavioural approach on Volvo employees with subacute low back pain. Patients were examined by an orthopaedic surgeon and a social worker and randomly assigned to an activity group ($n = 51$) or a control group ($n = 52$). The activity programme involved measurements of functional capacity, a work-place visit, back school education, and an individually tailored sub-maximal exercise programme. Tests of functional capacity included forward, lateral, and backward bending, active leg raising, spinal rotation, walking, stair-climbing, and pulling and pushing. Endurance time for back and abdominal muscles and endurance on a stationary bicycle were calculated. The operant principles advocated by Fordyce (1976) were used: The therapist chooses activity carefully and shows the patient that it is safe to do the exercise. Individual tailoring meant that most patients performed abdominal and back muscle exercises during treatment before return to work, and a fifth used jogging as well. The activity group had an average of 10.7 appointments with a physiotherapist. The average duration of sick leave attributable to low back pain in the second follow-up year was 12.1 weeks, compared with 19.6 weeks in the control group.

FEAR OF PAIN

This is the theory advanced by Lethem et al. (1983) to account for individual differences in low back pain. Many individuals confront pain, which usually results in progressive resumption of social activities as the organic basis of the back injury subsides. Avoidance, by contrast, promotes the development of invalid status and exaggerated pain perception. Several surveys have found an increased incidence of stressful life events prior to the injury, which tend to dispose the individual to avoidance. The back injury then entails time off work and fewer demands, so that confrontation of ordinary stressors becomes increasingly frightening.

Low back pain is also often associated with depression. It is not immediately clear whether the depressed mood is the consequence or cause of pain. Atkinson et al. (1988) investigated stressful life events and depressed mood in patients with chronic backache. The 15 patients with depression reported significantly more untoward life events and ongoing life difficulties than the 17 with back pain but no depression or the 19 controls. This finding would separate pain from depression, as the latter is well known to be associated with number of life events and chronic difficulties (Brown & Harris, 1978). A major reason for failure to resume normal activity after back injury is fear of pain. Many sufferers see the continuing pain as an indication of imminent fracture and are reluctant to continue. Several remedial approaches use paced activity and tolerance for pain as the basis of rehabilitation.

The *"school for bravery"* is a concept coined in the Doncaster physiotherapy department. Williams (1989) describes the current practice, which combines a carefully progressed gymnasium programme with behaviour modification. This approach regards much back pain as illness behaviour, though Williams also uses mathematical catastrophe theory to model the problem. Some of the observable chronic pain and illness behaviours reported by Williams are:

- use of *pain gestures* to indicate suffering—e.g. clutching the part, wiping brow
- *lack of eye contact*
- *stooping depressed postures*
- *expressionless, unsmiling faces*
- *look much older than their years*
- *overt badges of invalidism*—collars, sticks, wheelchairs
- *complaints of dizziness*, even staggering, without actually falling

Gait patterns are quite abnormal, and may be seen as a penguin waddle:

- *absence of rotation* of head, trunk, and body
- *arms held to the side*
- *no arm swing*

The school for bravery typically lasts three weeks. Most patients are expected to show normal movements by the end of the second week and are unlikely to achieve normalisation if they have not and the course is further protracted; however, some patients with "psychiatric background" seem to benefit in six weeks or so. The school has the following elements:

- *Reducing fear by authoritative suggestion.* To the complaint, "It hurts", the therapist may reply, "Yes, it should when you start using your muscles again". Pain is presented as a challenge, as it is to an athlete. Anatomy is not taught in this approach, as it is thought to heighten pain awareness.

- *Confidence building.* Tiny progressive exercise steps are prescribed. Verbal reinforcement is given by constant compliments on the patient's looks, bravery, and willingness to "have a go".

- *Reducing pain behaviours, increasing wellness behaviours.* This may include the staff keeping their hands in their pockets when the patient staggers, or playing badminton so that gait has to become freer.

In Salford, near Manchester, Christopher Main uses a pain management programme that includes paced activity and other elements appropriate to this chapter (Waddell & Main, 1984). Main's programme includes paced activity in combination with self-hypnosis and controlled use of analgesics. The main target is usually number of steps per day. This may be as few as 1000, which might include two or three times up the stairs in a day for basic self-care, and one walk to the shops. The principle is to try to maintain this level of activity independent of pain, rather than be guided by "good and bad days". Over a period of weeks muscle strength should build, without the relapses caused by overexertion when pain seems lower. The effects of such pain programmes may be to increase movement and independence, rather than pain per se. Spinhoven and Linssen (1989) used education and self-hypnosis with 45 back pain sufferers in a Dutch university hospital. Significant improvements in the 31 who persevered were found in depression, up-time, and medication use, but not in pain intensity.

OVERUSE (REPETITIVE STRAIN) INJURY

Intense use of particular muscles and tendons can give rise to problems that are currently referred to as overuse or repetitive strain injury (RSI). Commonly experienced symptoms are pain, fatigue, and weakness, and signs include tenderness, swelling, and a crackling sound accompanying movement. Most of these involve the fingers, wrists, and shoulder girdle, where the muscles and connective tissues are relatively weak and adapted for fixation rather than agonistic use. Overuse patterns have been described under a variety of terms. Ramazzini in 1713 first described a pattern of overuse of a particular joint, which came to be called "writer's cramp". The overuse pattern is usually associated with particular occupations and was identified as a major source of disability in Japanese keypunch operators in the 1950s. The "chicken-worker's wrist" is similar to the "data-processor's arm". Health and safety directives originating from the European Community in 1993 were extended to include a new regulation on repetitive use, but RSI does not constitute an industrial injury in the way "beat hand" and "beat arm" do. In Australia, there was a sudden increase in RSI complaints in the early 1980s, but the "epidemic" died off in the same decade (Ferguson, 1987). The "diagnosis" of RSI was given readily at the beginning of that period, which seemed to increase sick-role and compensation issues. Employers reacted by improving ergonomic practices and by screening potential employees for RSI risk. The Royal Australasian College of Physicians published a report in 1986 which cast doubt on the relationship between RSI and work practices. A journalist successfully faked an RSI claim in 1987, and published the account of how he had received compensation. The concept of RSI as an occupational disease declined dramatically thereafter.

Musicians make heavy use of wrist movements and are thus particularly prone to repetitive use injuries. More than a century ago, Dr G.V. Poore (1887) described an overuse pattern in 21 pianists with hand and wrist symptoms. Clinical description in the absence of controlled research still dominates in this field. Bird (1989) reviewed overuse syndrome in musicians and concluded that physiological, pathological, psychological, and psychosocial factors all have effects. The review includes a study of 29 women with chronic pain and loss of function in upper limb muscles. These muscles were found to have an increase in type-1 muscle fibres, decrease and hypertrophy in type-2 muscle fibres, and various cell changes. Rest is usually effective in relieving the pain and disability in the short term, but recurrence is likely in the person whose livelihood depends on wrist and hand use. Sataloff, Bradfornbrener, and Lederman (1990) attempt to give a systematic approach to overuse in the performing arts.

Rest and removal from the activity are the immediate remedies. Any of the many techniques in the physiotherapist's armamentarium may be helpful: cold or heat treatment, spray and stretch, ultrasound and TENS. Splinting will prevent aggravating movements in cases of severe discomfort. However, prevention of RSI will involve reduction of the pattern of abuse. Consideration of the ergonomics of the task should identify the main abuse movements: rapid small repetitive movements, excessively forceful movements, and static loading of fixator muscles. Keyboard users will benefit from work-tops and monitors at appropriate heights and wrist support, as described in the ergonomics section. Alternation of use of the preferred and non-preferred arm will distribute muscle use for many hand tools. Pauses for antagonistic stretching movements, which are generally extensor, will help in prolonged tasks. Full-range stretching movements will reduce RSI, which mainly arises from inner-range movements. Preparatory strengthening of the forearms before taking up work as a chicken-plucker has been shown to prevent overuse injury. A cognitive-behavioural approach to the management of RSI was reported by Spence (1989). Common psychological strategies for management of pain were used—cognitive restructuring of pain beliefs, relaxation as a way of breaking the pain–tension–pain cycle, and distraction imagery. Sufferers were also encouraged to resume reinforcing relationships and activities, and to assert themselves to reduce work demands. Patients were seen either individually, in a group, or assigned to a waiting list. After two months, both treated groups had improved in mood and social function, though they were not more likely to have returned to work.

MAINTAINING MOBILITY IN LATER LIFE

The effect of exercise in building skeletal and cardiac muscle declines with age but does not disappear. Exercise may have value in preventing problems associated with skeletal ageing, such as osteoporosis and fractures. Yoga confers various benefits in stress reduction and breathing, and the stretching of yoga may be protective against musculoskeletal stiffening. There is little direct evidence on the preventive value of suppleness exercise at present. The available animal evidence on osteoporosis prevention is reviewed by Smith, Smith, and Gilligan (1990). In these studies it was found that a few intermittent compressive mechanical stresses per day would reduce bone atrophy. Four repetitions at high strain seemed as effective as 36 or 1800 repetitions.

Blumenthal et al. (1991) report a study on the value of aerobic and yoga exercise in healthy older people, in which 101 men and women over 60 years were randomly assigned to aerobic exercise, a yoga and flexibility control group, or a waiting-list control group. A semi-crossover design was employed such that, following completion of the second assessment, all subjects completed 4 months of aerobic exercise and underwent a third assessment. Subjects were given the option of participating in 6 additional months of supervised aerobic exercise (14 months total), and all subjects, regardless of their exercise status, completed a fourth assessment. Aerobic subjects experienced a 10–15% improvement in aerobic capacity, with 4 months of aerobic exercise training producing an overall 11.6% improvement in peak VO_2 and a 13% increase in anaerobic threshold. Yoga subjects showed no increase in cardiovascular measures. The authors also claim a trend towards an increase in bone mineral content for subjects at risk for bone fracture. In general, there were relatively few improvements in cognitive performance associated with aerobic exercise, although subjects who maintained their exercise participation for 14 months experienced improvements in some psychiatric symptoms.

CONCLUSION

Good ergonomic design and the skilled use of the body should prevent many movement problems of the back, neck, and forearm. Formal evaluations of such strategies are difficult to find at present, except in the area of secondary prevention of low-back injuries. Back school education, activity pacing, and confronting fear have each been shown to be effective in restoring mobility. The suitable populations for each approach are probably somewhat different. Suppleness training can prevent overuse injury, especially in occupations with intensive forearm use.

REFERENCES

Atkinson, J.H, Slater, M.A., Grant, I., Patterson, T.L., & Garfin, S.R. (1988). Depressed mood in chronic low back pain: Relationship with stressful life events. *Pain, 35*, 47–55.

Bendix, T. (1986). Chair and table adjustments for seated work. In N. Corlett (Ed.), *The ergonomics of working postures* (chapter 31). London: Taylor & Francis.

Bird, H. (1989). Overuse syndrome. *British Medical Journal, 298*, 1129.

Blumenthal, J.A., Emery, C.F., Madden, D.J., Schniebolk, S., Walsh-Riddle, M., George, L.K., McKee, D.C., Higginbotham, M.B., Cobb, F.R., & Coleman, R.E. (1991). Long-term effects of exercise on psychological functioning in older men and women. *Journal of Gerontology, 46* (6), 352–361.

Brown, G.W., & Harris, T. (1978). *Social origins of depression: A study of psychiatric disorder in women*. London: Tavistock.

Ferguson, D.A. (1987). "RSI" putting the epidemic to rest. *The Medical Journal of Australia, 147*, 213–214.

Fordyce, K. (1976). *Behavioral methods for chronic pain and illness*. Chicago, IL: C.V. Mosby Co.

Forssell, M.Z. (1980). The Swedish Back School. *Physiotherapy, 66* (4) (April), 112–114.

Health Services Advisory Committee (1992). *Guidance on manual lifting of loads in the health services*. London: HMSO.

Klaber Moffett, J.A., Chase, S.M., Portek, I., & Ennis, J.R. (1986). A controlled prospective study to evaluate the effectiveness of a back school in the relief of chronic low back pain. *Spine, 11* (2), 120–122.

Lethem, J., Slade, P.D., Troup, J., & Bentley, G. (1983). Outline of a fear-avoidance model of exaggerated pain perception. *Behaviour Research and Therapy, 21* (4), 401–408.

Lindstrom, I., Ohlund, C., Eek, C., Wallin, L., Peterson, L., Fordyce, W., & Nachemson, A. (1992). The effect of graded activity on patients with subacute low back pain: A randomised prospective clinical study with an operant conditioning behavioral approach. *Physical Therapy, 72* (4), 279–293.

McKenzie, R. (1981). *The lumbar spine: Mechanical diagnosis and therapy*. Waikanae, New Zealand: Spinal Publications.

McKenzie, R. (1985). *Treat your own back*. Lower Hutt, New Zealand: Spinal Publications.

Poore, G.V. (1887). Clinical lecture on certain conditions of the hand and arm which interfere with the performance of professional arts, especially piano playing. *British Medical Journal, i*, 441–444.

Sataloff, R.T., Bradfornbrener, A.G., & Lederman, R.J. (Eds.) (1990). *Textbook of performing arts medicine*. New York: Raven.

Smith, Smith, & Gilligan (1990). In C. Bouchard, R.J. Shephard, T. Stephens, J.R. Sutton, & B.D. McPherson (Eds.), *Exercise, fitness, and health: A consensus of current knowledge*. Leeds: Human Kinetics Publishers.

Spence, S H. (1989). Cognitive-behaviour therapy in the management of chronic occupational pain of the upper limbs. *Behaviour Research and Therapy, 27*, 435–446.

Spinhoven, P., & Linssen, A. (1989). Education and self-hypnosis in the management of low back pain: A component analysis. *British Journal of Clinical Psychology, 28* (2), 145–154.

Stankovic, R., & Johnell, O. (1990). Conservative treatment of acute low back pain. A prospective randomized trial: McKenzie method of treatment versus patient education in "mini back school". Cited in C. Von Hagen & G. Hierholzer (1991), Back school for patients with orthopaedic fractures. *Archives of Orthopaedic Trauma and Surgery, 110* (6), 273–276.

Waddell, G., & Main, C. (1984). Assessment of severity in low-back disorders. *Spine, 9*, 204–208.

Williams, J.I. (1989). Illness behaviour to wellness behaviour—the "School for bravery" approach. *Physiotherapy, 75* (1), 2–7.

Wilson, J.R., & Corlett, E.N. (1990). *Evaluation of human work: Practical ergonomic methodology*. London: Taylor & Francis.

13

Alternatives to Pain

This chapter describes a variety of activities antagonistic to pain. Whereas other chapters of this book are concerned with maintaining function of particular organ systems, this one concerns maintenance of subjective experiences of attention, rational thought, and emotional well-being. Chapter 12 has already considered activities that maintain function, particularly of the spine. Intuitively, pain is a sensation of something unpleasant happening to a particular part of the body, and physiologists often consider pain phenomena alongside pressure, heat sensitivity, and other tactile sensations. Yet in many respects pain is more like an emotion: It is aggravated by worry or other unpleasant emotions and reduced by attention diversion. We need to distinguish between pain and "nociception"; the latter means the nervous impulses arising from tissue damage, and has a variable relation with the unpleasant subjective experience of "pain". In this chapter we shall consider pain as an experience that is the summation of nociception, modulating spinal and brain stem events, and higher mental processes.

Karoly and Jensen (1985) provide a psychological framework for describing the contributions to pain, which they call "multimodal assessment of chronic pain". They distinguish between several "contexts" of pain—biomedical, i.e. site and severity of nociceptive stimulus; psychological, e.g. avoidance or confrontation of life-events, and locus of control; sensory-affective, including illness behaviour; sociocultural, e.g. compensation claims accompanying prolonged pain, and religious or national values on the toleration of pain. There are additional influences between nociception and these higher mental processes, such as counter-irritation and motor activity. Many techniques may reduce pain, but few do so invariably. A pragmatic approach is therefore essential for those seeking to assist pain sufferers to regain mental functions that have been compromised by pain. This chapter presents factors in ascending order of influence on the pain experience. It should be noted that some inhibition of pain occurs through influences descending from brain to spinal column.

PATHWAYS FROM PERIPHERY TO BRAIN

There are specialised receptors in the skin, including corpuscles of Krause, which respond especially to cold, and corpuscles of Ruffini, which respond especially to warmth. The most abundant type are free nerve endings. Neurons from such receptors synapse close to their origin, and the interneurons receive bushy branching input from many receptor fields. Free nerve endings can be stimulated by histamine and other chemicals, collectively referred to as "algic substances". Most pain originates in stretch receptors in muscle. From the periphery, fibres enter the spinal column at the dorsal (back) side. The A and C fibres are two groups of nerves known to be maximally responsive to pain. Some investigators believe that A fibres mediate sudden sharp pain, while C fibres mediate slow, diffuse, dull, or aching pain. Fibres are differentiated by physiologists according to conduction velocity, which is a function of diameter and the presence of myelin sheaths (see Table 13.1).

Sensory fibres enter the spinal cord through narrow channels between the lumbar vertebrae. This anatomical fact means that nerves are fairly vulnerable to inflammation at these points. Referred pain in the legs, known as sciatica, can occur if nerves entering the lumbar spine are being pressed by inflamed surrounding tissue. Nerves in the dorsal horn of the spinal column are arranged in several layers, or "laminae". Two types of nociceptive cells have been proposed (Liebeskind & Paul, 1977): Class-1 nociceptive cells re-

Table 13.1 Proporties of nerve fibres

Fibre type	Diameter (mm)	Conduction velocity (m/sec)	Responds mainly to:
A-beta	5–15 myelinated	30–100	light pressure
A-delta	1–5 myelinated	6–30	pressure, chemicals, cooling
C	0.2–1.5 unmyelinated	1–2	pressure, chemicals, warming

ceive input from A-delta and C-fibres only; class-2 fibres can respond to many fibres, but their activity is maximal in the presence of input from A-delta and C fibres. Laminae II and III have a jelly-like appearance and are hence known as the substantia gelatinosa—important in Melzack and Wall's gate control theory, which is described later.

Within the brain stem there are medial and lateral tracts, named by their position in relation to the core of the brain stem. The lateral spinothalamic tract is thought to mediate sudden pain, and mapping of body surface is retained. Projections upward eventually reach the cerebral cortex. Brain areas are apportioned according to the sensory discrimination involved, so the hands, mouth, and genital areas take up a large brain volume in comparison to the trunk. The disproportionately large brain areas for these regions were shown by the neurosurgeon Penfield in his famous "sensory homunculus" (Penfield & Roberts, 1959). The body is mapped according to dermotomes, which are labelled by the space between the vertebrae where the sensory nerves enter. For example, the L3 dermotome involves leg areas whose nerves enter at the third lumbar vertebra. The medial tract conducts slowly along small fibres, is less clearly mapped, and has connections to the limbic system. These anatomical properties suggest that it mediates longer-term pain and may be influenced by emotions. The variety of influences of pain are summarised graphically in Figure 13.1.

SPECIFICITY AND PATTERN THEORIES

Von Frey proposed a century ago that the quality of a skin sensation such as touch, cold, or pain depends initially on the type of sensory receptor that is stimulated. These specialised nerve endings were supposed to transduce physical, chemical, or electromagnetic stimuli into nerve action potentials. Von Frey assigned free nerve endings the role of transducing pain. However, these free nerve endings have since been found to transduce other sorts of sensation: The pinna or ear lobe has basically only free nerve endings, but sensations of warmth, cold, touch, itch, or pain can all be felt with appropriate stimuli. Similarly, the cornea of the eye has only free nerve endings, but a similar range of sensation can be experienced. The simple mapping of sensations onto receptors proposed by specificity theory can be only partly true at best.

The alternative "pattern" theory, therefore, sees pain as excessive stimulation of any receptors; bright light, heavy pressure, or excessive heat can all cause pain by their excess. Receptors may adapt at different rates to stimuli, and the patterns of discharges reaching the central nervous system may represent a code; in the pattern view, it is the quantity rather than the type of stimulation that gives rise to the experience of pain.

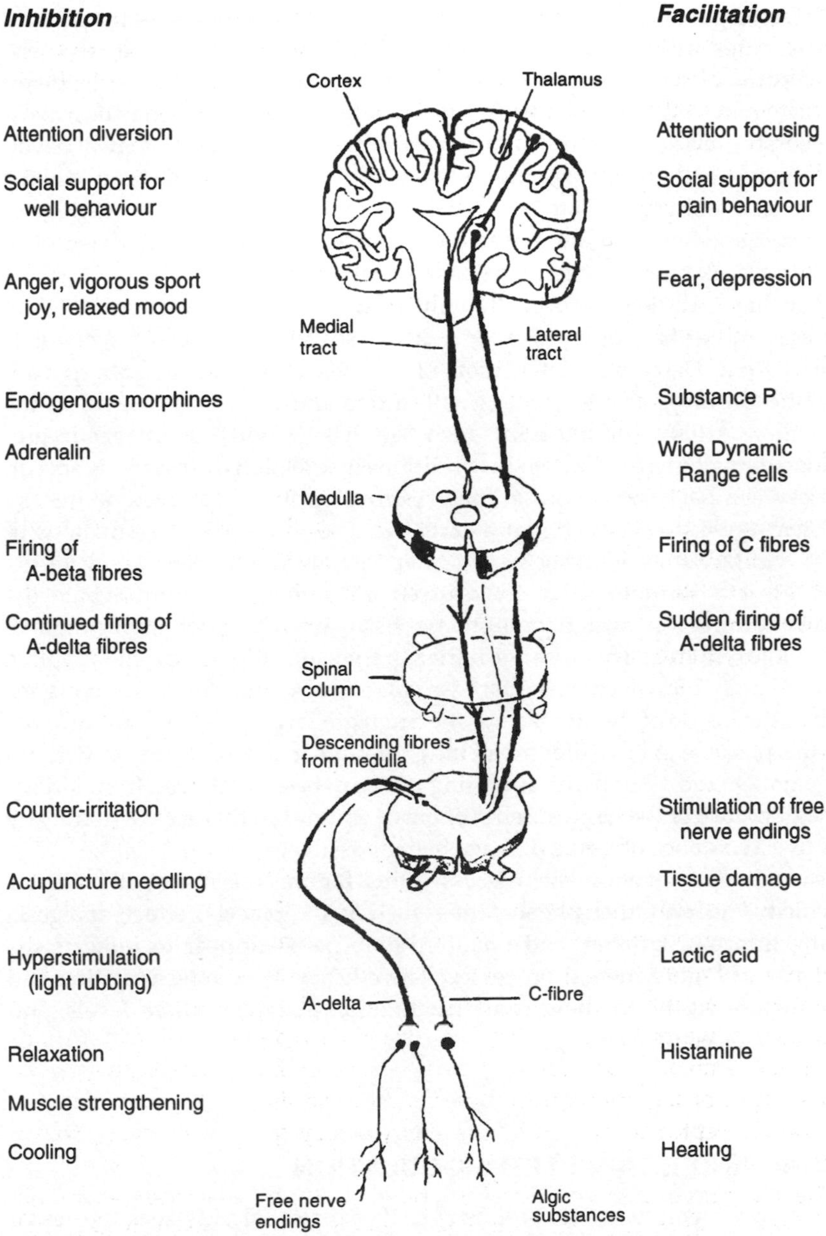

Figure 13.1 Facilitation and inhibition of pain

Referred pain is a phenomenon that appears strange but is relatively consistent with specificity theory. Pain is said to be referred when it is experienced some distance away from the presumed damage. For example, blood shortage to the myocardial muscle which characterises angina may be experienced in the left upper arm. This anomaly arises during embryological development, in which the heart migrates away from the arm, but the branch of the vagus nerve supplying both areas does not become similarly differentiated. Sciatica is another form of referred pain, in which inflammation of nerves in the lower back causes shooting pains to be felt in the legs.

Pain has traditionally been thought of as a warning to prevent tissue damage, and at first sight this seems obviously true. The classic account of pain is René Descartes' description of a boy's foot in a fire: Sharp pain indicates burning, and the foot is withdrawn and pain is registered at the same time. Although unpleasant, such pain has definite advantages in preventing damage, as can be seen in conditions where pain awareness is absent. Leprosy is a bacterial condition that destroys peripheral nerve-endings, so that damage can occur without awareness. The gruesome deformations of limbs and face that we associate with leprosy are not a direct result of the disease but of the injuries that are incurred and not treated. Without pain, the leprosy sufferer can crush fingers and not be aware of the process of gangrene in the injured area. This disease rather graphically illustrates the adaptive value of pain. However, this adaptive value is not consistent. Some organs such as the inside of the stomach or the brain are largely devoid of sensation, and it is possible to have life-threatening tumours grow in these sites without any pain. On the other hand, agonising pain can be experienced from kidney stones, because of the large number of nerve endings in this area, without any effective avoidance of tissue damage being possible.

Several apparent anomalies discussed thus far are consistent with receptor specificity theory. Other phenomena—such as the placebo effect, analgesia during trance or combat, and phantom-limb pain—appear to indicate the influence of higher mental processes. The efficacy of counter-irritation and acupuncture seems to show some modulation at intermediate levels, and these are examined next.

SPINAL AND BRAIN STEM MODULATION

Gate control theory was first proposed in 1965 by Ronald Melzack, professor of psychology at McGill University, and Patrick Wall, professor of physiology at University College London. Five stages were proposed:

1. Small-diameter (A-delta and C) fibres are stimulated by injury. They de-

liver impulses to transmission cells in the spinal cord, which can transmit upwards and trigger reflex withdrawal.

2. Facilitatory cells in the spinal column cause all cells in the spinal cord to fire after a brief input volley.

3. Other cell types in the spinal column include common "wide dynamic range cells", which receive inputs from both small- and large-diameter cells, and rarer "nociceptive specific cells", which respond only to small-diameter fibre input. Wide dynamic range cells are presumed to respond with pain impulses if triggering exceeds a critical threshold, but they can also be inhibited by input from large-diameter low-threshold inputs. Inhibitory effects occur if the input is at the edge of the receptor field, and excitatory effects if input is at the centre.

4. In the substantia gelatinosa (SG) of the dorsal laminae exist some densely packed small cells with short projections, which they believed to be the inhibitory interneurons. These are the "gates" that can be closed to reduce pain awareness. It has been found that opioids such as enkephalins and dynorphins are released by cells in the SG, and that the highest concentration of such opioids is in the SG.

5. Descending influences from the brain stem (midbrain and medulla) inhibit the firing of transmission cells. Ascending influences could also feed back to these descending structures.

Gate control theory tends to dominate theoretical accounts of pain at the present time (Melzack & Wall, 1988).

PHARMACOLOGICAL PAIN CONTROL

Analgesia is the reduction of pain that can be achieved with the aid of certain pharmacological substances. Of particular theoretical interest are the alkaloids derived from the opium poppy, quite small doses of which can reduce even intense pain. The opium derivative that is used most widely in medical analgesia is morphine. Papavaretum is another opium derivative containing about 50% morphine, and diamorphine or heroin is a stronger but more addictive preparation from morphine. The potency of these substances led to the suspicion that they must mimic some naturally occurring substance in the body and lock onto its receptor sites. Research eventually located a new class of endogenous opioids that lock onto receptor sites in exactly the way predicted. The well-known addictive properties of morphine discourage many physicians from prescribing it, but Melzack (1990) argues that morphine only becomes addictive when used for pleasurable recreation. Apart from addiction, these powerful analgesics have other dangers, such as the reduction of respiration and the cough reflex, so that they are properly used only under medical supervision.

Prescribed drugs are largely beyond our present scope but are well reviewed in texts on pharmacology for nurses, such as Hopkins (1983). A comprehensive account of family use of medicines may be found in the British Medical Association's (1991) guide to medicine and drugs. Pain-killers that are available without prescription are the most widely used strategy for self-control of pain. Some principles are worth mentioning here, especially those concerned with achieving appropriate dosages. The same considerations apply to recreational drugs (see chapter 5). Proprietary pain-relief compounds usually combine aspirin or paracetamol or one of the synthetic compounds, and perhaps accelerators such as caffeine. Three commonly used pain-killers are:

1. *Aspirin* or acetylsalicylic acid is the best-known of a group of substances sometimes referred to as coal-tar analgesics. It is probably the most popular and useful of the mild analgesics, often used in association with paracetamol. It is rapidly absorbed and excreted, so that administration every 4 to 6 hours is needed. In prolonged use it has a number of side-effects, which can include nausea, tinnitus, and allergic reactions. A small amount of blood is lost from the stomach with aspirin, but the effect of aspirin in reducing blood clotting makes it an important preventive drug for patients at risk of heart attack. The addition of chalk, as in Disprin, reduces the side-effects, as does taking the tablet with food.

2. *Paracetamol* is a mild analgesic with far fewer gastric side-effects than aspirin, but without its valuable anti-inflammatory properties. Prolonged use is hazardous to the kidneys and liver. Overdosing with this otherwise safe drug can cause serious liver damage, and this may not be evident until many hours after ingestion.

3. *Codeine* is one of the alkaloids present with morphine in opium, but with only one-sixth the analgesic potency of morphine. Dihydrocodeine (DF118) is a codeine derivative with increased analgesic potency. In excessive use it has risks to the liver, in aggravating asthma, in suppressing cough, and in nausea and constipation.

For the pain-sufferer to make maximum use of these self-administered drugs, some pharmacological principles should be learned:

• *Weight/dose.* Most drugs that are absorbed through the gut are distributed widely through the body, so their effect on the painful area is inversely proportional to the body mass. Number of units (tablets) should be directly proportional to weight, as is the case with alcohol. An average man might require three tablets to achieve about the same effect as an average-weight woman would achieve with two. (More precise estimates would be based on proportions of fat and lean body mass). This is most important in relation to overdose risk; the maximum adult dose of paracetamol might be 4 grams per day, but a child 6 to 12 should not exceed 2 grams in 24 hours.

- *Placebo effect.* Most families have patent remedies for hurt children, which may include cough medicine, plasters, or rubbing on some sort of cream. Application of sticking plaster or antiseptics will have no pharmacological effect on nociception but may reduce pain considerably. The value of these remedies is mainly through the child's belief in their value rather than their pharmacology. Provided that safe doses are not exceeded and the substance is used occasionally, these learned remedies form a useful part of pain control.

- *Scheduling.* Regular use of analgesic medication can itself become a pain behaviour. Fordyce (1975) has developed a drug-scheduling approach that separates the pharmacological and psychological aspects of pain-killing medication. The usual medical prescription is to tell the patient to take the drug when it hurts and not when it does not hurt. Fordyce's regime involves the taking of analgesics, and also exercise, at fixed times, so breaking the reinforcing relationship of pill use.

COUNTER-IRRITATION

Counter-irritation is the familiar and intuitive trick of using a little deliberately induced pain in one area to counteract a greater pain elsewhere. For example, on banging the "funny bone" at the elbow, we vigorously rub the tingling arm. This is called "hyper-stimulation analgesia", and it appears to work through stimulating pressure receptors, and hence A-beta fibres, which antagonise nociceptive transmission.

Transcutaneous electrical nerve stimulation (TENS), derived from gate theory, appears to use the same principle. TENS involves the application of electrical stimuli over the painful area. Katz and Melzack (1991) describe a method of auricular TENS to reduce phantom-limb pain. Small, but significant, reductions in the intensity of non-painful phantom-limb sensations were found. Experiments have been undertaken to try to stimulate low-threshold afferents in a painful region, and hence "close the gates". Application of a voltage just large enough causes the patient to feel a local tingling and a simultaneous reduction in general pain to tolerable levels. A surgical technique used an electrode implanted on the dura by means of an epidural catheter (Krainick & Thoden, 1984). The approach of applying voltages or counter-irritants to the skin generally has less analgesic effect than do invasive methods, but the technique is simpler.

ACUPRESSURE

Acupuncture is widely used in pain prevention in various European countries and, of course, in China. Traditional Chinese Medicine (TCM) is a comprehensive system involving macrobiotic diet, acupressure (Shiatsu), exercise (Tai chi), and other techniques. TCM may be used for all kinds of treatment in addition to pain reduction. Acupuncture anaesthesia is used routinely for surgery in those Chinese hospitals that specialise in TCM. A typical analgesic procedure involves the continuous twirling of a single needle in the forearm. For example, caesarean section for childbirth is routinely performed under acupuncture anaesthesia in China. Blood pressure, pulse rate, and respiration are said to be stable during the operation, and blood loss is less than in it is under epidural or local anaesthesia. Hormone and immune changes in 20 patients were investigated by Kho et al. (1990) during and for 6 days following thyroid surgery performed under acupuncture anaesthesia, during which the patients remained conscious. In the postoperative phase, immune changes were generally small and transient, except for large neutrophil changes. Levels of noradrenalin and beta-endorphin rose and remained elevated, whereas the other circulating hormones gradually returned to normal values. This suggests that the pain-reducing effects are similar to those achieved through combat analgesia.

Positive reinforcement for well behaviours certainly occurs in acupuncture surgery; for example the conscious patient may be applauded by theatre staff, and the surgeon can shake hands at the end of the operation. Patients usually report some pain, but of a bearable level, and can carry on a conversation. However, optimism and belief on the part of the patient is unlikely to be the principal mechanism, since acupuncture is effective with animals such as dogs and rabbits. Ear-point acupuncture was used in 30 dogs suffering from thoracolumbar disc disease by Still (1990), and 50% of the dogs recovered completely. Dogs with back pain only (Type I) and dogs with paresis (Type II) responded best, and the analgesic effects were especially impressive. Acupuncture failed in three (50%) of paralysed dogs, with more severe types III and IV disc disease. There was some relapse over the next few weeks. The mildly aversive method of acupuncture by an unfamiliar veterinary surgeon is moderately effective in pain relief, so the placebo effect is not likely to be the main reason for this effect.

Counter-irritation, or diffuse noxious stimulation, is a mechanism known to Western medicine, and it may be part of the explanation of acupuncture's pain-reducing effects. However, several effects seem to be more specific than the counter-irritation hypothesis would imply. Changes such as skin warming at remote sites seem to follow the meridians postulated by TCM. The effects of needling can be lost by misplacing the needle by a few millimetres. Acupuncture has local effects on electrical conductivity, and mediating effects, at least on C fibres. Stronger effects were achieved historically by warming the needle with smouldering moxa herb, or in modern times by applying an electrical potential to the needle. The effects of acupressure and laser stimulation are generally less than those of invasive methods.

Acupressure is of greater interest than are needling methods for our purposes, since it may be self-administered. It involves firm pressure by the thumbs applied to an acupuncture point. TCM acupressure remedies include pressure in the angle between thumb and forefinger to antagonise cardiac events, or pressure at the side of the temples to antagonise headache. One of the better-validated methods is the use of pressure at the wrist to counteract nausea, rather than pain. Pressure on the Neiguan point on the midline of forearm has been shown to relieve nausea of pregnancy (De Aloysio & Penacchioni, 1992; Dundee & McMillan, 1990). Reduction in nausea after surgery also occurs (Barsoum, Perry, & Fraser, 1990), but there is little effect on motion sickness.

Considerable difficulties, both linguistic and physiological, arise in evaluating acupressure. Key concepts, such as "chi" (or Qi), may be translated as "energy", though it has nothing to do with electromagnetic energy and might better be translated as "transport function". The more important difficulty is that the lines in the body along which chi moves, called meridians, do not correspond to known nervous, lymph, or other pathways. The Neiguan point used for nausea reduction is described in TCM as on the "Pericardium channel of Hand-Jueyin", which follows a line from the chest above the heart to the middle finger. Acupuncture points themselves can be objectively defined in modern terms as areas of low electrical resistance. The meridians may correspond to areas of rapid cell death or high numbers of mast cells. A full anatomical atlas, in English, of Chinese acupuncture points is given by the Cooperative Group of Shandong Medical College (1982). The beneficial effects of acupressure probably come from specific analgesic and anti-emetic effects, combined with counter-irritation and social reinforcement.

EMOTIONS AND PAIN

There are a number of well-documented reports of the absence of pain during highly aroused states that indicate that emotions can inhibit pain. The strongest motivational states, including fear, hunger, sex, and anger, involve the hypothalamus. Electrical stimulation of this brain area can produce extreme emotions in animals. Other emotions involve mid-brain structures including the limbic system and thalamus. The anatomical proximity of the medial pain pathway and the thalamus suggest that modulation of nociception may occur in these structures. It would be tempting to think of emotions as located in the thalamus, and consciousness as located in the cortex; in this view, the mid-brain would act as a middle-hierarchy sub-system censoring what reaches consciousness, including pain. However, psychological research on emotion has shown that higher-level processes such as memory and appraisal, as well as autonomic and other bodily changes, are involved in emotion. Therefore it would be rash to say where pain occurs—the seat of consciousness, and hence pain awareness, may be mid-brain rather than the cortex.

Various phenomena show behavioural analgesic effects, probably involving emotional inhibition of pain.

- *Trance analgesia:* Apparent insensitivity to pain during ceremonial rituals has been described in a variety of cultures, including Dervishes, Kalahari Bushmen, and various Indian communities. In the hook-swinging ceremony of South India, the celebrant has two steel hooks inserted into the muscles of the small of the back (Kosambi, 1967). He is carted from village to village, and at times his weight is entirely suspended from the hooks while he blesses each child and farm field. The crowds cheer at each swing, and the celebrant is in a state of exaltation and shows no sign of pain. Social support for the celebrant is also evident in Dervish and Bushmen rituals. Rhythmic dancing for some hours is another common feature of several rituals and seems to be essential for achieving analgesia.

- *Combat analgesia:* Various anecdotes from war situations indicate that soldiers frequently feel little or no pain from intense injuries. Israeli soldiers injured in the Yom Kippur war often used neutral terms like "bang" or "thump" to describe the first sensation and volunteered their surprise that it did not hurt. They were mostly depressed—an emotion that usually accompanies increased pain—but felt no pain until hours later. Beecher (1959) made a previous observation on American casualties from the Anzio landings in 1944. He was astonished to find that only one out of three complained of sufficient pain to warrant morphia. Reports of sports injuries may reflect the same trend: During very intense combative activity, injuries may be noted but become painful only later. Combat involves high levels of adrenalin, and there is an obvious adaptive value for animals antagonising pain awareness during struggles for food or with predators. However, fear also involves adrenergic effects, and fear is usually associated with increased pain awareness, so analgesia during combat cannot be a simple result of adrenalin antagonism. Fight involves a willingness to confront and a diminished perception of risk of damage to the self. Flight, by contrast, involves the perception that the adversary is powerful enough to inflict pain.

Neither trance nor combat states can be prescribed deliberately as a way of reducing pain, but some voluntary activities may work the same way. Regular runners often experience considerable aching in the middle stages of their run, but the pain diminishes if they continue to push themselves. This has been referred to as "the runner's high". It has been speculated that endogenous opioids may be produced to counteract the pain of lactic acid, but adrenalin may also be the anatagonist to nociception. Some European patients report pain reduction during rock music or sustained dancing.

REPRESENTATION OF THE BODY IN THE BRAIN

Phantom limb

The phenomenon that most clearly shows that pain is a higher mental state is the occurrence of phantom-limb pain. This remarkable phenomenon is persisting awareness of an arm or leg months or years after its surgical removal. Amputees usually describe the phantom as a tingling feeling, having a definite shape, which moves through space appropriately for sitting, standing, or lying; later on, the arm or leg may fade, leaving the foot "in midair". A week after surgery, 72% have phantom limb pain, and seven years later 60% still complain of it (Krebs et al., 1984). Pain in the phantom, if it occurs, has a specific location. For example, Livingston (1943) gives a vivid description of a doctor who accidentally broke a test tube in his hand and contracted gangrene. Amputation was necessary to save his life, but he was left with the awareness of the last movement he made—a painfully clenched hand. Melzack (1992) gives some recent extraordinary anecdotes of phantom experiences. One girl with a congenitally deformed lower leg had several operations, culminating when the foot was surgically removed early in her school years. She adapted so well to the prosthesis that she became a skilled dancer in her teens. However, she continued to experience phantom toes at three different levels, though this was not greatly troubling, as she could wiggle all fifteen toes together! Phantom limb may involve specific mental representations, in which central processes are uncorrected by new peripheral impulses. A quite different explanation comes from bereavement theory and postulates grieving for the lost body part.

Procedures that relieve phantom pain are equally surprising: Injection of a local anaesthetic in the stump should wear off after a few hours, but relief sometimes persists for months. Saline injections in the stump, which would normally irritate, sometimes relieve phantom pain. Thermal biofeedback has been reported as one of the more effective relieving procedures in Vietnam veterans.

Placebo effect

The role of higher mental processes is also revealed in the placebo effect. This literally means "I shall please" and is the reduction of pain through suggestion rather than pharmacological action. Volygesi (1954) studied the effects of placebo injections on hospitalised patients with intense pain from bleeding duodenal ulcers. In one treatment condition, injections of distilled water were given by a doctor who described the procedure as a "new cure" for ulcers. In the other procedure, a nurse gave the injection with the message that it was an "experimental procedure". In the first condition, an excellent result was obtained in 70% of cases, while in the second only 25% experienced pain reduction to an "excellent" level. More recent studies have compared a mechanical pump controlled by a computer timer with injections by a dentist. Again the suggestion of pain relief by a person of high credibility has been shown to be the effective agent, sometimes comparable with that of the drug. Jerome Frank (1973) has described the placebo responses as part of a more general "non-specific treatment effect". The person trapped in a state of suffering may be released from it by procedures arousing optimism and a belief in change.

SOCIAL REINFORCEMENT OF PAIN AND WELL BEHAVIOURS

The response of others provides one important context for pain and its inhibition, and some authors distinguish these effects by the term "pain behaviours", which include grimaces, vocalisations, alterations in posture, etc. (see chapter 12). Sickness or injury usually entail some response from others, and the sociologist Talcott Parsons (1972) has described this as the "sick role". While some illnesses are obvious to other people, complaints such as low back pain are noticed only because of pain behaviours. Fordyce (1975) has espoused the view that pain behaviours are "shaped" by the responses of others, and operant conditioning effects maintain pain longer than the underlying injury would require. Differential reinforcement of well behaviour at the expense of pain behaviour has already been described in the "School for Bravery" approach. Social reinforcement is also quite strong in some acupuncture procedures—for example, where the surgical team applaud the conscious patient at the completion of surgery under acupuncture anaesthesia.

HYPNOSIS

Hypnosis is an ancient procedure involving the combined use of relaxation, imagery, and sensory withdrawal or fatigue to produce a suggestible state. The effect is often called a hypnotic "trance", viewed as an altered state of consciousness, like the twilight state before sleep. Debate continues about an alternative view that the hypnotic subject is actually using exaggerated role-play in compliance with the hypnotist's suggestion. Hypnosis is of interest because some dramatic effects on pain reduction have been reported. In 1842, a Doctor Ward amputated a leg while a patient was hypnotised and reported this to the Royal Medical and Chirurgical Society in London. The society refused to believe that the patient had experienced no pain, and a motion was put to remove the record of the paper from the society's minutes on the grounds that the patient must have been an impostor. Eight years later, a rumour was put to the society that the patient had admitted having falsely denied his pain. At this time, witnesses came forward, and a signed declaration from the patient was produced that the operation had been painless.

In the laboratory such dramatic effects cannot easily be reproduced, but laboratory analogue studies can resolve some questions. Hilgard and Hilgard (1983) report that involuntary aspects of pain (such as a rise in pulse and BP) remain unaltered during deep hypnosis, but voluntary aspects (such as grimacing or crying) are reduced. One hypothesis of hypnotic pain reduction equates it with suggestibility. McGlashan (1983) used a tourniquet-exercise method, in which the subject kept working as long as possible after the tourniquet cuff was inflated. The exercise was to squeeze a bulb to pump water, and outcome was measured by time and pumping effect, to the point when the subject announced some pain (threshold pain), and then to the point when no further pumping was possible (tolerance). Placebo suggestions of pain reduction did not increase tolerance time in 12 low-hypnotisable subjects, but 12 high-hypnotisable subjects increased their tolerance by a mean of about 30 seconds. "Natural trance" may occur with prolonged immobility such as motorway driving or in ceremonial rituals.

Analgesia for pain seems to occur only in strong hypnotic subjects. Strong subjects comprise 20% of the population in most reports, but 10% of the population according to Spiegel (1974). Strongly hypnotisable subjects are described as having "Grade V syndrome" by Spiegel because they occupy the fifth point of a hypnotic induction profile and have the following attributes:

1. high eye roll, unaffected by practice
2. innocent expectation of support, lack of cynicism
3. suspension of critical judgement, willingness to accept new beliefs
4. high degree of empathy—e.g. nausea in sympathy

5. exclusive time focus—e.g. recall childhood as real

6. tolerance of logical inconsistency—e.g. army logic: "We had to destroy the village to protect it"

7. excellent eidetic and rote memory, enhancing ability to regress under hypnosis

8. intense concentration—e.g. an author describes writing as "the character created himself"

9. a fixed core underlying changeable exterior

10. role confusion and sense of inferiority

The simulation of hypnotic trance because of social compliance has attracted interest from researchers who take a role-playing view of hypnosis. Subjects who are refractory to hypnosis are instructed to act as if they were hypnotised. If the non-hypnotised can act like the truly hypnotised, the hypnotist must have given suggestions about his expectations. The hypnotist must not know which subject is which. In the version described by Orne (1971), 12 subjects were hypnotised and 12 non-hypnotisable subjects were asked to imitate hypnotic behaviour. However, in the debriefing it was clear that pressure to comply was a factor only for the non-hypnotisables, because they did not actually reduce their felt pain. Faking has also been of interest since the defendant in the "Hillside strangler" case in California apparently faked a hypnotic trance (see chapter 3).

COGNITIVE TECHNIQUES

Some pain reduction can occur without hypnotic induction, but simply by the induction of a conscious cognitive set. Pain control can be made available to those who are not deep hypnotic subjects. Wardle (1985) reports that this "waking analgesia" was found equally effective in some studies, notably by Scott and Barber (1977). They used distraction, coping imagery, dissociation, and imaginative transformation, all to some effect in pain reduction. Holzman and Turk (1986) describe a cognitive–behavioural strategy for pain reduction, which uses many of the principles of Meichenbaum's stress inoculation training described in chapter 2.

It is difficult at present to evaluate the effect of cognitions alone on pain reduction. Tan (1980) reviewed 27 studies of cognitive coping strategies, compared with those spontaneously generated by patients. Taught strategies gave superior pain control in 15 of these. Attention diversion is potentially a very powerful technique, because of the way pain "seizes" the attention. One stage performer of Indian origin allowed himself to be repeatedly impaled by swords; asked how he could tolerate this, he said, "I think about something else". As a child, he had had a very painful illness, and he had learned to distract himself very effectively. Tan describes the following techniques that can be taught to pain sufferers to counteract their own pain:

- *Imaginative inattention.* Subjects are trained to ignore pain by evoking imagery incompatible with the pain—e.g. imagining themselves are on a beach (in the country, etc.)

- *Imaginative transformation.* Subjects are instructed to interpret the experience in terms other than "pain"—e.g. to transform it into tingling or other purely sensory qualities or to minimise the experience as trivial or unreal.

- *Imaginative transformation of context.* The patient is trained to acknowledge the pain but to transform the setting or context—e.g. if the arm is hurting, the patient can imagine being a fighter pilot wounded in battle.

- *Attention-diversion—internal:* The subject focuses on self-generated thoughts—e.g. mental arithmetic or composing a limerick.

- *Attention diversion—external:* This focuses attention on events such as counting ceiling tiles or concentrating on the weave of a fabric.

- *Somatisation.* Subjects are trained to focus attention on the painful area, but view it in a detached manner—e.g. analyse the pain sensations as if preparing to write a magazine article on pain.

CONCLUSION

Sudden pain may serves as a warning to prevent tissue damage, but much chronic pain has no such adaptive value. Nociceptive impulses are processed through emotions and social context to give the subjective sense of pain. Modulatory processes probably occur at spinal, brain stem, and cortical levels. Nociceptive impulses can be antagonised in the spinal column by counter-irritation and acupuncture, in the brain stem by activity, social reinforcement, and emotion, and in the middle and higher brain by cognitions and trance.

REFERENCES

Barsoum, G., Perry, E.P., & Fraser, I.A. (1990). Postoperative nausea is relieved by acupressure. *Journal of the Royal Society of Medicine, 83* (2), 86–89.
Beecher, H.K. (1959). *Measurement of subjective responses.* Oxford: Oxford University Press.

British Medical Association (1991). *Guide to medicine and drugs* (2nd ed.). London: Dorling Kindersley.

Cooperative Group of Shandong Medical College. (1982). *Anatomical atlas of Chinese acupuncture points*. Oxford: Pergamon.

De Aloysio, D., & Penacchioni, P. (1992). Morning sickness control in early pregnancy by Neiguan point acupressure. *Obstetrics and Gynecology, 80*, 852–854.

Dundee, J.W., & McMillan, C.M. (1990). Clinical uses of P6 acupuncture antiemesis. *Acupuncture and Electro-Therapeutics Research, 15* (3–4), 211–215.

Fordyce, W.E. (1975). *Behavioral methods for chronic pain and illness*. Saint Louis, MO: C.V. Mosby.

Frank, J.D. (1973). *Persuasion and healing*. Baltimore, MD: Johns Hopkins University Press.

Hilgard, E.R., & Hilgard, J.R. (1983). *Hypnosis in the relief of pain*. CA : William Kaufmann.

Holzman, A.D., & Turk, D.C. (Eds.), (1986). *Pain management*. Oxford: Pergamon.

Hopkins, S.J. (1983). *Drugs and pharmacology for nurses* (8th ed.). London: Churchill Livingstone.

Karoly, P., & Jensen, M.P. (1985). *Multimethod assessment of chronic pain*. Oxford: Pergamon.

Katz, J., & Melzack, R. (1991). Auricular transcutaneous electrical nerve stimulation (TENS) reduces phantom limb pain. *Pain Symptom Management, 6* (2), 73–83.

Kho, H.G, van Egmond, J., Zhuang C.F., Zhang, G.L., & Lin, G.F. (1990). The patterns of stress response in patients undergoing thyroid surgery under acupuncture anaesthesia in China. *Acta Anaesthesiol Scand, 34* (7), 563–571.

Kosambi, D.D. (1967). Living prehistory in India. *Scientific American, 216* (2), 105–114.

Krainick, J.U., & Thoden, U. (1984). Dorsal column stimulation. In P.D. Wall & R. Melzack (Eds.), *Textbook of pain*. Edinburgh: Churchill Livingstone.

Krebs, B., Jensen, T.S., Kroner, K., Nielsen, J., & Jorgensen, H.S. (1984). Phantom limb phenomena in amputees 7 years after limb amputation. *Pain* (suppl. 2), S85.

Liebeskind, J.C., & Paul, L.A. (1977). Psychological and physiological mechanisms of pain. *Annual Review of Psychology, 28*, 41–60.

Livingston, W.K. (1943). *Pain mechanisms*. New York: Macmillan.

McGlashan (1983). Cited in E.R. Hilgard, & J.R. Hilgard, *Hypnosis in the relief of pain*. CA: William Kaufmann, 1983.

Melzack, R. (1990). The tragedy of needless pain. *Scientific American, 262* (2), 19–25.

Melzack, R. (1992). Phantom limbs. *Scientific American, 266* (4), 90–96.

Melzack, R., & Wall, P.D. (1965). Pain mechanisms: A new theory. *Science, 150*, 971.

Melzack, R., & Wall, P.D. (1988). *The challenge of pain* (2nd ed.). Harmondsworth: Penguin.

Orne, M. (1971). Cited in E.R. Hilgard & J.R. Hilgard, *Hypnosis in the relief of pain*. CA: William Kaufmann, 1983.

Parsons, T. (1972). Definitions of health and illness in the light of American values and social structure. In E.G. Jaco (Ed.), Patients, physicians, and illness (2nd ed., pp. 107–127). New York: Free Press.

Penfield, W., & Roberts, L. (1959). *Speech and brain mechanisms*. Princeton, NJ: Princeton University Press.

Scott, D.S., & Barber, T.X. (1977). Cognitive control of pain: Effects of multiple cognitive strategies. *Psychological Record, 27,* 373–383.

Spiegel (1974). Cited in R. Aldridge-Morris, *Multiple personality: An exercise in deception*. Hove: Lawrence Erlbaum Associates Ltd., 1989.

Still, J. (1990). A clinical study of auriculotherapy in canine thoracolumbar disc disease. *Journal of South African Veterinary Association, 61* (3), 102–105.

Tan (1980). Cited in A.D. Holzman & D.C. Turk (Eds.), *Pain management.* Oxford: Pergamon, 1986.

Volygesi (1954). Cited in J.D. Frank, *Persuasion and healing.* Baltimore, MD: Johns Hopkins University Press, 1973.

Wardle, J. (1985). Pain. In F. Watts (Ed.), *New developments in clinical psychology.* Leicester: British Psychological Society.

14

Immunity

The general function of the immune system is to identify and eliminate foreign, "non-self" materials that contact or enter the body. These foreign materials are called "antigens" and include bacteria, viruses, parasites, and fungi. Components of the immune system are also capable of identifying and destroying cells that have undergone alterations associated with malignancy, and of directing responses against non-self agents such as donated organs. A reductionistic approach to medicine has tended until recently to see the immune system as autonomous and unaffected by brain states. However, the effects of life events and behaviour on proneness to disease are appearing in an increasing number of studies.

It is folk wisdom that people are most vulnerable to illness when they are "run down", but this had not been demonstrated convincingly until quite recently. A general demonstration of the effect of life-events on vulnerability to disease was made by Holmes and Rahe (1967, see chapter 3). Life-change units (LCUs) are scored consensually: Death of spouse has the highest LCU of 100, while marriage scores 50, and Christmas 12. In the 1975 study, they asked navy personnel to count their LCUs during 6-month blocks over the previous four years. The life-change total for blocks where an illness occurred was found to average 174 LCUs, and in the 6 months prior to the illness period the average was 125 LCUs. This study was retrospective, so there is probably some tendency to recall adverse life events selectively alongside illness, but a similar effect was found in a prospective study (Rahe, 1975). This type of research indicates a general relation between both positive and negative events and illness, but this is not very useful prophylactically. This chapter

258

attempts to find *specific* connections between life events or psychological processes and illnesses.

A number of studies have shown a relationship between upper respiratory tract infections and psychological processes. For example, Evans and Edgerton (1991) asked 100 clerical workers to keep diaries of life-events, moods, and cold symptoms; 55 life-events could be recorded, along with 12 mood adjectives, and 6 questions concerning symptoms of the common cold. Events rated by the subjects as desirable were categorised as "uplifts" and undesirable events as "hassles". Uplifts were found to decrease in frequency in the four days prior to cold onset, and there was a less significant tendency for hassles to rise during the same period. Subjects' ratings also indicated that they had been feeling more angry, tense, and sceptical during this period. Such findings might indicate that the proliferation of the cold virus in humans is a result of lowered levels of the T cells and antibodies that mediate immunity. However, changes in breathing behaviour creating inflammation might also be a mediating factor (See chapter 10). Persistent viral illnesses have often been shown to recur during emotional stress. For example, in the case of genital herpes, the proportions of cytotoxic and suppressor T cells were found to be negatively related to an aggregate index of negative mood (Kemeny et al., 1989).

PHYSIOLOGY OF IMMUNITY

The immune system is extremely complex, and detailed understanding of it requires knowledge of biochemistry and classification based on microscopic appearance. The present account is concerned only with function. The immune system is composed of specialised cells that originate in the bone marrow and that mature and are sequestered in particular organs, such as the thymus, the peripheral lymphoid organs, the spleen, and the lymph nodes. From these organs, the specialised cells are released into the blood; they may also return to these organs from the blood. In most human research, cells are collected from the peripheral blood for laboratory analysis. Most cells with immune effects are to be found in the broad class of leucocytes ["leuco" = white; "cytes" = cells]. Lymphocytes comprise roughly 20% of the circulating leucocyte pool and are predominantly of the two types, B and T cells. The immune system is shown schematically in Figure 14.1.

Antibody-mediated immunity. The humoral arm of the immune response is mediated by B cells. These are one type of lymphocyte and are responsible for the production and secretion of antibodies. These highly specific molecules (immunoglobulins) recognise and combine with antigens, which are non-self substances. B cells are so called because they are released from the bursa in chickens, or the bone marrow in humans. When a B cell encounters its target

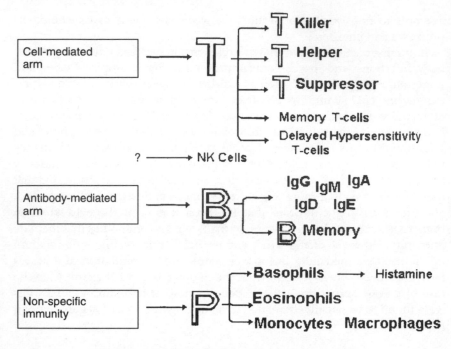

Figure 14.1 Physiology of the immune system

antigen, it develops into an antibody-producing plasma cell and also reproduces and multiplies (proliferates), so that the infection can be managed rapidly. This process is referred to as clonal expansion or blastogenesis. Antibody–antigen complexes are presented to and destroyed by phagocytes. There are five classes of immunoglobulins: IgG, IgA, IgM, IgD, and IgE. Immunoglobulins comprise the predominant response to bacterial infection and provide specific defence against some viruses. IgA has been frequently assessed in psychoneuroimmunology (PNI) research. It is present in mucous secretions, such as saliva and nasal and genitourinary fluids. After an initial response to a specific antigen, "memory B cells" are created, which produce more rapid and efficient response to repeated exposure; this is the basis for the effectiveness of inoculation, as small numbers of memory B cells persist for many years and can multiply rapidly upon re-exposure to an infection.

Cell-mediated immunity. This is carried out by T cells, so called because they mature in the thymus. They make direct or close contact with the antigen, which may be a virus, parasite, or cancerous cell. There are three general types of T cells (although it is possible to identify many more specific types within and between these categories). Cytotoxic T cells are capable of destroying target cells. The other two types function primarily as regulators of the immune response. Helper T cells (T4 cells) enhance the immune response, whereas suppressor T cells reduce it. Helper T cells are the primary target of the human immunodeficiency virus (HIV). This actions of this virus have been compared to a military strategy that selects only the enemy's sergeants and turns them traitor. Other immune "troops" are then aroused by the virus but are unable to target it. Another lymphocyte-like cell, whose origins are unclear but of considerable importance, is the natural killer or NK cell; it destroys virally infected cells and certain types of tumour cells and micro-metastases.

Non-specific response. There are two other categories of leucocytes apart from lymphocytes: granulocytic cells, and monocytes/macrophages. The most familiar aspect of the non-specific response is the swelling associated with a graze, nettle rash, or allergic response. Histamine serves as the first-line, non-specific response to injury and is produced by basophils, which are one type of granulocytic cell. Basophils release histamine and other substances to increase vascular permeability during inflammatory responses, thus facilitating the migration of other immune cells to the region. Other leucocytes involved in the non-specific response are neutrophils and eosinophils. Neutrophils (also called polymorphonuclear leucocytes or PMNs) are phagocytes (literally, "eating cells") that engulf and destroy bacteria in a non-specific manner. Eosinophils similarly engulf antigen–antibody complexes formed when immunoglobulins attach to a non-self substance, and defend against some parasites. The monocyte/macrophage is a cell that achieves a more specifically targeted phagocytosis. Monocyte is the name given the cell in its less mature form, when it resides in the blood stream. When it enters tissue, the cell is referred to as a macrophage. These cells recognise certain carbohydrates on the surfaces of microorganisms, as well as the immuno-globulins that are present during the immune response. In addition to phago-cytosis of microorganisms, monocyte/macrophages play other roles, such as "presenting" antigen to lymphocytes.

Assays of immunity

The efficiency of the immune system is estimated by enumeration, and two measures are generally derived: absolute numbers of cells within a given volume of blood, and percentages of cells constituting each subtype. Counting of cells that have become activated in response to an antigen, and redistribution of cells to lymphoid organs, are also sometimes important. In addition to the use of enumeration measures, immune function can be assessed in a variety of ways. Rate of proliferation can be assessed by exposing lymphocytes (separated from the rest of the blood) to relatively non-specific antigens (mitogens) such as phytohemaglutinin, to which a radioactive protein has been added. As the cells proliferate, they take up the radioactive source, which can be identified in the cells. Some immune cells secrete soluble factors, called "interleukins" or "lymphokines". Interleukins are produced by cells that have become activated by contact with an antigen, so it is possible to assess immune function by assaying levels of these soluble factors following lymphocyte stimulation.

PSYCHONEUROIMMUNOLOGY

Stress and emotions have been known for some time to be associated with substantial physiological changes, including activation of the sympathetic adrenal–medullary (SAM) system, the hypothalamic–pituitary–adrenocortical (HPAC) system, and other endocrine systems. O'Leary (1990) provides an excellent review of these interactions for psychologically trained readers. The two major stress systems (SAM and HPAC), which have previously been described as the fight/flight and conservation/withdrawal systems, affect numerous aspects of immunity.

The SAM system tends to increase most, but not all, immune functions. Injections of adrenalin result in redistribution of lymphocytes out of areas of storage and into circulation while reducing the lymphocytes' functional efficacy. Direct sympathetic innervation of lymphoid organs has been demonstrated in the mouse. In addition, injection of noradrenalin has been shown to increase NK cell activity. On the other hand, cortisol and pharmacological glucocorticoids from the HPAC system seem to be primarily suppressive. Administration of corticosteroids results in reductions of lymphocyte numbers in the bloodstream that are primarily T-cell and monocyte-specific and due mostly to redistribution of cells, an exception to this being neutrophils, whose numbers increase following corticosteroid administration. In general, cortisol seems to have greater suppressive effects on the cellular (T-cell-mediated) than the humoral (B-cell-mediated) arm of the immune response. The effects differ according to whether the stress hormones are generated endogenously by stress, administered medically, or added exogenously in vitro. Some immune functions can be classically conditioned to simple environmental cues. For example, Buske-Kirschbaum et al. (1993) showed that rise in numbers of mononuclear cells in rats could be conditioned to peppermint odour.

Pain has complex interactions with immune function: In vitro, endogenous opiates most often facilitate immune activity, but in vivo, opiates appear to inhibit immune responses and impair tumour rejection (Dunn, 1989). Opioids are produced in response to pain, and evidence of their effect on immune function comes from animal studies, which show suppressive effects of electric-shock–induced opioid activation on lymphocyte response to non-specific antigens and NK cell activity. In addition, people who are addicted to exogenous opiates (e.g. heroin) display reduced lymphocyte response to such non-specific antigens, have fewer helper T cells, and display poor phagocytosis by neutrophils. In vitro addition of opioid peptides to immunologic assays has been shown to enhance NK cell activity, and this has led to the use of metenkephalin as a treatment for cancer and acquired immune deficiency syndrome.

Pathways exist for bidirectional communication between the neuro–endocrine and immune systems. Most hormones have been shown both to be stress-responsive and to have immunologic effects. A variety of neuropeptides, or proteins that modulate neural activity, have been found to influence immune function. Interestingly, receptors for most hormones and neurotransmitters have been found on the surfaces of lymphocytes, and these cells themselves secrete neuroendocrine precursor cytokines. Interleukin-1 (IL–1) produced by immune cells may be the mediator of these effects, thus acting as an "immunoneurotransmitter". The cerebral responses suggest that the brain can monitor the progress of immune responses. IL–1 and the glucocorticoids together may form a regulatory feedback mechanism for immune responses. Certain immunologic treatments, such as the infusion of interferon in the treatment of cancer, have been shown to have neurologic effects.

Examination stress has been shown to affect immunity in all the following reports. Glaser et al. (1990) explored the expression of the interleukin–2 receptor (IL–2R) in medical students experiencing examination stress in three independent studies. The peripheral blood leucocytes obtained at low-stress baseline periods had significantly higher percentages of IL–2R-positive cells when compared with cells obtained from the same individuals during examinations. The stress of final examinations on students was studied by Kiecolt-Glaser et al. (1984). Blood was drawn twice from 75 first-year medical students, with a baseline sample taken one month before their final examinations and a stress sample drawn on the first day of exams. Natural killer cell activity declined significantly from the first to the second sample. High scorers on stressful life events and loneliness had significantly lower levels of NK activity. Total plasma IgA increased significantly from the first to second sample, but other antibody measures did not. Tomei et al. (1990) demonstrated an association between taking examinations and the induction of substantial changes in the response of blood leucocytes to biological hazards.

Natural killer cell activity may increase during brief stresses but decrease if they are protracted. Persistently low NK activity in relation to "hassles" was studied by Levy et al. (1989). Age and the perception of environmental stressors or "hassles" predicted persistently low NK activity in healthy people. Younger subjects, who perceived environmental events to which they were exposed as more serious in nature, were more likely to exhibit a persistently low NK profile over time than were older individuals who perceived daily events as less important to them. Naliboff et al. (1991) found that young female subjects (21–41 years) showed increases in NK cell activity and in the numbers of circulating suppressor T cells and NK cells following a 12-minute stressful mental-arithmetic examination. Older female subjects (65–85 years) failed to show the stress-related increase in NK activity.

Controllability has often been shown to affect stress hormones, so the effects of control on immunity were examined by Weisse et al. (1990). Mild electric shock and loud (100-dB) white noise were administered in an unpredictable, intermittent fashion. During stress sessions, only half of the subjects were able to control the stressor. Subjects with control were yoked to subjects who could not control the stressor, so that both groups were exposed to identical intensities and durations of noise and shock. Immunologic function was assessed across stress and non-stress conditions by measuring changes in lymphocyte proliferation to antigens. Exposure to the uncontrollable stressor altered mood but did not affect immune function. By contrast, exposure to controllable stress did not alter mood but did result in lowered lymphocyte proliferation. Post-stress percentages of monocytes were also lower in subjects exposed to the controllable stressor. Controlling a stressful stimulus may, therefore, be accompanied by lowered levels of lymphocytes, though the adaptive value of findings such as this is unclear.

Uncontrollable chronic stress associated with living near the damaged nuclear power plant at Three Mile Island (TMI) was studied by Schaeffer and Baum (1984). Relative to control subjects, TMI subjects had higher levels of urinary cortisol, as well as urinary catecholamines, self-report of physical and mental symptoms, and decrements in task performance. TMI males had higher urinary cortisol levels than did females. No significant relationship between coping style and urinary cortisol was detected. Levels of stress response among TMI area residents, though significantly greater than among control subjects, were within normal ranges, but had persisted over 17 months.

The immune system may respond adaptively according to the major challenge facing the organism, rather than simply becoming less efficient during stress. The role taken in conflict in rat communities has been shown to affect immune responses differentially (Bohus et al., 1991). Like humans, rats live in hierarchical social structures. A newly forming community has struggles for dominance between the males, which settle into a hierarchy after a few days. After this point, the subdominant animals continue to be chased by the dominant, and also to fight each other. Subordinates, by contrast, do not initiate interaction, but freeze when another male approaches. If the dominant male is defeated, he becomes an outcast who is attacked by all members of the colony and is likely to die quickly. Bohus induced dominance conflicts by housing rats in a laboratory cage; the observed immune changes according to the animal's role in conflict are presented in Table 14.1.

Table 14.1

Immune parameter	Dominant	Subdominant	Subordinate	Outcast
B lymphoctyes	+ +	+	–	– –
T lymphocytes	–	–	+	–
T helper	+ +	+	–	– –
T suppressor	–	–	+	+
Interleukin-2 production	+	+	–	0
Proliferation to PHA mitogen	+ +	+	– – – –	
Thymus size	normal	involuted	normal	involuted

Note: + = increase; – = decrease; 0 = no change

There is a sharp contrast between those who fight and lose and those who avoid fighting. Subdominants experience an increase in antibody immunity but a decline in cytotoxic immunity. Subordinate animals have poor immune response to infection, as indicated by the diminished proliferation in response to challenge with the antigen phytohaemagglutinin. Offering no social challenge is therefore associated having little resistance to infection following injury in combat. However, subdominant animals have some compensation in the form of normal thymus response and some increase in T-cell numbers, whereas the outcasts have no such compensation. Contrasting ways of coping with conflict are of interest when cancer is examined later in this chapter.

Extensive pathways and mechanisms for the influence of psychological processes on immune function have been identified in the above research. Their significance for behavioural prevention of disease remains unclear. Dantzer (1993) argues that the psychoneuroimmunologic pathway is mainly from immune system to brain, not in the other direction. Temperature rise and lethargy are part of the response to infection, and these are adaptive in energy terms. The lethargy may be induced as a brain state in the hypothalamus by cytokines secreted by rapidly proliferating immune cells, rather than simply a lack of energy. At present we are a long way from a comprehensive view of psychoimmunological phenomena. Hopefully, this will eventually include specification of the size and direction of associations between specific subjective states, neuroendocrine processes, and immune processes.

One perspective on psychoneuroimmunology which may be helpful is in the cognitive reframing of long-term infections such as glandular fever, which have a very demoralising effect. Some improvement in morale can be obtained by positive framing of the adaptive nature of the immune response. The author has used rationales such as the following:

> *"Your body has been invaded by a powerful alien virus. It has mobilised a huge defensive effort against this threat. Every minute armies of antibodies are seeking out the invader, and marking them. Tens of thousands of fresh troops of white cells are following them, organised into platoons by their sergeants, the helper T cells. They are relentlessly attacking the invader, and will eventually overcome it. To concentrate your energy for your immune system, your body has turned up its temperature and wants you to rest your muscles. Concentrate on the fight inside. Your need to withdraw and be still is a strength."*

AUTOIMMUNE DISEASE

Autoimmunity involves inappropriate attacks by the immune system on self cells. It differs from infectious disease in that it is characterised by enhanced activity in some components of immunity, and thus prognosis is improved when the immune response targeted against self-agents is reduced. Consequently, if negative affective states are associated with worse disease outcome (and the evidence that exists seems to indicate that this is generally the case), then positive affect ought to be associated with greater response in the relevant immunologic parameters, and psychological improvement ought to be associated with reduced response. In fact, for rheumatoid arthritis and multiple sclerosis, there is suggestive evidence for underresponse (in the suppressor T-cell system), associated with failure to control autoimmune processes.

Rheumatoid arthritis

Rheumatoid arthritis (RA) is the most common polyarthritis, with prevalence estimates ranging from 1% to 4% of the population. It can be a severely painful and disabling disease. RA is an autoimmune disorder whose precise aetiology is not yet clearly understood, but it seems to have its basis in an inflammatory response, possibly initiated by a virus. Many, although not all, patients demonstrate rheumatoid factor in their serum, a type of immunoglobulin that is directed against other immunoglobulins; that is, rheumatoid factor attacks other antibodies as though they were pathogens. Inadequate functioning of the suppressor T-cell system has been observed and may be causally implicated (Abdou, Pascual, & Racela, 1979; Decker et al., 1984).

Effects of psychological factors on immunologic activity in RA have been studied in several ways. Early research reviewed by Solomon (1981) indicated the prevalence among RA patients of a personality pattern characterised by inhibition of emotional expression and dependence. Other research (reviewed in Anderson et al., 1985) indicated that stressful life events tended to precede the onset of RA. In a study of stress and coping in female RA patients, Zautra et al. (1989) found that greater psychological distress was associated with lower proportions of T cells, and major life events with lower helper/suppressor T-cell ratios. Both of these results were unexpected; however, subjects with greater numbers of small stressors had higher percentages of B cells (which are elevated during inflammatory phases in the disease). No relationship between immune indices and disease activity was observed.

A cognitive–behavioural intervention for RA was tested by Lawrence Bradley and colleagues (Bradley et al., 1987). Subjects were assigned to one of three treatment groups: (1) a cognitive-behavioural programme that included thermal bio-feedback at painful joints, training in deep muscle relaxation, and behavioural goal setting; (2) a non-directive social-support condition; or (3) a no-treatment control. Only the cognitive–behavioural intervention was effective, resulting in increased joint temperature, reduced pain behaviour during a videotaped 10-minute movement sequence, less pain, a lower assessment of disease activity, and lowered levels of rheumatoid factor. A measure of "arthritis helplessness"—a hypothesised psychological mediator of treatment effects—did not change as a result of treatment.

A similar study (O'Leary, 1990) evaluated results at a cellular level. A cognitive–behavioural treatment, which included pain- and stress-management training and behavioural goal setting, was compared with a bibliotherapy (literature provision) control. Treated subjects demonstrated reduced pain and improved joint condition, as determined by examinations conducted by rheumatologists who were blind to the patients' treatment groups. No changes in numbers of T-cell subjects or lymphocyte response to mitogens were observed. The hypothesised psychological mediator of change in this study was perceived self-efficacy. This is a person's self-perceived ability to cope effectively with particular stressors—in this case, pain, physical functioning, and general arthritis symptoms. Self-efficacy variables correlated with the relevant outcome variables, supporting the mediating role of the construct. Furthermore, perceived ability to manage pain was positively correlated with number of suppressor cells and negatively correlated with helper/suppressor T-cell ratios at the end of treatment, although the meaning of this association in the absence of treatment effects on cellular immunity remains unclear.

In summary, evidence from psychosocial RA interventions suggests that, although serum measures of immune function may not be related to psychological factors, local inflammatory processes may be. Psychological treatment has been shown to result in lower sedimentation rates and reductions in joint impairment, both of which are indices of local inflammation. That local factors are more closely associated with psychosocial ones is not surprising in view of the possibly low correlation between serum and local measures of immunologic functioning in the disease.

Multiple sclerosis

Multiple sclerosis (MS) is a chronic neurological illness in which the myelin sheaths of nerve cells are destroyed. It is accompanied by immunologic changes, although it is not known whether the changes are causes or effects of demyelination. As with RA, there is evidence of dysregulation of the suppressor/cytotoxic lymphocyte population. Steinman (1993) argues that T cells become sensitised to attack myelin protein following infection by adenovirus, which conceals itself by mimicking myelin protein. Groen (1982) claims that there are some common personality features of the MS sufferer: a tyrannical father, evoking both strong attachment and intense fear; an ineffectual mother; taboos on sex; consequent difficulty in expressing aggression. However, he offers no explanation of how this might affect the neurological changes.

The role of psychological factors in the immunologic as well as neurologic manifestations of the disease were recently explored by Foley et al. (1988). Patients were divided into low and high groups for both anxiety and depression on the basis of median splits. Because anxiety and depression were highly correlated in the study, there was presumably considerable overlap between both high groups and both low groups. Those who were more depressed had higher absolute numbers and percentages of T4 (helper) cells; high-anxiety patients had higher absolute numbers of T4 cells. However, there was no difference between groups in numbers or percentages of suppressor/cytotoxic lymphocytes. Furthermore, no relationship between psychological distress and physical impairment was observed. The significance of these findings remains unclear, although further explication of psycho-immunological relationships is warranted because the immunologic aspects of multiple sclerosis are not yet understood.

AIDS

The possibility of psychoimmunological influences on Acquired Immune Deficiency Syndrome is of obvious importance for research, but there are formidable problems in controlling the variables involved. HIV, the presumed aetiologic agent of AIDS, produces its immune-suppressing effects by destroying the helper T cells. The virus also enters, but does not always destroy, the monocyte/macrophage, which thus may become a reservoir for the virus, and which is the probable route of transport to the brain. HIV is spread through sexual contact or infected blood, or perinatally from infected mother to infant. As the immunologic aspects of HIV become better understood, the prospects for managing the disease will doubtless improve. In the meantime, it is widely believed that the mortality rate from AIDS, and even from HIV infection, will approach 100% over the course of several years. Infected persons, following asymptomatic periods that typically last for years, will eventually develop any of a variety of symptoms and opportunistic diseases making up the AIDS-related complex (ARC). AIDS is likely to be diagnosed when any one of several conditions develop; these include pneumocystis carinii pneumonia, an opportunistic neoplasm such as Kaposi's sarcoma or non-Hodgkins lymphoma, dementia, or wasting syndrome in the presence of HIV infection.

The multiplication of helper T cells will presumably also cause the HIV to proliferate, while increase in NK cells, cytotoxic T cells, and some others may inhibit the development of AIDS. Several pathways for possible effects of psychosocial factors on AIDS progression exist (reviewed by O'Leary, 1990). They include reactivation of latent viruses (e.g. herpes viruses), causing proliferation of helper T cells and subsequently of HIV; reduction of numbers and functioning of peripheral lymphocytes due to neuroendocrine processes (e.g. cortisol); and more productive initial infection due to host condition at the time of infection. Solomon (1989) and Temoshok and colleagues (1985) have conducted a series of studies in San Francisco and reported effects of psychosocial factors on immune function in persons with AIDS and ARC. Some of the trends reported by Solomon (1989) were:

- *Helper T cell* numbers in 18 persons shortly after diagnosis (pneumocystis carinii pneumonia or Kaposi's sarcoma) were found to be associated with less tension and anxiety. Later studies found higher levels of helper T cells associated with lower depression–dejection, fatigue–inertia, and anger–hostility on the Profile of Mood States (POMS). In a longitudinal study of 100 seropositive, symptomatic gay men at two points in time, findings were at odds with those obtained by the same investigators in subjects with AIDS. At the first assessment, absolute numbers of T4 (helper) cells were associated with more POMS tension–anxiety, trait anxiety, anger–hostility, and loneliness. In addition, more reported control of emotion was associated with more T4 cells and more NK cells. Percentages of T4 cells were positively correlated with more anxiety, less emotional control, and greater loneliness. At the second assessment greater loneliness was associated with higher percentages of T4 cells.

- *Cytotoxic T cells* may in theory compensate for losses of helper T cells. Correlates of cytotoxic T-cell levels were less stress from illness, less fatigue–inertia, less stress due to factors other than illness, not doing unwanted favours, and less tension–anxiety. When stress from illness was controlled, only the variable of not doing unwanted favours remained significant.

- *Suppressor T-cell* numbers were positively associated with more fitness and regular exercise, not doing unwanted favours, less POMS fatigue–inertia, and withdrawing to nurture the self.

- *NK cell* numbers were related to nurturing the self, less preoccupation with AIDS, and less POMS fatigue–inertia. NK cell activity was increased in subjects who regularly exercised. Autonomic reactivity during the reliving of emotional events revealed that subjects who evinced greater skin conductance and finger temperature responses had superior NK cell cytolytic capacity. At a three-year follow-up, autonomic reactivity predicted survival after disease (months since diagnosis, and number of helper T cells at the initial interview were controlled). NK cell activity was marginally predictive of survival, suggesting that it may have mediated the effects of reactivity on survival. Greater peripheral arousal was interpreted to reflect a more autonomically reactive temperament, which ought to be associated with greater and more frequent release of catecholamines. Sudden bursts of adrenalin are associated with enhanced NK cell activity.

- *Virucidal cells* are among several less important immune factors considered to be possibly able to compensate for lost helper T cells. Greater absolute numbers of virucidal cells were associated with not doing unwanted favours, less POMS fatigue–inertia, less POMS tension–anxiety, less stress from factors other than sickness, and higher scores on an "upness" scale. Levels of an antigen associated with the HIV virus were associated with more depression, less vigour, more fear, less of a self-rated sense of humour, and less active coping.

- *Serum cortisol* failed to demonstrate significant associations with any of the immunologic parameters. Antoni et al. (1990) found that persisting intrusive thoughts about risk of HIV–1 infectivity (after seronegativity notification) were consistently associated with higher plasma cortisol levels.

- *Beta-endorphin* levels did not change significantly across the 10-week observation period of Antoni et al. (1990), were not associated with psychological variables, and were inconsistently associated with immune functioning.

- *Bereavement.* The contribution of grief was assessed by Kemeny et al. (1994) based in Los Angeles: 45 seropositive gay men who had lost one or more close friends to AIDS during the preceding year were compared to 45 age- and serostatus-matched non-bereaved men. No differences between bereaved and non-bereaved groups were found for any immune parameters among either the seropositive or seronegative subjects, but depression was associated with immune changes consistent with HIV progression.

- *HIV test.* The effects of taking the test seems to be to increase in advance the NK-cell level, which declines by 72 hours later, irrespective of whether the results were positive or negative. Lymphocyte proliferation remained unchanged in the face of significant increases in state anxiety and intrusive thoughts following serostatus notification. Correlational analyses suggested that individual differences in anxiety responses at the time of notification of seropositivity predicted subsequent (1-week lag) declines in NK cell cytotoxicity, but not in other functional markers. (Ironson et al., 1990).

Preventing morbidity in HIV-positive people

Stress management

Efforts to improve immune status through stress management or aerobic fitness have been disappointing thus far. In a controlled study, Coates et al. (1989) failed to demonstrate effects on lymphocyte subset enumeration, NK cell activity, or mitogen response in a group of men given training in relaxation and other stress-management skills. A research group in Florida has begun to examine the efficacy of physical exercise as a behavioural intervention to improve immune function in HIV-spectrum illness (LaPerriere et al., 1990). Subjects were healthy gay men, some of whom were found to be positive for HIV antibody during the study. They were randomly assigned to three sessions of aerobic exercise per week or to a control condition. Initial assessments were conducted after 4 weeks of training. In subjects who were not infected with HIV, exercise produced increases in T4 helper cells and B cells, as well as enhancement of lymphocyte response to mitogens. Only a modest increase in numbers of T4 cells was observed in subjects whose antibody status was positive.

Psychotherapy for depression

Most people told that they are HIV-positive become depressed and tend to withdraw socially, mainly through fear of contaminating others. Markowitz, Klerman, and Perry (1991) argue that this depression is a separate condition, which can be treated. The person carrying the virus can anticipate several years of good health, and spans of 10 years before symptoms develop are quite common. Markowitz and colleagues treated 23 HIV-positive males with brief psychotherapy, and 20 were judged to be free from depression after a mean of 16 sessions. The approach used was Interpersonal Therapy, a method of brief psychotherapy that focuses on three problem areas: grief, role transition, and interpersonal dispute.

Drug adherence

Medical strategies at the time of writing concentrate on treating the intercurrent infections that take hold in the person with impaired immunity, and in obstructing the proliferation of the virus. Some HIV-positive men in San Francisco continue to be healthy a decade after infection, presumably because other aspects of health have been well managed. Intercurrent infections are doubly damaging, as they cause proliferation of T4 helper cells as part of the healthy immune response, which, incidentally, increase the HIV virus. The common infections are pneumocystis carinii pneumonia and tuberculosis, and a skin cancer called Kaposi's sarcoma is also found. Tuberculosis (TB) is an old epidemic illness, which is becoming re-established in undernourished and immune-compromised communities in Africa, in some American cities, and in immune-impaired people. It can be treated effectively with antibiotics, but these need to be taken regularly over many months, and the tendency not to adhere is strong. Incentive schemes for antibiotic adherence have been used as part of a strategy to control the development of TB. Drugs such as AZT are sugars to which the virus mistakenly attaches during RNA replication, so that the copy is unsuccessful. These drugs can defer the spread of the virus by periods of about 18 months, though eventually they cease to have much effect. Adherence to AZT was initially high, as HIV-carriers saw this as the main way in which AIDS could be prevented. A different sort of adherence problem sometimes arises when withdrawal of the drug is proposed on the grounds that it is no longer having an effect, and side-effects no longer justify its prescription.

CANCER

Pathophysiology

Cancers develop when some of the body's cells multiply without control; the normal limits on cell reproduction are overridden, and an "immortal" line of cells proliferates. The commonest cancers are those of the breast, lung/bronchus, prostate, and colon/rectum, and these all carry high mortality. First-line treatment of cancer is to a large extent by surgery, and the survival rate of people with cancers mainly reflects the ability of the surgeon to detect and remove the tumour at an early stage. Skin cancer has a 97% survival rate at five years, while lung cancer has only a 7% survival rate. People with cancers of reproductive tissue, which is operable but not easily detected, have intermediate five-year survival rates: prostate 43%, cervix 58%. Cytotoxic drugs are proving increasingly effective against some leukaemias, and selective radiation is very effective against thyroid cancers. Despite these improvements, cancer death rates are probably increasing: Age-adjusted mortality in the United States went up by 7% between 1975 and 1990 (Beardsley, 1994).

Causes of cancer are predominantly environmental and therefore in principle highly preventable. Tobacco smoking is the major cause of lung cancer, which is the biggest contributor to the increase in cancer deaths. Male rates have remained nearly constant. However, smoking became more prevalent in women after the Second World War and has nearly doubled in the last 15 years. Smoking has caused lung cancer to overtake breast cancer as the commonest cause in women under the age of 30. Smoking also increases risk for upper-airway cancers and those of the pancreas and bladder. Diet is the second major preventable cause, and dietary factors have been estimated by the US National Cancer Institute to be involved in one-third of cancers. The circumstantial evidence for high fat consumption was described in chapter 5, and alcohol and some fermented and smoke-cured foods may also contain carcinogens. The role of synthetic oestrogens in water as a cause of cancers of reproductive tissue is currently under investigation. There are many carcinogens in the environment, including asbestos fibres, ionising radiation, and chemicals found in engine oil or rubber, though most of these have been well controlled by public health measures. Many substances in food may in principle be carcinogenic, but only at high doses, so the arguments for controlling tiny quantities remain to be established. Ionising and ultra-violet radiation have caused concern in recent years, and limits on the mutations in skin cells from sun-bathing are now recommended. Hereditary vulnerability is strong in the case of breast cancer, and the detection of an oncogene, provisionally dubbed BRCA1, would allow prophylactic treatment in women at high risk.

Psychophysiology

The influence of psychological processes on cancer is initially implausible, so it is necessary to see how "escape pathways" to normal immunity might occur. Antibodies play little role in detection of cancers, so destruction of tumour cells is mainly by the following cell-mediated mechanisms: cytotoxic T lymphocytes, NK cells, macrophages, and K cells. Cancers are antigenic, though weakly so. Immune mechanisms routinely destroy small tumour colonies, which have been estimated to occur at a frequency of about once a week in normal humans, but are less effective against large tumours. By the time it reaches detectability, a tumour may already contain a thousand million cells, and at this stage it exceeds the cytotoxic capacity of the body. The development of a tumour to this size is thought to occur when an escape pathway occurs, when the immune surveillance is temporarily reduced. Cortisol is one of the substances that reduce cell-mediated immunity, and NK cell levels are lower when cortisol level is raised. It is the influence of long-term stress hormones that provides the most plausible, if unproven, link between psychological state and cancer.

Apoptosis is the name given to genetically programmed alterations of cell structure that lead to a failure of proliferation and differentiation, and eventual cell death. It is induced by a variety of toxic insults, including growth-factor deprivation and ionising radiation. The failure of normal cell death is argued by Tomei and others to result in the immortal cell lines of cancer. The concept of "programmed cell death" was identified decades ago as a result of observations on rare squamous cell tumours that regress spontaneously, but it has recently been seen as a universal part of human development. A flurry of research in the 1990s on apoptosis includes that of Suda et al. (1993), who identified a substance that binds to a cell surface receptor, known either as Fas or Apo–1, and triggers its death. The theory of programmed cell death views cancer proliferation as a "failure of cellular suicide".

Prognostic studies of cancer involving psychosocial risk factors have identified various predictive factors. The most frequently reported is "emotional calm or repression"; other trait factors include "disturbed upbringing", and "conflicts over sexuality". Situational factors that have been reported concentrate on "poor social support" and "loss of an important relationship". Early reports by LeShan (1977) and others tended to focus on traumatic life-events, especially bereavement, but attention shifted to the pattern of emotional calm, or repression, that some people showed in the face of such disasters. The personality characteristics associated with cancer vulnerability have been defined as the "saintly personality", or by Morris and Greer (1980) as "Type C" (by analogy with types A and B), and by Grossarth-Maticek and Eysenck (1990) as "Type 1: rational and anti-emotional". The last-named authors report on prediction of physical illness using their personality–stress inventory. On this occasion the sample was 1600 men and 3000 women from the German town of Heidelberg, starting in 1974. In this part of the study 36 extreme scorers on Type 1 were followed to see which, if any, of the target diagnoses were applicable at 13-year follow-up. Of the 36, 11 had cancer, while none of the other six types exceeded 2 cancer cases.

Temoshok et al. (1985) investigated the relationship between prognosis in cutaneous melanoma (a skin cancer) and a comprehensive set of physical risk and demographic, psychosocial, and situational variables in 50 patients from two melanoma clinics in San Francisco. Variables significantly correlated with tumour thickness were: darker skin/hair/eye colouring, longer patient delay in seeking medical attention, two correlated dimensions within an operationally defined "Type C" constellation of characteristics, two character-style measures, and less previous knowledge of melanoma and understanding of its treatment. Of these variables, delay was the most significant in a hierarchical multiple-regression analysis in which tumour thickness was the dependent variable. Associations between tumour thickness and psychosocial measures of Type C were considerably stronger for subjects less than age 55. This suggests that the role of behavioural and psychosocial factors in the course of malignant melanoma is more potent for younger than for older subjects, as also reported in heart disease.

Not all psychology researchers have found psychosocial predictors of cancer. Cassileth, Walsh, and Lusk (1988) reported on a prospective investigation of 359 patients with malignant diseases, 8 years after diagnosis. Two groups of patients were studied: 204 patients with advanced, prognostically poor malignant disease at diagnosis; and 155 patients with intermediate or high-risk melanoma or breast cancer. Shortly after diagnosis, patients completed a self-report questionnaire that assessed seven psychosocial factors previously reported to predict longevity in the general population. Factors included social ties and marital history, job satisfaction, use of psychotropic drugs, general life-satisfaction, subjective view of adult health, hopelessness, and perception of amount of adjustment required to cope with the new diagnosis. Whilst clinical factors (performance status and extent of disease at diagnosis) predicted clinical outcome, no psychosocial factor was consistently associated with length of survival or remission.

Reactions to the diagnosis of cancer

Greer and Watson have taken diagnostic disclosure as a focus, in that they looked at patients' reaction to see whether subsequent prognosis was affected by such psychological reactions. In their first study (Pettingale et al., 1984), they interviewed people at three months after surgery, categorised reactions in one of four ways, and followed up these patients after 5 and 10 years. The results are shown in Table 14.2. This seemed to show that "fighting spirit" had a positive effect in preventing the recurrence (metastasis) of the tumour. Greer, Moorey, and Watson (1989) have refined their four categories into five, using a questionnaire measure called the Mental Adjustment to Cancer (MAC) Scale. Five responses identified here were:

• *fighting spirit*
• *helplessness*

- *fatalism (ex-stoic acceptance)*
- *avoidance (ex-denial)*
- *anxious preoccupation*

In a validation study, patients with various cancers were given the MAC scale. The patient's adjustment to cancer was also rated clinically by two psychiatrists who had no knowledge of the MAC scale scores, and ratings by the spouse were also used as a validation measure. Reliability within scales ranged from alpha coefficients of 0.84 for fighting spirit to 0.65 for fatalistic; correlation with spouse measures ranged from 0.76 for fighting spirit to 0.38 for fatalistic; avoidance was the least clear scale, with only one item and weak agreement.

Complementary therapy

Many people with cancer view it as a psychosomatic complaint, whatever their medical advisors may say. A rather negative finding on "alternative therapies" for cancer emerged from the findings of a study of survival (Bagenal et al., 1990), based on the Bristol cancer help centre. In comparison with other hospital series, survival was apparently only half as good in those following the centre's recommended practices, which included vegan diet, meditation, healing, and so forth. However the comparison was made with other clinical series, and patients who sought out the Bristol centre had had somewhat more surgery, so the degree of cancer progression at the beginning of the study may not have been adequately controlled. Most commentators who thought the poorer survival was a genuine effect have focused on the vegetable diet. Advanced cancer is accompanied by loss of appetite and of

Table 14.2

| Response | Outcome at 10 years | | | |
	Alive, no recurrence (n = 19)	Alive with metastases (n = 2)	Dead (n = 36)	Total (n = 57)
Denial	5	—	5	10
Fighting spirit	6	1	3	10
Stoic acceptance	7	1	24	32
Helpless/hopeless	1	—	4	5

the ability to metabolise food, called cachexia. It requires planning to take in adequate protein on a vegan diet, and patients changing suddenly from a meat diet may have become undernourished. It is also possible that reduced compliance with radiotherapy and other unpleasant treatments was having an effect.

Creative visualisation

The possibilities of psychological prevention of cancer are now being explored. Carl and Stephanie Simonton (1978), a radiation oncologist and a psychotherapist, respectively, at Dallas Cancer Counselling and Research Center, describe methods of guided imagery for increasing immune response. Patients are asked to draw images of their immunity, the tumour, and the chemotherapy. A typical case is that of Jennifer, who drew white cells tumbling to waste over a waterfall, while an unrelated chemical tap dripped onto the tumour. Six months later her imagery was of small greyish tumour cells, similar-size chemotherapy tablets, and large Natural Killer sharks foraging through them. The hope is that such positive images bring about an actual increase in immune cells.

Supportive group therapy

Spiegel et al. (1989), working in the Stanford University Medical School psychiatry service, reported some surprising results with patients whose cancers had advanced beyond the point of surgical removal. In this study, 86 patients with metastatic breast cancer had a weekly support group, which also involved self-hypnosis for pain. There was random allocation to the intervention group ($n = 50$) and the control group ($n = 36$), both of which had routine oncological care. At the 10-year follow-up, the survival time from onset of intervention was:

Intervention   36.6 months (SD 37.6)

Control   18.9 months (SD 10.8)

Divergence in survival started 20 months after entry, or 8 months after intervention ended. Only three patients were still alive at 10 years.

Fawzy et al. (1990) evaluated the immediate and long-term effects on immune function measures of a six-week structured psychiatric group intervention for patients with malignant melanoma. Along with a reduction in levels of psychological distress and greater use of active coping methods, the following immune changes were seen at the six-month assessment point in the intervention-group patients (n = 35) compared with controls (n = 26): significant increases in the percentage of large granular lymphocytes and NK cells along with indications of increase in NK cytotoxic activity; and a small decrease in the percent of CD4 (helper/inducer) T cells. At the six-week follow-up point, the majority of these changes were not yet observable. The results indicate that a short-term group intervention in patients with malignant melanoma with a good prognosis was associated with longer-term changes in affective state, coping, and the NK cell system. Affective rather than coping measures showed some significant correlations with immune cell changes.

Changing the cancer-prone personality

Grossarth-Maticek et al. (1986) used a cognitive–behavioural approach in an attempt to change the putative cancer-prone personality. One hundred subjects from the Heidelberg "stressed" group (see chapter 3) were randomly assigned to a cognitive–behavioural treatment or a control group. Therapy was intended to increase emotion expression—a process that has been translated into English as "hysterising" by "creative novation therapy". These initially healthy subjects have been followed up over more than 10 years, and Eysenck (1988) reports that all 100 were traced. In the control group, 19 were reported as still living and 16 to have died of cancer. Of those who had had cognitive–behavioural therapy, 45 were still living and none had died of cancer.

This is a startling claim, and Eysenck's advocacy of Grossarth-Maticek's work is discussed at length in a special issue of the journal *Psychological Inquiry* in 1991. Unfortunately, therapeutic enthusiasm seems to have overcome scientific detachment in several areas, and initial data have been retrospectively interpreted in the light of the theory. The initial typology of the probands was rated after the disease results were available. Fox (1991) notes that the percentages for cancer diagnoses seems to have changed at various points in the history of the study. Cooper and Faragher (1991) strongly rebut Eysenck's claim that smoking and personality type operate synergistically and argue that if multiple logistic regression analysis is applied, the two factors appear as independent (but still strong) predictors. Vetter (1991), who collaborated on the projects, acknowledges his own increasing scepticism about the data, though he still believes that improved survival as a result of therapy has occurred.

Immunity is generally higher during SAM activation, so a "fighting" response might theoretically be more effective in promoting immune responses to cancer. However, palliative coping, in the form of support groups and affect expression, also seem to be helpful. Bohus described immune advantages of both dominant and subordinate status, by comparison with outcast and subdominant status, and it may be necessary to model cancer prevention in a more ethological way. The case for the psychological prevention of cancer seems quite strong, though Grossarth-Maticek's reports have not met scientific criteria to date. Kiecolt-Glaser and Glaser, who have undertaken much work on psychoneuroimmunology at Ohio State University, tentatively concluded in 1992 that the case that psychological interventions can alter the incidence, severity, or duration of disease is promising, but that no strong evidence was yet available.

CONCLUSION

There has been a rapid accumulation of evidence that immunity is affected by psychological processes. Immune responses include antibodies, T cells (cytotoxic, helper, and suppressor), and others including NK cells. Many—but not all—immune processes increase during SAM activity and reduce during HPAC activation. Many common infections are more likely after adverse life-events. Auto-immune diseases may be aggravated if stress increases T-cell activity. There is considerable interest in behavioural influences on immunity in AIDS: The psychological response can be improved considerably, but there is as yet little evidence of strong effects on proliferation of the disease. Evidence that cancers become established during an immune escape pathway seems to be related to suppressed emotion during adverse life events. Evidence is accumulating that psychological prevention may affect the course of cancers.

REFERENCES

Abdou, N.I., Pascual, E., & Racela, L.S. (1979). Suppressor T-cell function and anti-suppressor antibody in active early arthritis. *Arthritis and Rheumatism*, 22, 586.

Anderson, K.O., Bradley, L.A., Young, L.D., McDaniel, L.K., & Wise, C. (1985). Rheumatoid arthritis: Review of psychological factors related to aetiology, effects, and treatment. *Psychological Bulletin, 98*, 358–387.

Antoni, M.H, August, S., LaPerriere, A., Baggett, H.L., Klimas, N., Ironson, G., Schneiderman, N., & Fletcher, M.A. (1990). Psychological and neuroendocrine measures related to functional immune changes in anticipation of HIV-1 serostatus notification. *Psychosomatic Medicine, 52* (5), 496–510

Bagenal, F.S., Easton, D.F., Harris, E., Chilvers, C.E.D., & McIlwain, T.J. (1990). Survival of patients with breast cancer attending Bristol cancer help centre. *The Lancet* (8 September), 606–610.

Beardsley, T. (1994). Trends in cancer epidemiology: A war not won. *Scientific American, 270* (1), 118–126.

Bohus, B., Koolhaas, J.M., De Ruiter, A., & Heijnen, C. (1991). Stress and differential alterations in immune system functions: Conclusions from social stress studies in animals. *Netherlands Journal of Medicine, 39*, 306–315.

Bradley, L.A., Young, L.D., Anderson, K.O, Turner, R.A., Agudelo, C.A., McDaniel, L.K., Pisko, E.J., Semble, E.L, & Morgan, T.M. (1987). Effects of psychological therapy on pain behaviour of rheumatoid arthritis patients: Treatment outcome and six-month follow-up. *Arthritis and Rheumatism, 30*, 1105–1114.

Buske-Kirschbaum, A., Grota, L., Kirschbaum, C., Bienen, T., Moynihan, J., Ader, R., Hellhammer, D.H., & Felten, D.L. (1993). Classically conditioned increase in white blood cell counts and glucocorticoid secretion in rats. *Paper Presented at the Seventh Conference of the European Health Psychology Society*, Brussels (1–3 September).

Cassileth, B.R, Walsh, W.P., & Lusk, E.J. (1988). Psychosocial correlates of cancer survival: A subsequent report 3 to 8 years after cancer diagnosis. *Journal of Clinical Oncology, 6* (11), 1753–1759.

Coates, T., McKusick, L., Kuno, R., & Stites, D. (1989). Stress reduction training reduced number of sexual partners but not immune function in men with HIV. *American Journal of Public Health, 79*, 885–887.

Cooper, C.L. (1984). *Psychosocial stress and cancer*. Chichester: John Wiley.

Cooper, C.L., & Faragher, E.B. (1991). The interaction between personality, stress, and disease: Throwing the baby out with the bath water. *Psychological Inquiry, 2* (3), 236–237.

Dantzer, R. (1993). Stress and disease: Where do we stand? *Paper Presented at the Seventh Conference of the European Health Psychology Society*, Brussels (1–3 September).

Decker, J.L., Malone, D.G., Haraoui, B., Wahl, S., Schreiber, L., Klippel, J.H., Steinberg, A.D., & Wilder, R.L. (1984). Rheumatoid arthritis: Evolving concepts of pathogenesis and treatment. *Annals of Internal Medicine, 101*, 810–824.

Dunn, A.J. (1989). Psychoneuroimmunology for the psychoneuroendocrinologist: A review of animal studies of nervous system–immune system interactions. *Psychoneuroendocrinology, 14* (4), 251–274.

Evans, P.D., & Edgerton, N. (1991). Life-events and mood as predictors of the common cold. *British Journal of Medical Psychology, 64* (1), 35–44.

Eysenck, H.J. (1988). Personality, stress and cancer: Prediction and prophylaxis. *British Journal of Medical Psychology, 61*, 57–75.

Fawzy F.I., Kemeny M.E., Fawzy N, W., Elashoff, R., Morton, D., Cousins N., & Fahey, J.L. (1990). A structured psychiatric intervention for cancer patients. II. Changes over time in immunological measures. *Archives of General Psychiatry, 47* (8), 729–735; also 221–232.

Foley, F.W., Miller, A.H., Traugott, U., LaRocca, N.G., Scheinberg, L.C., Bedell, J.R., & Lennox, S.S. (1988). Psychoimmunological dysregulation in multiple sclerosis. *Psychosomatics, 29*, 398–403.

Fox, B.H. (1991). Quandaries created by some unlikely numbers in some of Grossarth-Maticek's studies. *Psychological Inquiry, 2* (3), 221–232.

Glaser, R., Kennedy, S., Lafuse, W.P., Bonneau, R.H., Speicher, C., Hillhouse, J., & Kiecolt-Glaser, J.K. (1990). Psychological stress-induced modulation of interleukin 2 receptor gene expression and interleukin 2 production in peripheral blood leukocytes. *Archives of General Psychiatry, 47* (8), 707–712.

Greer, S., Moorey, S., & Watson, M. (1989). Patients' adjustment to cancer: The Mental Adjustment to Cancer (MAC) scale vs. clinical ratings. *Journal of Psychosomatic Research, 33* (3), 373–377.

Groen, J.J. (1982). *Clinical research in psychosomatic medicine.* Assen: Van Gorcum.

Grossarth-Maticek, R., & Eysenck, H.J. (1990). Personality, stress and disease: Description and validation of a new inventory. *Psychological Reports, 66,* 355–373.

Grossarth-Maticek, R., Eysenck, H.J., Vetter, H., & Frentzel-Beyme, R. (1986). The Heidelberg prospective intervention study. *Paper Presented at the International Conference of Health Psychology,* Tilburg University (3–5 July).

Holmes, T.H., & Rahe, R.H. (1967). The social readjustment rating scale. *Journal of Psychosomatic Research, 11,* 213–218.

Ironson, G., LaPerriere, A., Antoni, M., O'Hearn, P., Schneiderman, N., Klimas, N., & Fletcher, M.A. (1990). Changes in immune and psychological measures as a function of anticipation and reaction to news of HIV-1 antibody status. *Psychosomatic Medicine, 52* (3), 247–270.

Kemeny, M.E., Cohen, F., Zegans, L.S., & Conant, M.A. (1989). Psychological and immunological predictors of genital herpes recurrence. *Psychosomatic Medicine, 51,* 195–208.

Kemeny, M.E., Weiner, H., Taylor, S.C., Schneider, S., Visscher, B., & Fahey, J.L. (1994). Repeated bereavement, depressed mood, and immune parameters in HIV seropositive and seronegative gay men. *Health Psychology, 13* (1), 14–24.

Kiecolt-Glaser, J.K., Garner, W., Speicher, C., Penn, G.M., Holliday, J., & Glaser, R. (1984). Psychosocial modifiers of immunocompetence in medical students. *Psychosomatic Medicine, 46* (1), 7–14.

Kiecolt-Glaser, J., & Glaser, R. (1992). Psychoneuroimmunology: Can psychological interventions modulate immunity? *Journal of Consulting and Clinical Psychology, 60* (4), 569–575.

LaPerriere, A.R., Antoni, M.H., Schneiderman, N., Ironson, G., Klimas, N., Caralis, P., & Fletcher, M.A. (1990). Exercise intervention attenuates emotional distress and natural killer cell decrements following notification of positive serologic status for HIV-1. *Biofeedback Self Regulation, 15* (3), 229–242.

LeShan, L. (1977). *You can fight for your life.* Philadelphia, PA: Lippincott.

Levy, S.M., Herberman, R.B., Simons, A., Whiteside, T., Lee, J., McDonald, R., & Beadle, M. (1989). Persistently low natural killer cell activity in normal adults: Immunological, hormonal and mood correlates. *Nat. Immun. Cell Growth Regul., 8* (3), 173–186.

Markowitz, J.C., Klerman, G., & Perry, S.W. (1991). Interpersonal therapy of depressed HIV-positive outpatients. (Address: Payne Whitney Clinic, 525 East 68th. Street, New York, NY 10021.) *Paper Presented at Society for Psychotherapy Research Conference,* Lyons, France.

Morris, T., & Greer, S. (1980). A "Type C" for cancer? Low trait anxiety in the pathogenesis of breast cancer. *Cancer Detection and Prevention, 3* (1), Abstract No. 102.

Naliboff, B.D., Benton, D., Solomon, G.F., Morley, J.E., Fahey, J.L., Bloom, E.T., Makinodan, T., & Gilmore, S.L. (1991). Immunological changes in young and old adults during brief laboratory stress. *Psychosomatic Medicine, 53* (2), 121–132.

O'Leary, A. (1990). Stress, emotion, and human immune function. *Psychological Bulletin, 108,* (3), 363–382.

Pettingale, K.W., Morris, T., Greer, S., & Haybittle, J.L. (1985). Mental attitudes to cancer: An additional prognostic factor. *The Lancet, i,* 750.

Rahe, R.H. (1975). Life changes and near-future illness reports. In L. Levi (Ed.), *Emotions—Their parameters and measurement.* New York: Raven.

Schaeffer, M.A., & Baum, A. (1984). Adrenal cortical response to stress at Three Mile Island. *Psychosomatic Medicine, 46* (3), 227–237.

Simonton, C., & Simonton, S. (1978). *Getting well again.* New York & Toronto: Bantam Books.

Solomon, G.F. (1981). Emotional and personality factors in the onset and course of autoimmune disease, particularly rheumatoid arthritis. In R. Ader (Ed.), *Psychoneuroimmunology* (pp. 159–182). San Diego, CA: Academic Press.

Solomon, G.F. (1989). Psychoneuroimmunology and human immunodeficiency virus infection. *Psychiatric Medicine, 7,* 47–57.

Spiegel, D., Bloom, J., Kraemer, H.C, & Gottheil, E. (1989). Effect of psychosocial treatment on survival of patients with metastatic breast cancer. *The Lancet* (Oct. 14), 888–890.

Steinman, L. (1993). Autoimmune disease. *Scientific American* (Special issue: Life, Death and the Immune System), *269* (3).

Suda, T., Takahashi, T., Goldstein, P., & Nagata, S. (1993). *Cell, 75,* 1169–1178. Cited by S. Cory, in "Fascinating death factor". *Nature, 367* (27 January 1994).

Temoshok, L., Heller, B.W., Sagebiel, R.W., Blois, M.S., Sweet, D.M., DiClemente, R.J., & Gold, M.L. (1985). The relationship of psychosocial factors to prognostic indicators in cutaneous melanoma. *Journal of Psychosomatic Research, 29* (2), 139–153.

Tomei, L.D, Kiecolt-Glaser, J.K., Kennedy, S., Glaser, R., & Arthur, G. (1990). Psychological stress and phorbol ester inhibition of radiation-induced apoptosis in human peripheral blood leukocytes. *Psychiatry Research* (1), 59–71.

Vetter, H. (1991). Some observations on Grossarth-Maticek's Data Base. *Psychological Inquiry, 2* (3), 286–287.

Weisse, C.S., Pato, C.N., McAllister, C.G., Littman, R., Breier, A., Paul, S.M., & Baum, A. (1990). Differential effects of controllable and uncontrollable acute stress on lymphocyte proliferation and leukocyte percentages in humans. *Brain Behav. Immun., 4* (4), 339–351.

Zautra, A.J., Okun, M.A., Robinson, S.E., Lee, D., Roth, S.H., & Emmanual, J. (1989). Life stress and lymphocyte alterations among patients with rheumatoid arthritis. *Health Psychology, 8,* 1–14.

15

Maintaining Health

This book has presented evidence that positive health can be thought of in broad terms as fitness, which includes psychological resources. This general conception resolves into about two dozen specific health behaviours. The first part of the book showed how these skills can be developed in particular areas of life, and the second part showed which health behaviours are needed to maintain particular physical functions. A brief discussion of some strategic issues is now needed. These issues are: To what extent can skills be disseminated? Are benefits achievable at reasonable cost?

SKILL DISSEMINATION

The principles of primary prevention are deceptively easy to describe. For example, a pamphlet of the "Look After Yourself! Project" provides the following exhortations:

Weight control	Eat well, be well
Sugar	Food labels
Exercise	Stress
Smoking	Know your drink
Mind your back	

Improvements in general health will depend on the extent to which such health behaviours become general throughout the population. The hypotheses about the fit person described in chapter 1 have been supported by abundant epidemiological information presented in this book. Knowledge and behaviour are not the same thing, and many people with accurate knowledge continue to act in risky ways. Many smokers acknowledge the hazards of cigarettes but find them outweighed by stress reduction or social conformity. Information alone can sometimes have an effect: Food information has the quickest effect on behaviour, though this also goes with food scares and with scepticism about food messages that are seen as contradictory: "They used to tell us that milk was good food, then they said it was bad for your heart, now they're saying it's good again!"

Knowledge can be established by health education, though skills usually cannot. For primary health education to be effective, both audience and message need to be properly analysed. The discrepancy between knowledge and behaviour arises in the clash between health knowledge and other belief systems. Health promotion by information alone is clearly inadequate for the establishment of health behaviours, so skills and attitudes must also be appraised. Preventive health strategies using media need to consider the audience, the medium, the source, and the interactions between source and audience.

Secondary interventions for people who have developed a health problem are mainly psycho-educational. The incentive to take health behaviour seriously often follows alarm about illness, and health promotion at this secondary level is considerably more effective. Each remedial profession, such as physiotherapy or clinical psychology, has a repertoire of teaching techniques. Although knowledge can be acquired by lay people without professional input, it is doubtful whether most health behaviours can be established by clients without this specialised teaching input. The benefits of such teaching need to be audited, preferably several years later, to monitor the level of smoking abstinence, back care, or dietary fat. Rather little data is available as yet from such audits.

Promoting health behaviours in adolescents creates a particular challenge. Health is generally good at this point in life, so perceived susceptibility is low, and costs of health behaviour are high. Health-oriented information sometimes even creates a backlash, particularly if the target audience is adolescent. A series of TV advertisements under the slogan "Heroin screws you up!" used the supposedly aversive image of a weary-looking teenager who turned out to be a positive role-model for some viewers. Promoting behaviour that is not immediately connected with health, especially fitness and attractiveness, are likely to be more effective.

Poverty constitutes a severe limitation of the dissemination of health behaviours. Morbidity from virtually all illnesses increases disproportionately with lower socio-economic status, but the efficacy of treatment and prevention programmes declines in the same proportion. Smoking, diets high in starch and fat, and poor stress coping are much more prevalent in unskilled workers and long-term unemployed people. This effect applies to remedial education programmes as well as to health promotion, and Bronfenbrenner's (1976) conclusions about Project Headstart in the United States are salutary. After reviewing the efficacy of nursery and home-based programmes for the most deprived pre-school children, he concluded that:

> The critical forces of destruction lie neither within the child nor within his family but in the desperate circumstances in which the family is forced to live. What is called for is intervention at the ecological level, measures that will effect radical changes in the immediate environment of the family and the child.

The disproportionate allocation and uptake of health resources in higher socio-economic groups has been referred to as "the inverse care law". The difficulty in disseminating health behaviours to people suffering from poverty does not, of course, mean that services should not be provided. It does mean that the strategies have to be effectively targeted. The examples of "outreach" and the influence of work patterns in reducing heart disease risk have been described in chapter 6 and give some clues to the achievement of health behaviours in people in poverty.

COST AND BENEFIT

The spiralling cost of healthcare is most industrialised countries has led to calls for lower-cost healthcare. In the United Kingdom, hip replacement was taken as the paradigm of a standard procedure that could be made cheaper and more accessible by good commercial practice. However, a 1993 report by the NHS management executive (*The Guardian*, 23 February) indicates problems with this approach. According to research by Dr Chris Bulstrode of Oxford, the number of primary failures of replaced hips had risen to 12% in the 1980s and is probably still rising. Revision operations are much less successful, and more costly. Reasons for the rising failure rate include the proliferation of commercially available prosthetic hips (currently 34), and the drafting-in of non-specialist surgeons to reduce waiting lists. In the United States huge costs of medical treatment have led to cost–benefit analyses (e.g. by Weinstein and Stason, 1976). By comparing the age at death of treated and untreated patients, it is possible to work out the average increase in life expectancy, and hence "cost per year gained." An even harder-nosed approach costs this in terms of "quality-adjusted years of life added", allowing for the fact that some treatments prolong life but with disabilities such as congestive heart failure.

Secondary prevention of heart disease provides us with the best information on cost and benefit. Estimates for coronary care by Weinstein and Stason (1976) are included in the review by Goldman (1988), who converted costs in US dollars at 1985 prices. Antihypertensive treatment costs used data from the Framingham study. They concluded that the direct care costs for stroke and CHD would offset 22% of the costs of treating where diastolic BP at screening was above 105 mm, and 15% of the costs where BP was 95–104 mm. The annual cost per quality-adjusted year of life gained by screening and/or treating was $15,000 for severe and $31,000 for moderate hypertension.

The costs of preventing heart disease by lifestyle means alone fall partly to the healthcare provider and partly to the client. Provision of a programme such as Lifestyle Heart would require training input from dietitians, exercise physiologists, psychologists, and others. Exercise tests, serum measures, and BP monitoring would be required to achieve a careful regime, and facilities such as a gymnasium would be required on a long-term basis. The client would need to be able to commit at least eight hours a week, negotiate various situations incompatible with eating a specialised diet, and have the commitment to acquire the necessary calm and fitness. These are not trivial costs, but they are much less than those of surgical procedures and may give the same level of benefit.

Regular evaluation is an integral part of a healthcare service designed to increase health behaviours. An audit of health behaviours after a heart attack has already been mentioned (see chapter 9). In summary, the prevalence of health behaviours seven months later was found to be:

- *Smoking:* 70% of the smokers at time of MI had quit completely
- *Fat:* 50% "hardly ever" eat high-fat foods (1% eat "every day")
- *Stress coping:* 38% felt "calm and constructive" (but 16% felt "often agitated")
- *Exertion:* 59% felt "more tired" (8% "more energetic")
- *Aspirin use:* 37% were well informed
- *Antihypertensives:* 42%–51% were well informed

Such data is relatively soft, but it has allowed skills in controlling health to be more effectively disseminated since the audit. The gain in health behaviours in this programme is very large in relation to the professional time involved.

"Quality of life" is increasingly being used as a way of comparing outcomes of medical, surgical, and behavioural methods. The Quality of Well-

Being (QWB) scale (Kaplan & Anderson, 1988) attempts to express benefits and side-effects of a programme in terms of completely well years of life. Scores on the QWB scale are obtained by classifying people into steps on scales for mobility, physical activity, and social activity, and also by classifying the symptom/problem complex that bothered the patient most on a particular day. Steps are weighted by consensus ratings from community surveys, to give a quality varying between 0 (dead) and 1.0 (optimum function). A score of 0.64 would indicate that the individual was achieving 64% of optimum function. The use of QWB analyses gives some surprises—for example, the finding that more quality-adjusted years of life are lost in the United States through arthritis than through murder. Both health gain and cost-benefit approaches to well-planned preventive health strategies have strong cases, and should be pursued energetically. It is hoped that this book will provide a source of inspiration and reference in that process.

REFERENCES

Bronfenbrenner, U. (1976). Is early intervention effective? Facts and principles of early intervention: A summary. In A. M. Clarke & A.D.B. Clarke (Eds.), *Early experience: Myth and evidence*. London: Open Books.

Goldman, E. (1988). Cost-effective strategies in cardiology. In E. Braunwald (Ed.), *Heart disease: A textbook of cardiovascular medicine* (Chapter 52). London: W.B. Saunders.

Kaplan, R.M., & Anderson, J.P. (1988). A general health policy model: Update and applications. *Health Serv. Res., 23*, 203–234.

Weinstein, M.C., & Stason, W.B. (1976). *Hypertension : A policy perspective*. Cambridge, MA: Harvard University Press.

Glossary

A–B–C principle: behavioural principles used to achieve control of an appetitive behaviour such as smoking or alcohol use; Antecedents may cue the Behaviour, and Consequences may reinforce it.

Acetylcholine: one of the substances that mediate the transmission of nerve impulses from one nerve to another, or from a nerve to the organ it acts on, such as muscles.

Acupressure: a pain-control technique in which pressure is applied to the skin at certain locations.

Adherence: the extent to which a person implements healthcare recommendations without direct supervision.

Adrenalin: secretion of the adrenal medulla. Among its effects are raising of blood pressure, increasing the amount of glucose in the blood, and constricting the smaller blood vessels. Also known as epinephrine.

Adrenergic receptors: the sites in the body on which adrenalin and comparable transmitters of the sympathetic system act.

Aerobic exercise: physical activities that involve the heart in replacing energy at the muscles.

AIDS [Acquired Immune Deficiency Syndrome]: infectious disease characterised by reduced immune resistance to opportunistic infections. It is apparently caused by the Human Immunodeficiency Virus.

Aldosterone: a hormone secreted by the adrenal cortex. It plays an important part in maintaining the electrolyte balance of the body by promoting the re-absorption of sodium and the secretion of potassium.

Alexander technique: a method of training posture and voice.

Alexithymia: "having no words to express emotion" (Taylor, Sifneos).

Anaerobic exercise: a high level of muscle exertion, which entails breakdown of glucose to lactic acid without metabolising oxygen.

Angina pectoris: pain originating from heart muscle when its blood supply is restricted, often felt as a crushing sensation or a pain in the left arm.

Anorexia nervosa: an eating disorder marked by distorted body image and self-starvation.

ANS [Autonomic Nervous System]: a division of the peripheral nervous system that carries messages between the central nervous system and the internal organs largely without voluntary action; divides into the sympathetic and the parasympathetic arms.

Antibody: protein molecule created by the immune system to protect against non-self antigens.

Antigens: foreign substances that stimulate the immune system to respond.

Arousal: the level of mental alertness of an individual, and the levels of activity of the sympathetic–adrenal system and reticular system in the brain.

Assertiveness: to promote one's rights or opinions while respecting the rights of another.

Asthma: a disorder of the bronchi in the respiratory system characterised by spasms, with episodes of breathing difficulty, wheezing, and coughing.

Atherosclerosis: a form of arteriosclerosis, in which there is a fatty deposition on the arterial wall.

Autoimmune disease: a disease characterised by tissue injury caused by the immune system attacking the person's own tissue.

Back School: educational approach to the restoration of optimal use of the lower thorax (Forssell).

Bereavement: morbidity and grief following death of a valued person; more generally, reaction to any loss.

Beta-blockade: interruption of the effects of adrenalin on adrenergic beta-receptors, particularly in the heart.

Beta-endorphins: endogenous morphines, or hormones that reduce pain awareness.

Biofeedback: a process by which individuals can acquire voluntary control over a physiological function by monitoring its status.

Blood clotting time: time taken for platelet aggregation and other clotting processes after a wound.

Blood pressure: the name given to the pressure that must be applied to an artery in order to stop the pulse in the vessel beyond the point of pressure.

BMI [Body Mass Index]: weight in kilos divided by square of height in metres (Quetelet); insurers regard ideal body weight as having indices between 20 and 25.

Body image: perception of one's own body.

Bronchodilation: the dilation of the air passages in the lungs, usually in response to adrenalin or related chemicals.

Bulimia Nervosa: a disorder characterised by overpowering urges to eat large amounts of food followed by induced vomiting or abuse of laxatives to avoid weight gain.

COAD: Chronic Obstructive Airways Disease.

Capillaries: minute vessels that join the ends of the arteries and the commencement of the veins.

Carbon monoxide: a gas that is a constituent of cigarette smoke.

Cardiac arrest: cessation of normal pumping activity of the heart, usually as a result of abnormal electrical stimulation.

Catecholamines: hormones produced in the body from the dietary amino acids, including adrenalin, noradrenalin, and dopamine.

Cholesterol: a waxy material derived from animal and vegetable tissues, widely distributed throughout the body, especially in the brain, nervous tissue, adrenal glands, and skin.

Cognitive restructuring: an approach to therapy that emphasises the modification of thoughts and images to obtain psychological and behavioural changes.

Combat analgesia: lack of awareness of pain during battle or vigorous activity.

CHD [Coronary Heart Disease]: a dramatic manifestation of ischaemic heart disease resulting in narrowing of the arteries until transport of blood to the heart leads to noticeable drop in performance.

Compliance: the degree to which patients participate in medical procedures; also extended to mean following the recommendations of practitioners.

Conversion reaction: process in which an emotion is converted into a bodily state, such as motor impairment or sensory reduction.

Correlation coefficient: a statistic that reflects the degree and direction of relationship between two variables. Correlations near zero indicate no relationship, while correlations of 0.7 to 0.9 indicate a strong but not perfect relationship.

Coping behaviours: the way in which people try to cope with stressful situations.

Counter irritation: : administering a small aversive stimulus to reduce awareness of a larger pain.

Corticosteroids: the generic term for the group of hormones with a cortisone-like action, including cortisol, secreted by the adrenal glands.

Cortisol: a hormone of the adrenal cortex that is secreted under protracted stress.

Creative visualisation: therapeutic procedure used to imagine immune responses to a cancer (Simonton).

Cynicism: avoidance or hostility thought to contribute to heart disease (Cook–Medley).

Diaphragmatic breathing: inspiration of air by downwards movement of the muscle which divides the chest from the abdomen; may be compared with costal breathing.

Diastolic BP: blood pressure during diastole, i.e. between heartbeats.

Duodenum: the first part of the intestine immediately beyond the stomach, so named because its length is about 12 finger breadths.

ECG [Electrocardiograph]: device for amplifying voltages from the heart muscle, used to diagnose cardiac problems.

Emphysema: an abnormal presence of air in certain parts of the body, it is generally employed to designate an infection of the lungs.

Endogenous opioids: opiate-like substances the body produces naturally that reduce the sensation of pain.

Enkephalins: peptides that have the same action as endorphins.

Ergonomics: the design of workplaces and physical environments to harmonise effectively with human strengths and proportions.

Fats: food substances including oils with high energy yield.

Fear of pain: inhibition of activity following an injury, particularly of the lower back, which tends to prolong disability.

FEV [Forced Expiratory Volume], often in 1 second (FEV1): measure of the resistance of the airways to expiration.

Fitness: capacity for physical work; used in this book to describe preparedness for challenges of all kinds.

Gastric secretions: acids etc. secreted by the stomach lining to digest food.

Gate control theory: postulated mechanisms in the spinal column which can diminish or enhance ascending nociceptive influences (Melzack & Wall).

Globus: sensation of a lump in the throat without detectable physical abnormality; the words "hystericus" or "pharyngeus" are often appended.

Glucocorticoids: the group of steroid hormones produced by the adrenal cortex, which includes cortisol and cortisone.

Glue ear: thickening of the mucus in the middle ear, which causes temporary hearing loss in children; associated with passive smoking.

Glycogen: food store in the body, which is broken down to glucose.

Gonadotrophins: hormones that control the activity of the testes and the ovaries.

GSR [Galvanic Skin Response]: electrical conductivity of the skin related to activity of the sweat glands; has some correlation with arousal.

HBM [Health Belief Model]: theory of behaviour that connects severity, susceptibility, benefits, and barriers for a health behaviour (Becker).

Hierarchy of needs: the model of needs such as self-esteem and curiosity according to their prepotency (Maslow).

HIV [Human Immunodeficiency Virus]: a virus found in humans that probably leads to AIDS; reproduces itself in human T-helper cells.

Hostility: psychological traits such as suspicion, cynicism, avoidance, and overt aggression.

HPAC [Hypothalamo–Pituitary–Adrenocortical Axis]: the hormonal system mainly involved in conservation and withdrawal.

Hypercholesterolaemia: having a regular level of the lipid cholesterol in circulation at a level statistically associated with heart disease risk.

Hyper-stimulation analgesia: reduction of pain awareness by rubbing

Hypertension: high blood pressure associated with a statistically increased risk of stroke or other illness.

Hyperventilation: overbreathing, a common reaction to stress or anxiety; lowers the amount of carbon dioxide in the arterial blood and increases its acidity.

Hypnosis: process involving relaxation and suggestion, which induces altered state of consciousness, or perhaps exaggerated role-playing ability.

Hypochondriasis: preoccupation with bodily sensations that are wrongly interpreted as signs of illness (Greek: below the breast bone).

IBD [Inflammatory Bowel Disease]: tendency of the large bowel to bleed easily (ulcerative colitis) or thickening of any part of the GI tract (Crohn's Disease)

IBS [Irritable Bowel Syndrome]: a motility disorder of the gut giving pain and defaecation problems without major pathological changes.

Immunoglobulins: the antibody-mediated arm of the immune system; five different types of immunoglobulin are identified by the initials IgG, IgA, IgM, IgD, IgE; also known as antibody globulin.

Instrumental coping: way of dealing with an external demand that has some effect on that demand and thereby reduces unpleasant states in the individual.

Insulin: the internal secretion of the pancreas formed by groups of cells called the Islands of Langerhans in this organ. It acts by enabling the muscles and other tissues that require sugar for their activity to take up this substance from the blood.

Interleukins: chemical messengers secreted into the blood by white cells.

Isotonic solution: fluids that have similar ionic concentration to fluids in the human body.

Leukocytes: white (Greek: *leuko*, or *leuco*) blood cells (*cyto*); by contrast with erythrocytes (red cells).

LCUs [Life Change Units]: Amount of adjustment necessary for specified life events, using consensus ratings obtained by Holmes and Rahe.

Lipoprotein: proteins that bind with lipids such as cholesterol found in blood.

Locus of control: a belief people have about the internal or external causes of events in their lives; internal are related to self, and outside may be powerful others or chance (Rotter).

Lordosis: increased curvature of the spine convex towards the front; mainly defined in the lumbar region.

Lymphokines: substances produced by T lymphocytes; promote phagocytosis and also influence the activity of B lymphocytes.

Lymphocytes: a variety of white blood corpuscle produced in the lymphoid tissues and lymphatic glands of the body.

Midlife transition: the process of adjustment to challenges such as ageing parents and awareness of limited life-expectancy.

Morphine: the chief alkaloid upon which the action of opium depends.

Motivation-hygiene: a model of motivation that contrasts satisfaction through the achievement of motivators and dissatisfaction through the absence of hygiene factors.

MI [Myocardial Infarction]: occurs when a blockage of blood flow causes damage to the muscle tissue of the heart; medical name for a heart attack.

Narcissistic vulnerability: tendency to perceive criticism and other threats; a consequence of low self-esteem.

Nicotine: the active chemical in tobacco.

NK cell [Natural Killer cell]: cell of uncertain origin, found in human blood, which tends to digest non-self organisms.

Nociception: peripheral registration of tissue injury; one component of subjective awareness of discomfort and displeasure known as pain.

Noradrenalin: a precursor of adrenalin in the medulla of the suprarenal glands. It is also present in the brain. Known as norepinephrine in United States.

Nuclear conflict theory: theory of psychosomatic influence, in which an organ defect is directly connected with a specific unconscious mental conflict.

Obesity: an excessive accumulation of fat in the subcutaneous tissues located immediately beneath the skin; BMI above 30.

Oestrogen: the term applied to the substances that induce the changes in the uterus that precede ovulation; also responsible for the secondary characteristics in women.

Operational thinking: tendency to see concrete detail, rather than the emotional significance of events; one component of alexithymia (Taylor).

Overarousal: maintaining a higher level of SAM activity than appropriate to demand conditions or good health.

Pain behaviours: actions such as limping or grimacing which indicate to others that one is in pain.

Palliative skills: coping skills that improve the subjective state of the person without altering the external situation; also called emotion-focused coping.

Pancreatitis: inflammation of the pancreas, associated with gallstones and possibly with abuse of alcohol.

Parasympathetic nervous system: division of the ANS which promotes digestion and repair; includes the vagus and sacral nerves.

Passive smoking: being exposed to tobacco smoke from sidestream of smokers.

Pepsin: ferment found in the gastric juice, which digests proteins by converting them into peptides and amino acids.

Peristalsis: the worm-like movement by which the stomach and bowels propel their contents downwards.

Personality trait: stable characteristic of an individual, viewed as a position on a continuum.

Phantom-limb pain: occurs when people who have lost limbs experience pain in the missing limb, despite adequate healing of the stump area.

Placebo effect: feeling physically and emotionally more healthy as a result of suggestion, e.g. after taking "dummy" tablets or medication.

PNI [Psychoneuroimmunology]: scientific study of relationships between mental states and nervous and immune processes.

Psychosomatic illness: disease with observable physical changes but predominantly psychological causes.

RA [Rheumatoid Arthritis]: autoimmune disease causing thickening of the synovial lining of the joint; cartilage may becomes ulcerated and ultimately destroyed in severe cases.

RCPP [Recurrent Coronary Prevention Programme]: for heart disease.

RDA [Recommended Daily Amounts]: minimum quantity of a vitamin or other nutrient necessary to maintain health.

Respiratory alkalosis: low partial CO_2 in the blood due to hyperventilation.

RSI [Repetitive Strain Injury]: disorder due to overuse or abuse, characterised by musculoskeletal pain; often associated with occupational use of particular muscles and connective tissue.

Rumination syndrome: regurgitation of food into the mouth where it is chewed or spat out.

Safer sex: the use of barriers during penetrative sex, i.e. condoms or femidoms, or masturbation, to reduce risk of sexually transmitted diseases.

SAM [Sympathetic Adrenal–Medullary Axis/Sympathetic Adrenal–Medullary System]: nervous and endocrine structures which prepare the body for urgent action such as fight or flight.

Sciatica: pain in the distribution of the sciatic nerve, often accompanied by pain in the back; originates from pressure on the nerve in the spinal column.

SD [Standard Deviation]: a measure of the spread of data around its mean.

Self-efficacy: theory that our beliefs about our capabilities of meeting some challenge determines our choice of activities and the amount of effort we put into them.

Self-esteem: the sense of one's own worth which allows criticism and other challenges to be endured.

SES [Socio-Economic Status]: *see* social class.

Sick role: the adoption of a less independent role, giving a patient rights to specialist treatment, freedom from blame, and reduced responsibilities (Parsons).

Social class: a measurement of socio-economic status of a family; census data commonly utilises employment of head of household: professional/managerial, white-collar, skilled, semi-skilled, and unskilled manual.

Social isolation: the state of a person unable to have sufficient interaction with others socially, due to reduced mobility, lack of family or friends, or an inability to join groups or social events.

Stages of change: theory of the acquisition of new health behaviours (Prochaska and DiClemente).

STD: sexually transmitted disease.

Stress: unpleasant internal state associated with the perception that demands exceed one's coping resources.

Stress management: training the ability to cope sufficiently with physical, social, and psychological problems through skills including relaxation and instrumental skills.

Steroids: the group name for compounds that resemble cholesterol chemically; includes the sex hormones, the hormones of the adrenal cortex, and bile acids.

SI [Structured Interview]: for assessing Type A behaviour, which includes cues such as stammering and observations of motor signs, as well as formal questions (Friedman).

Sudden cardiac death: death caused by ventricular fibrillation, mechanical dissociation or other cause which prevents effective cardiac output; may be contrasted with myocardial infarction and heart failure.

Suppleness: ability to move body with ease and fluency; may be contrasted with stamina and strength.

TABP [Type A Behaviour Pattern]: traits of hostility, time-urgency and competitiveness thought to predispose heart attacks (Friedman and Rosenman).

T cell: type of lymphocyte (70% of total) responsible for cell-mediated immunity.

TENS [Transcutaneous Electrical Nerve Stimulation]: procedure using electrical stimulation of the skin for pain control.

Testosterone: hormone responsible for development of secondary sexual characteristics of males, and sexual arousal and assertive behaviour in both sexes.

Thrombogenesis: process of blood clot formation.

Time management: instrumental coping skill in which time is deployed according to priority of goals.

Trait anxiety: the long-term disposition of an individual to perceive threats and show strong autonomic reactivity; may be contrasted with short-term states, which may follow trauma (Spielberger).

Trance analgesia: relative insensitivity to pain after an hypnotic induction procedure or some rhythmic activity such as dancing.

Typologies: psychological approaches to personality, which divide people into discrete categories; may be contrasted with trait and psychodynamic approaches.

U-Curve: theoretical relationship between performance and arousal or anxiety, which proposes that best performance occurs at moderate arousal (Hebb).

Ulcer: erosion of skin or mucous membrane; may be found in stomach (gastric ulcer), duodenum (duodenal ulcer), or elsewhere in gut.

Vasoconstriction: constriction of blood vessels, commonly in response to adrenalin or angiotensin.

VF [Ventricular Fibrillation]: very rapid and irregular action of ventricles of heart, with no mechanical effect.

Vital exhaustion: state of fatigue and hopelessness thought to predispose myocardial infarction (Appels).

Vocal folds/cords: folds of muscle in larynx, whose vibration produces voice.

VSI: videotaped structured interview for Type A.

Index